Lupus Nephritis

Oxford Clinical Nephrology Series

Chronic Kidney Disease: A practical guide to understanding and management
Edited by Meguid El Nahas and Adeera Levin

Treatment of Primary Glomerulonephritis (Second Edition)
Edited by Claudio Ponticelli, and Richard J. Glassock

The Spectrum of Mineral and Bone Disorders in Chronic Kidney Disease (Second Edition)
Edited by Klaus Olgaard, Isidro B. Salusky, and Justin Silver

Cancer and the Kidney: The frontier of nephrology and oncology (Second Edition)
Edited by Eric P. Cohen

Lupus Nephritis (Second Edition)
Edited by Edmund J. Lewis, Melvin M. Schwartz, Stephen M. Korbet, and Daniel Tak Mao Chan

Lupus Nephritis

SECOND EDITION

Edited by

Edmund J. Lewis

Melvin M. Schwartz

Stephen M. Korbet

Daniel Tak Mao Chan

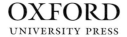

OXFORD
UNIVERSITY PRESS

OXFORD
UNIVERSITY PRESS

Great Clarendon Street, Oxford OX2 6DP

Oxford University Press is a department of the University of Oxford.
It furthers the University's objective of excellence in research, scholarship,
and education by publishing worldwide in

Oxford New York

Auckland Cape Town Dar es Salaam Hong Kong Karachi
Kuala Lumpur Madrid Melbourne Mexico City Nairobi
New Delhi Shanghai Taipei Toronto

With offices in

Argentina Austria Brazil Chile Czech Republic France Greece
Guatemala Hungary Italy Japan Poland Portugal Singapore
South Korea Switzerland Thailand Turkey Ukraine Vietnam

Oxford is a registered trade mark of Oxford University Press
in the UK and in certain other countries

Published in the United States
by Oxford University Press Inc., New York

First published 1999
Second edition published 2011

British Library Cataloguing in Publication Data
Data available

Library of Congress Cataloging in Publication Data
Data available

Typeset in Minion by Glyph International Bangalore, India
Printed in Great Britain
on acid-free paper by
CPI Antony Rowe, Chippenham, Wiltshire

ISBN 978–0–19–956805–5

10 9 8 7 6 5 4 3 2 1

Preface

"Here you see the beginning of philosophy, in the discovery of the conflict of men's minds with one another, and the attempt to seek for the reason of this conflict, and the condemnation of mere opinion, as a thing not to be trusted; and to search to determine whether your opinion is true, and an attempt to discover a standard...thus things are judged and weighed if we have standards ready to test them; and in fact the work of philosophy is to investigate and firmly establish such standards; and the duty of the good man is to proceed to apply the discussions arrived at."

With these words Epictetus (Book II Chapter XI) described the obligation of those who live in a world which requires convincing data to form the basis of their knowledge. Only recently have those who work in the field of lupus nephritis been exposed to the intellectual underpinnings which are required in order to develop and test the potential efficacy of new therapies. The classification of lupus nephritis has been scrutinized and critically analyzed in order that therapeutic approaches be properly applied. While not perfect, current classifications liberate us from the Babel of loosely descriptive terminology which has had been the basis of much confusion. Agents which interrupt the immune response in highly specific ways are being scrutinized for their value in lupus nephritis. Clinical trials can now be designed in a patient population appropriate for the interruption of the specific immunopathogenetic step associated with the kidney lesion encountered. We are on the threshold of treating specific lesions responsible for renal damage. No longer will the treatment of "lupus nephritis", "severe lupus nephritis", "diffuse lupus nephritis", "proliferative lupus nephritis" suffice. On the basis of careful analysis of morphologic, immunologic and ultrastructural features, it is clear that multiple immune mechanisms are responsible for renal injury and any given patient can experience a combination of these mechanisms. On the basis of this knowledge, specific therapies can be tested. Indeed, "mere opinion" is "not to be trusted". Therapeutic regimens which only represented strategies proposed by influential clinicians and were not the result of controlled trials are no longer acceptable. It is our work to determine the standards and remove "the conflict of men's minds". A decade has passed all too quickly since the first volume of *Lupus Nephritis*. The discipline of medicine has experienced some revolutionary changes in the pharmacologic approach to immune diseases. Our ability to interfere with aspects of autoimmunity prevalent in patients with SLE has only begun. Our goal in this book is to review and update the scientific information currently available in order that therapeutic measures in our patient population be carried out utilizing the latest knowledge available. Our present exceeds our past. Look at the horizon, the future indeed appears ever brighter.

Edmund J. Lewis, M.D.

Contents

Contributors *xi*

Abbreviations *xiii*

1 Clinical manifestations of lupus nephritis *1*
Mary Anne Dooley

Introduction *1*

Historical perspective *1*

Definitions of lupus *3*

Clinical factors in the genesis of lupus *5*

Sex and age in the presentation of lupus *8*

Differential diagnosis *9*

The clinical manifestations of lupus *10*

Clinicopathological correlations *22*

Summing up *23*

2 Autoantibodies and lupus nephritis *35*
Anisur Rahman, Jessica J. Manson and David A. Isenberg

Introduction *35*

Anti-DNA antibodies in lupus nephritis *37*

Anti-DNA antibodies and mechanisms of glomerular damage *39*

The importance of DNA–histone complexes *44*

Antibodies to protein components of chromatin *45*

Antibodies to other nuclear antigens *46*

Antibodies to cytoplasmic antigens *47*

Antibodies to complement component C1q *48*

Antiphospholipid (APL) antibodies *48*

The origin of pathogenic autoantibodies in SLE *49*

Conclusions *50*

3 T cells and B cells in lupus nephritis *59*
Mary H. Foster

Introduction *59*

Initiation of nephritogenic autoimmune responses *59*

T cells and cellular immunity in lupus nephritis *64*

B cells and humoral immunity in lupus nephritis *69*

Summary and conclusion *73*

4 The many effects of complement in lupus nephritis *83*
Lihua Bao and Richard J. Quigg

    Why complement in human SLE? *86*

    Mouse models of human SLE *88*

    Functional studies of complement in experimental lupus models *89*

    What we've learned from animals can be used in the treatment
        of humans *93*

5 Pathways of cellular adaptive immunity in autoimmune crescentic
glomerulonephritis and lupus nephritis *105*
Stephen R. Holdsworth and Peter G. Tipping

    Introduction *105*

    T helper pathways in experimental crescentic GN *106*

    T helper cells in autoimmune human GN *110*

    T regulatory cells in crescentic GN *113*

    NK cells and NKT cells in crescentic GN and lupus *114*

    Dendritic cells, TLRs, and type I interferons *116*

    Conclusion *118*

6 Pathology, pathogenesis, and clinical features of severe lupus
nephritis *129*
Stephen M. Korbet and Melvin M. Schwartz

    The definition of severe lupus nephritis (SLN) *129*

    The glomerular pathology of SLN *136*

    The pathogenesis of SLN *148*

    Clinical features and prognosis of SLN *153*

    Insights from the Lupus Nephritis Collaborative Study Group *153*

    Insights from the International Society of Nephrology and
        Renal Pathology Society classification *157*

    Why do the clinical observations differ? *159*

    Conclusion *161*

7 Lupus membranous nephropathy *169*
Howard A. Austin III, Gabor G. Illei, and James E. Balow

    Introduction *169*

    Historical perspective on lupus membranous nephropathy *169*

    Pathogenesis *170*

    Renal biopsy features and classification *174*

    Clinical presentation *177*

    Prognosis of lupus membranous nephropathy *178*

    Supportive therapies *180*

    Immunosuppressive therapies *182*

Experimental therapies *187*

Current treatment recommendations *189*

8 Lupus podocytopathy *199*

Edmund J. Lewis

Introduction *199*

Clinical association of active systemic disease of lupus with the onset of nephrotic syndrome *200*

Nephrotic syndrome and acute renal failure *203*

Minimal change glomerulopathy: a manifestation of lupus *204*

Mesangial lupus nephritis *205*

SLE and podocytopathy: not a coincidence *206*

Glomerular epithelial cell damage and the nephrotic syndrome *207*

Clinical recommendations *208*

9 Renal vascular involvement in SLE *211*

Ben Sprangers and Gerald B. Appel

Introduction *211*

Immune complex deposits *211*

Noninflammatory necrotizing vasculopathy *213*

Inflammatory vasculitis *216*

Thrombotic vascular lesions *218*

Conclusions *227*

10 Mycophenolate mofetil as treatment in lupus nephritis *237*

Daniel Tak Mao Chan

Introduction *237*

Mycophenolate mofetil as induction treatment for lupus nephritis *238*

Mycophenolate mofetil as maintenance treatment for lupus nephritis *242*

Impact of mycophenolate mofetil treatment on renal and patient survival *244*

Mycophenolate mofetil and membranous lupus nephritis *245*

Effects of mycophenolic acid on resident kidney cells *246*

Other issues related to mycophenolate mofetil treatment *246*

Conclusions *249*

11 Lupus nephritis and pregnancy *257*

Kate Bramham, Sarah Germain, and Catherine Nelson-Piercy

Introduction *257*

Numbers affected *257*

Fertility *257*

Normal renal physiological changes in pregnancy *258*

Lupus and pregnancy hormones *258*

Effect of pregnancy on lupus and renal disease *259*

Effect of lupus nephritis on pregnancy outcome *261*

Factors influencing pregnancy outcome *262*

Management *265*

Conclusion *272*

12 The treatment of severe proliferative lupus nephritis *281*
Richard J. Glassock

Introduction *281*

General considerations in developing a therapeutic plan for severe
lupus nephritis *282*

Induction therapy for severe proliferative lupus nephritis *284*

Maintenance therapy for severe proliferative lupus nephritis *295*

Treatment of refractory severe lupus nephritis *299*

Treatment of renal and systemic relapses in severe lupus nephritis *300*

Special issues in treatment of severe lupus nephritis *301*

Summary of the therapy of severe lupus nephritis *303*

Index *317*

Contributors

Gerald B. Appel
Division of Nephrology
Columbia University College of
Physicians and Surgeons
Columbia University Medical Center
New York-Presbyterian Hospital
New York, USA

Howard A. Austin, III
National Institute of Diabetes and
Digestive and Kidney Diseases
National Institutes of Health
Bethesda, Maryland, USA

James E. Balow
National Institute of Diabetes and
Digestive and Kidney Diseases
National Institutes of Health
Bethesda, Maryland, USA

Lihua Bao
The Section of Nephrology
Department of Medicine
The University of Chicago
Chicago, Illinois, USA

Kate Bramham
Guy's & St. Thomas' Hospitals and
King's College London
London, UK

Mary Anne Dooley
Department of Medicine
University of North Carolina
Chapel Hill, North Carolina,
USA

Mary H. Foster
Department of Medicine,
Division of Nephrology
Duke University Medical Center
Durham, North Carolina, USA

Sarah Germain
Guy's & St. Thomas' Hospitals and
King's College London
London, UK

Richard J. Glassock
The David Geffen
School of Medicine
UCLA Los Angeles,
Los Angeles, California, USA

Stephen R. Holdsworth
Centre for Inflammatory Diseases
Department of Medicine
Monash University
Clayton, Victoria, Australia

Gabor G. Illei
National Institute of
Arthritis and Musculoskeletal
and Skin Diseases and National Institute
of Dental and Craniofacial Disorders
National Institutes of Health
Bethesda, Maryland, USA

David A. Isenberg
Centre for Rheumatology
UCL Division of Medicine
Windeyer Building
London, UK

Stephen M. Korbet
The Lester and Muriel Anixter
Professorship in Nephrology
Rush University Medical Center
Chicago, Illinois, USA

Edmund J. Lewis
Muehrcke Family Professor
of Nephrology
Rush University Medical Center
Chicago, Illinois, USA

Jessica J. Manson
Centre for Rheumatology
UCL Division of Medicine
Windeyer Building
London, UK

Catherine Nelson-Piercy
Guy's & St. Thomas' Hospitals and
King's College London
London, UK

Richard J. Quigg
The Section of Nephrology
Department of Medicine
The University of Chicago
Chicago, Illinois, USA

Anisur Rahman
Centre for Rheumatology
UCL Division of Medicine
Windeyer Building
London, UK

Melvin M. Schwartz
The Otho S.A. Sprague Chair of
Pathology
Rush University Medical Center
Chicago, Illinois, USA

Ben Sprangers
Division of Nephrology
Columbia University College of
Physicians and Surgeons
Columbia University Medical Center
New York-Presbyterian Hospital
New York, USA
and
Division of Nephrology
University Hospital, Leuven
Univesity of Leuven
Leuven, Belgium

Daniel Tak Mao Chan
Department of Medicine
University of Hong Kong
Queen Mary Hospital
Hong Kong

Peter G. Tipping
Centre for Inflammatory Diseases
Department of Medicine
Monash University
Clayton, Victoria, Australia

Abbreviations

ACE	angiotensin converting enzyme
ACEI	angiotensin converting enzyme inhibitor
ACL	anticardiolipin (antibodies)
ACR	American College of Rheumatology
ADAMTS	A Disintegrin-like And Metalloprotease with ThromboSpondin type
ALMS	Aspreva Lupus Management Study
ANA	antinuclear antibody
ANCA	antineutrophil cytoplasmic antibody
APC	antigen presenting cell
APL	antiphospholipid (antibodies)
APS	antiphospholipid syndrome
APSN	antiphospholipid nephropathy
APTT	activated partial thromboplastin time
ARB	angiotensin receptor blocker
AZA	azathioprine
BAFF	B cell activating factor
BILAG	British Isles Lupus Assessment Group
BLK	B-lymphoid tyrosine kinase
BLyS	B lymphocyte stimulator
BUN	blood urea nitrogen
C1-INH	C1 esterase inhibitor
c-ANCA	cytoplasm-staining antineutrophil cytoplasmic antibody
CAT	computed axial tomography
CDR	complementarity determining regions
CFH	complement factor H
CKD	chronic kidney disease
CLASI	Cutaneous Lupus Erythematosus Disease Area and Severity Index
CNI	calcineurin inhibitors
CNS	central nervous system
COX II	cyclooxygenase II
CRP	C-reactive protein
Crry	CR1-related gene/protein y
CSA	cyclosporine
CT	computed tomography
CTD	connective tissue disease
CTLA	cytotoxic T lymphocyte antigen
CTX	cyclophosphamide
DAF	decay accelerating factor
DC	dendritic cells
DGGN	diffuse proliferative glomerulonephritis
DHEA	dehydroepiandrosterone
DPGN	diffuse global glomerulonephritis
dsDNA	double-stranded DNA
DTH	delayed type hypersensitivity
EAE	experimental autoimmune encephalomyelitis
EBV	Epstein–Barr virus
eGFR	estimation of glomerular filtration rate
ELISA	enzyme-linked immunosorbent assay
ENA	extractable nuclear antigen
ERK	extracellular signal-related kinase
ESRD	end stage renal disease
FDA	(US) Food and Drug Administration
FSGN	focal segmental glomerulonephritis
FSGS	focal and segmental glomerulosclerosis
FTA	fluorescent treponemal antibody
GBM	glomerular basement membrane
GFR	glomerular filtration rate
GN	glomerulonephritis

GPI	glycosylphosphatidylinositol	MCP	membrane cofactor protein
GVHD	graft-versus-host-disease	MCTD	mixed connective tissue disease
HAE	hereditary angio-edema	MDRD	modification of diet in renal disease
HMG	high-mobility group protein		
HSP	Henoch–Schönlein purpura	MHC	major histocompatibility complex
HUS	hemolytic uremic syndrome		
IC	immune complex	MMF	mycophenolate mofetil
ICAM	intercellular adhesion molecule	MN	membranous nephropathy
ICC	intraclass correlation coefficients	MPA	mycophenolic acid
ICGN	immune complex glomerulonephritis	MPO	myeloperoxidase
		MRA	magnetic resonance angiography
ICOSL	inducible co-stimulator ligand	MRI	magnetic resonance imaging
IFN	interferon	NAT	N-acetyltransferase
Ig	immunoglobulin	NIH	National Institutes of Health
IL	interleukin	NK	natural killer (cells)
IMN	idiopathic membranous nephropathy	NKT	natural killer T (cells)
		NP	neuropsychiatric
IMPDH	inosine monophosphate dehydrogenase	NSAIA	nonsteroidal anti-inflammatory agents
INR	international normalized ratio	NSAID	nonsteroidal anti-inflammatory drugs
ISN	International Society of Nephrology		
		PAH	pulmonary arterial hypertension
IVCP	intravenous cyclophosphamide	PAMPS	pattern associated molecular patterns
IVCY	intravenous pulse cyclophosphamide		
		p-ANCA	perinuclear-staining antineutrophil cytoplasmic antibody
IVMP	intravenous methylprednisolone		
LA	lupus anticoagulant		
LACC	Lupus Activity Criteria Count	PAPS	primary antiphospholipid syndrome
LAMP	lysosome-associated membrane protein		
		PAS	periodic acid–Schiff
LDH	lactate dehydrogenase	p/c	urine protein to creatinine ratio
LFA	leukocyte function-associated antigen	PD	programmed death
		PET	position emission tomography
LMN	lupus membranous nephropathy	PKC	protein kinase C
LMWH	low molecular weight heparin	PML	progressive multifocal leukoencephopathy
LN	lupus nephritis		
LNCSG	Lupus Nephritis Collaborative Study Group	PNH	paroxysmal nocturnal hemoglobinuria
		PR3	proteinase 3
MAC	membrane attack complex	PTEC	proximal tubular epithelial cells
MAP	mitogen activated protein	RA	rheumatoid arthritis
MASP	mannose-binding lectin-associated serine proteases	RCA	regulators of complement activation
		RCT	randomized, controlled clinical trials
MBL	mannose-binding lectin (pathway)		
MCG	minimal change glomerulopathy	RNP	ribonucleoprotein

RPGN	rapidly progressive glomerulonephritis
RPS	Renal Pathology Society
RT-PCR	reverse transcriptase polymerase chain reaction
RVT	renal vein thrombosis
SCID	severe combined immunodeficiency
SCR	short consensus repeats
SGA	small for gestational age
SLE	systemic lupus erythematosus
SLEDAI	systemic lupus erythematosus disease activity index
SLN	severe lupus nephritis
SMR	standardized mortality ratio
SNP	single nucleotide polymorphism
STAT	signal transducer and activator of transcription
TGF	transforming growth factor

Th	helper (T cell)
Tfh	T follicular helper (cell)
TLR	toll-like receptor
TMA	thrombotic microangiopathy
TNF	tumor necrosis factor
TPMT	thiopurine methyltransferase
TRAIL	tumor necrosis factor apoptosis-inducing ligand
Treg	regulatory T cells
TTP	thrombotic thombocytopenic purpura
U1RNP	U1ribonucleoprotein
VDRL	venereal disease research laboratory (test)
VWF	von Willebrand factor
WHO	World Health Organization
WHOQOL	World Health Organization Quality of Life

Chapter 1

Clinical manifestations of lupus nephritis

Mary Anne Dooley

Introduction

Systemic lupus erythematosus (SLE) is a systemic autoimmune disorder characterized by a striking female predominance and frequent development of glomerulonephritis. Renal involvement in SLE remains the strongest predictor of overall patient morbidity and mortality. Renal involvement occurs in 20–49% of patients during their disease course, but lupus nephritis must be seen in the context of the characteristic multi-system involvement. Renal disease may be the first manifestation of lupus, or may come many years later in the clinical course. Although survival in lupus overall has improved with >90% 10-year survival, the survival in patients with nephritis remains lower at 83%.[1] Despite improvements in control of co-morbidities, such as diabetes, hypertension, and hyperlipidemia, the incidence of end stage renal disease (ESRD) from lupus nephritis in the USA between the years 1996 and 2004 has not declined.[2] Renal involvement from lupus occurs most frequently among children, in males, and among racial and ethnic groups including African Americans and Hispanics.[3] Although mortality rates from SLE have been stable among Caucasian patients since the 1970s, throughout 1995 the rate continued to increase among African American women, particularly those aged 35–44.[1] Recently, an international multi-center group reported a standardized mortality ratio (SMR; ratio of deaths observed to deaths expected). Estimates for 23 participating centers (9547 patients) noted that the overall SMR was 2.4. The highest SMR estimates were seen in patient groups characterized by female sex, younger age, SLE duration <1 year, or African ancestry.[4]

Historical perspective

The history of lupus was elegantly reviewed by Cameron in the prior edition of this book.[5] The term "lupus" (Latin: wolf) has been used for centuries in medicine to denote any skin condition including ulceration and tissue destruction, without specific disease connotations. Rudolf Virchow[6] noted the use of lupus for disease as early as the thirteenth and sixteenth centuries by Rogerius and by Paracelsus. *The Oxford English Dictionary* (2nd edn 1993) notes Lanfranc, in *c.* 1400 "Summen clepen [call] it cancrum & summen lupum," and Barrough writing of lupus in 1590 as "a malignant ulcer quickly consuming the neather parts; and it is very hungry like unto a woolfe."

Talbott[7] reviewed the history of lupus in detail; several disease states might have been considered as "lupus" up to the beginning of the nineteenth century, including cancers and lymphogranuloma and tuberculosis.

In the early nineteenth century, Robert Willan in London, Pierre Rayer in Paris, and Thomas Bateman first distinguished Lupus erythematodes from other forms of "lupus" such as lupus vulgaris. In 1833, Cazenave, following a suggestion by Biett, introduced the term "lupus erythemateux." In the 1870s, Moritz Kaposi of Hebra's clinic in Vienna first noted that the condition could be systemic, identifying pleuropericarditis, neurological problems, coma, and death as features of the condition. This paper, published with Hebra, was translated almost immediately into English[8] and became widely known. Although, in 1895, Brooke noted albuminuria in lupus,[9] it was the writings of Sir William Osler in the 1890s that led to the widespread recognition of visceral involvement, including renal disease.[10] Important early papers in the study of renal disease in lupus were those of Keith and Rowntree in 1922,[11] and Baehr and colleagues in 1935,[12] which reported the post-mortem histopathology of lupus nephritis with wire-loop lesions at autopsy in 13 of 23 patients with lupus and associated these findings with the disease. The modern definition of lupus nephritis awaited the seminal papers of Klemperer *et al.*[13] in 1941, again based on post-mortem results, and finally, in 1957, the complete description by Muehrcke, Kark, and colleagues of the renal biopsy appearances.[14] In the late 1950s, Dixon, Holman, Mellors, Kunkel, and Muller-Eberhard, among others[15–17], noted that positive lupus erythematosus (LE)-cell preparations often were found in patients who had immune deposits in renal tissue. Introduction of the LE-cell preparation in 1948[18] allowed investigators to evaluate the prevalence of SLE in patients with idiopathic nephritis.[19,20]

Prior to the development of corticosteroid therapy and nitrogen mustard in the late 1940s and hemodialysis in the 1960s, onset of lupus nephritis was associated with a significant risk of death within 2 years.[21] Survival has greatly improved with the availability of renal replacement therapy. Because ESRD may be managed by dialysis or transplantation, treatment should cause the patient as little harm as possible. Mortality rates among lupus patients on dialysis do not differ from the overall dialysis population, although lupus patients are younger, more frequently female, and have fewer co-morbidities.[22] Lupus patients do not have shorter overall graft survival, but clotting in the acute post-transplant period is a concern in patients who are antiphospholipid antibody (APL) positive at time of transplantation.[23] Recent evaluation gives the risk of recurrence of lupus nephritis following transplant at <10%.[24] Activity of lupus after renal failure appears diminished, although this can occur, particularly hemolytic anemia or thrombocytopenia.

The immunohistopathology of lupus glomerulonephritis is defined by the International Society of Nephrology (ISN) classification developed by nephropathologists in conjunction with nephrologists and rheumatologists.[25] This classification must be compared with the pre-existing World Health Organization (WHO) classification system and the National Institutes of Health (NIH)-developed activity and chronicity indices, as prognosis and therapeutic guidelines have been based on the prior systems. Few studies have evaluated the relationship of the ISN scoring system with long-term clinical outcomes to date,[26–28] but the ISN/Renal Pathology Society (RPS) classification has been used successfully in a number of clinicopathological studies. The critical changes in the ISN classification were the exclusion of "normal" from the system and the division of proliferative nephritis into "global versus segmental" involvement and "active versus chronic" features. Importantly, the 2003 ISN/RPS classification has achieved its goal of improved inter-observer reproducibility.[26] However, reproducibility of the assessment of disease activity and chronicity remained suboptimal ($\kappa = 0.33$). Several studies addressing the relationship between lupus nephritis (LN) IV-S (Class IV diffuse segmental) and LN IV-G (Class IV diffuse global) have failed to identify a significantly worse outcome in IV-S than IV-G, although there were some differences in presenting clinical and pathological features.[27] In a recent study of 92 adults with lupus nephritis, renal biopsies were predominantly proliferative (Class III (focal LN) 17%, Class IV (diffuse LN) 60%), with Class V (membranous LN) represented only in 10%.[26] Within Class IV, Class IV-S was 25% and Class IV-G 75%. Over time, renal function was more likely to deteriorate in Class IV-G cases than in Class IV-S cases. Importantly, Class IV-G (A/C) versus IV-G (A), had persistent proteinuria in spite of intensified therapies; loss of renal function was related to greater chronicity.[28] The relationships between lupus nephritis classifications and patient or renal outcomes are fully discussed in Chapter 6.

A false-positive Wasserman reaction in patients with lupus was noted as early as 1922 by Gennerich.[29] In 1948, Hargreaves and his colleagues reported phagocytosis of nuclear material in bone marrow preparations from patients with lupus,[18] and in 1957 several workers,[30–32] almost simultaneously, described antibodies directed against DNA, which have become an essential part of the definition of lupus. In 1959, Bielschowsky and colleagues[33] noted that New Zealand African ancestry/Caucasian (NZB/W) cross F_1 mice developed a disease resembling lupus. Comparison and studies of these and other animal models of lupus have yielded major insights into its pathogenesis.

Definitions of lupus

Lupus as a diagnosis requires the combination of characteristic clinical and laboratory findings. Systemic lupus erythematosus is best regarded as a syndrome, in which a number of varying immunological events may lead to a similar clinical picture. The presence of antibodies directed against components of the cellular nucleus is detected in the serum of >95% of patients. However, lupus patients typically express a plethora of autoantibodies, including rheumatoid factor, by up to 50%, antilymphocyte antibodies, and APL in 30% of patients to specify a few.[30] There are few disorders in which the patient's sex, race, and ethnicity so strongly impact the incidence of the disease, the frequency of disease manifestations, and the response to therapy. Separate clinical phenotypes can be grouped, yet it remains unclear whether these represent subsets of a single disorder or several diseases. Clinical and serological phenotypes identified to date have large overlaps between patients.

The criteria of the American College of Rheumatology (ACR), revised in 1982,[34] have been widely applied for the diagnosis of lupus, although they were introduced to discriminate the disease from other closely related clinical conditions. In 1987,[35] the

LE-cell preparation was replaced with APL testing, with few institutions performing the LE-cell preparation today. The presence of four or more criteria is usually taken as establishing the diagnosis with about 96% sensitivity and specificity. Patients may manifest more than four criteria at onset, or may accumulate criteria over different time points. However, other systemically ill patients may appear to display four criteria, whereas lupus patients may manifest fewer than four established criteria. In particular, some patients begin with single organ involvement, such as nephritis or thrombocytopenia, but later develop a full clinical and immunological picture.[17] These patients may be antinuclear antibody (ANA) negative at outset, but have hypocomplementemia and positive anti-Ro antibody. Recently, attention has focused on revising the ACR criteria to include tests not commonly performed 20 years ago, including renal biopsy and determinations of serum levels of complement components. The 1987 criteria include four cutaneous features, some difficult to standardize such as photosensitivity. More specific criteria for lupus skin involvement have been developed and published as the Cutaneous Lupus Erythematosus Disease Area and Severity Index (CLASI).[36] This instrument has been validated and may be incorporated into new ACR criteria.

Although the presence of ANA is crucial to the diagnosis of lupus, these proteins may be present in other disorders.[17] Positive ANA tests may be seen in a host of other disorders, such as other rheumatic diseases, treatment with certain biological agents, infection, or malignancies, especially lymphoreticular malignancies. Approximately 15% of normal aging individuals above age 65 will have positive ANA tests. The majority of these individuals are female and the antibody levels are low titer.[37] Many healthy family members of patients with lupus have detectable serum ANA and other autoantibodies.[37–40] Increased incidence of positive ANA tests in spouses of lupus patients[41] and in laboratory workers handling lupus sera has been observed.[42] The presence of anti-Sm antibody is highly specific for SLE, but is detected in only 15–30% of patients, more frequently in African American patients than in Caucasians.[43] Antibodies against double-stranded DNA (dsDNA) and the Smith (Sm) antigen are particularly useful tests as they are strongly associated with the presence of nephritis. Antibodies to Ro (SSA), La (SSB) and RNP are not unique to SLE. In the past, the various patterns of ANA (diffuse, speckled, etc.) were thought to associate with particular disease manifestations. These immunofluorescence patterns are now recognized as providing little help in distinguishing SLE from other ANA positive disorders. Increasingly, large commercial laboratories are abandoning tissue-based immunofluorescence assays for bead assays. Although these are less expensive and less subjective, there are concerns that some ANA positives may be missed. Anti-dsDNA antibodies once thought to be highly specific for SLE may occur in patients receiving a number of biological therapies, including antitumor necrosis factor (TNF) α inhibitors and interferon α. Typically these drug-induced dsDNA antibody titers are low and renal involvement is rare.[44]

Hypocomplementemia and anti-dsDNA antibodies can vary with disease activity in many, although not all, patients with lupus. Serologically active but clinically quiescent patients are well recognized.[45] Defining patients with unequivocal SLE (four or more ACR criteria, with positive anti-Sm or dsDNA antibodies) excludes many patients who satisfy current ACR criteria and who are as important to recognize and to treat as those with "classical" lupus. Similarly, some patients with SLE may not manifest four criteria but exhibit many less common clinical features consistent with lupus. There is no established terminology for such patients. A small number of patients with lupus nephritis but a negative ANA may have low titers of anti-Ro antibody; this subset of patients rarely has significant renal disease.[46] This group is frequently APL positive with associated thromboses,[47] cardiovascular events, and spontaneous abortions, as well as inherited complement deficiencies.[48,49] Patients may fall along a spectrum between SLE and APL syndrome. Up to 30% of SLE patients have measurable APL, yet only a third will develop any clinical consequences. To date, no clinical or laboratory features predict clinically significant APL.

Clinical factors in the genesis of lupus

Genetics

Patients with lupus have defects in all arms of the immune system. Multiple gene involvement in the etiology of lupus[52,53] is suggested by the increased risk of SLE or other autoimmune disorders in certain families. In children with lupus, a positive family history may be seen in 12–15% of cases.[54–56] Monozygotic twins with one twin diagnosed with lupus show a 25% concordance rate.[57] Major histocompatibility complex (MHC) associations have not had a strong impact in human lupus nephritis,[58,59] or with various specific autoantibodies, the strongest being C4A or C4B nul.[60] Low TNF production is associated with greater susceptibility to the disease. Other candidate genes have been examined for associations with susceptibility to lupus, including the interleukin (IL)-1 receptor antagonist, IgGm allotypes, T cell receptor genes, and drug hydroxylation—but none have yet been described independent of linkage disequilibrium with known associations.[62,63] Initial genetic analyses focused on the association of single genes affecting immune function with developing lupus. These candidate gene approach studies implicate the IL1 gene cluster, as well as cytotoxic T lymphocyte antigen (CTLA)4 in disease susceptibility. Additional gene/environment interactions have been described for CTLA4/Epstein–Barr virus (EBV) interactions, N-acetyltransferase (NAT) polymorphisms, and sun exposure in Caucasians.[64]

In SLE, adaptive CD4(+)CD25(+)Foxp3(+) regulatory T cells have been shown to suppress B cell activity *in vitro* and *in vivo* through cell contact-mediated mechanisms.[65] A meta-analysis of published candidate variants from genome-wide association scans, including data from 1310 cases and 7859 controls indicate an important role for B cell development and signaling through toll-like receptors 7 and 9, and neutrophil function.[66]

Ironically, lupus appears to be rare in West Africa, whereas the incidence and prevalence in descendants of West Africans is increased in the Caribbean, North America, and Europe.[67] This pattern may reflect genetic admixture, as well as possible environmental factors.

Immunodeficiency

A proportion of patients with lupus have inherited immunodeficiencies. Inherited deficiencies of complement components,[47–51] Clq-esterase inhibitor deficiency, and acquired deficiency of C3 from nephritic factors have also been found to be associated with SLE, so that a deficiency of functional complement rather than a genetic linkage appears to be most likely, with an inability to clear organisms and/or immune aggregates as a secondary result. In these individuals, SLE occurs early in life[47,51] and often ANA and anti-dsDNA antibodies are negative with extractable nuclear antigen (ENA) antibodies. In Clq-esterase inhibitor deficiency, episodes of angio-edema may precede SLE. Occasional deaths have been recorded.[49] It may be difficult to define deficiency versus consumption, but lupus patients receiving corticosteroids without heritable deficiency develop detectable or increased measured complement component levels. A deficiency of the complement receptors, CR-1, has also been described, thought to be inherited,[64] but recognized now as acquired.[48,50]

The C1QA gene is associated with subphenotypes of lupus in African American and Hispanic subjects.[68] Further studies with higher single nucleotide polymorphism (SNP) densities in this region and other complement components may elucidate the complex interactions between complement components and SLE.

Immunoglobulin (Ig)A deficiency is associated with lupus nephritis more often than would be expected by chance.[69] These individuals are prone to a variety of sinopulmonary and gastrointestinal infections, implicating greater antigenic stimulation of a susceptible subject in etiopathogenesis. Defective Fc receptor function has also been implicated, and is MHC-linked.[70]

Environmental factors

The earliest hypotheses for the pathogenesis of SLE suggested an inciting infection of tubercular, viral, or bacterial origin. Infections, including retroviruses, have been evaluated as candidates for inducing the lupus syndrome. However, there has been no convincing evidence of a single infectious agent in the pathophysiology of human lupus. As SLE is recognized to occur in countries around the world, such an agent would have to be ubiquitous among human populations. The chronic viral infection, EBV, has been considered as such a candidate infection.[71] In an inception cohort of newly diagnosed lupus patients from southeastern USA, a history of shingles and frequent (more than once per year) cold sores in the 3 years before diagnosis were significantly associated with risk of the disorder.[72]

Some medicines and chemicals—such as hydralazine, procaineamide, propylthiouracil minocycline, and a growing list of biological drugs—are known to precipitate drug-induced lupus. Hydralazine-induced lupus was thought to be related to slow acetylator status plus exposure to the drug.[73] More recent studies have shown that acetylator status does not affect susceptibility to drug-induced SLE.[74] Potential gene–environment interactions highlight the need to consider environmental exposures when assessing genetic susceptibility. An interaction between NAT genotypes and use of black hair dyes (a source of arylamines), with higher risk of SLE was noted among hair dye-users who had both the *10 NAT1 allele and the NAT2 slow-acetylation genotype.[75] A threefold increased risk of SLE was noted among Caucasians with the glutathione S transferase M1 (GSTM1) null genotype and 24 or more months' occupational sun exposure.[76]

Cigarette smoking may be associated with an increased risk of SLE, but the underlying mechanism of this association remains unclear. N-acetyltransferase 2 is highly variable and detoxifies aromatic amines. Among 152 SLE cases and 427 controls in a female Japanese population, cigarette smoking was associated with an increased risk of SLE.[77] A gene–environment interaction, with a combination of the NAT2 slow acetylator genotype and smoking conferred significantly higher risk compared with the NAT2 rapid acetylator genotype and no history of smoking.[77]

In a recent study, country of birth was shown to affect the risk of rheumatic disease. First-generation immigrants from Iraq and Africa had a higher risk of lupus than did native-born Swedes; these increased risks were also seen in the second generation.[78] These findings support the concept that both genetic and environmental factors are involved in the etiology of SLE.

Incidence and prevalence

A number of studies have examined the incidence of SLE, giving figures varying from 1.8 to 7.6 new cases per 100,000 per year. The overall prevalence of lupus in the USA has varied in different studies from 15[79] to 51[80] per 100,000 individuals, with an average of about 40/100,000.[81,82] The prevalence is highest in African American females during their reproductive years (approximately 1/250). Incidence figures for African ancestry females were 25 times greater than Caucasian males (0.3–0.4 versus 8–11), and three to four times greater for African ancestry females than Caucasian females.[83] The incidence peaked in African ancestry women either from 15 to 44 or from 25 to 34 years of age, but in Sweden the incidence was highest in the oldest age group, 45–64 years.[84] An intriguing aspect of the increased incidence of lupus among individuals with African ancestry is the relative rarity of lupus in their progenitors in West Africa.[85] Data for Asians are conflicting: in Hawaii, Serdula and Rhoads[86] and Maskarinec and Katz[87] found more than twice the prevalence of lupus amongst Orientals than Caucasians, but Fessel noted no difference in San Francisco, and other studies have noted a relatively low prevalence in mainland China, Taiwan, and Japan.[88] In the relatively small populations of Singapore and Hong Kong, lupus is more commonly identified.

The incidence and prevalence of SLE and SLE nephritis differs among patients of different racial/ethnic backgrounds. Despite continued investigation, these differences remain poorly understood. African American patients develop lupus three times more frequently than Caucasians, have onset of SLE at younger ages, and develop nephritis more frequently than Caucasians. They also have onset of nephritis earlier in the course of their SLE.[79] In an inception cohort of lupus patients in southeastern USA, 31% of African American patients versus 13% of Caucasian patients met ACR renal criteria within 18 months of diagnosis.[89] Hispanic and Asian patients also have greater frequency and severity of nephritis compared with Caucasians.[83] Once they have nephritis, African Americans and Hispanics are more likely to progress to ESRD than Caucasians.[90–91] The lupus nephritis plasmapheresis trial by Lewis et al was the first US clinical trial to include a significant minority participation; race made a significant impact on patient and renal survival.[92] Worse renal outcomes in patients with African ancestry have also been noted in lupus cohorts based in London and Toronto, both with national health-care systems.[93,94] Lupus nephritis is only one of many kidney diseases in which African American patients suffer more frequent adverse consequences. African ancestry may also be associated with a non-lupus-related predisposition towards kidney failure following renal injury. African American patients with hypertension, diabetes mellitus, HIV nephropathy, or focal segmental sclerosis develop renal failure significantly more often than Caucasian patients, and a family history of ESRD from any cause is associated with increased risk of ESRD from lupus nephritis.[95] Despite the greater frequency of nephritis in Asians, generally good outcomes of cytotoxic therapy have been observed.[96–100]

Mortality data from the USA give a similar picture, with figures from one to two deaths per million per year for Caucasian males and up to 10–20 for African ancestry females.[79] Again, in the important study of Lopez-Acuna et al.[100] of over 11,000 deaths attributed to lupus in the USA from 1968 to 1978, mortality for African ancestry peaked at 30–60 years of age, whereas for Caucasians the peak mortality appeared at over 75 years of age. Kaslow[101] examined data from 12 US states with major Oriental populations, and noted three times as many deaths among African ancestry and twice as many among Orientals as Europeans. The incidence of SLE is much lower in children. Levy and colleagues[102] studied a racially mixed, but predominantly Caucasian, population in Paris and its environs, and found an incidence of 0.22 cases/year per 105 children aged less than 16, girls showing 0.36 cases, boys 0.08 cases, per year.

Sex and age in the presentation of lupus

Female sex is a major risk factor for the development of lupus. The female:male ratio rises from 3:1 in pre-pubertal children up to 4.5:1 throughout older childhood and adolescence (see Table 1.1), to the 8–12:1 reported in series of adult-onset patients, falling back to 2:1 in those patients over 60 years of age.[103] Increased estrogen exposure has long been postulated to explain this female predominance. Studies to date have not shown uniform results. Pregnancy is not uniformly associated with lupus flare, although pregnant women are always considered at higher risk. A recent analysis of risk of lupus among participants in the Nurses' Health study, predominantly Caucasian women, reported an increased risk with estrogenic exposures.[104] However, a population-based case–control study of incident cases of lupus from university and community

Table 1.1 Presentation of children with lupus nephritis, collected from the literature

No.	NS 3 g	Prot < 3 g/25 h	Hematuria	Macro/micro	BPup	GFR <80 P_{creat}up	ARF
208	114	89	4	125/159	48/121	103	3
	55%	43%	1.4%	79%	40%	50%	1.4%

ARF, acute renal failure requiring dialysis; BPup, blood pressure more than 2 SD above normal for age; GFR, glomerular filtration rate or creatinine clearance of <80 ml/min; NS, nephrotic syndrome; P_{creat}up, plasma creatinine of above 125 μmol/l; prot, proteinuria.
For details of sources see Cameron.[116]

settings reported fewer estrogenic exposures—later onset of menarche, fewer pregnancies, and earlier naturally occurring menopause associated with risk of developing lupus.[89] Recent clinical trials have shown no increased risk of flare in women with lupus receiving estrogen-containing oral contraceptives [105,106] or post-menopausal hormone replacement therapy.[107,108] It is interesting that the clinical trials demonstrating safety of estrogen exposure have been largely in minority populations, whereas increased risk has been seen in Caucasian cohorts. An interesting hypothesis is that the female second X chromosome, inactive after Lyonization, may become demethylated, leading to greater expression of CD40 ligand[109]—a co-stimulatory molecule increasing activation signaling between T and B cells. Notably, men with Klinefelter's (XXY) are at increased risk of lupus.[79] In the past, researchers described elderly-onset lupus as "milder" lupus, with lower frequency of nephritis. However, race confounds the relationship between age of SLE onset and severity of disease. Studies controlling for race do not show an age-related reduction in risk of nephritis with lupus onset,[110] and suggest that older age of onset is a poor predictor for survival,[111] largely due to the accumulation of more co-morbidities.

Differential diagnosis[112]

The most common other diagnoses made in patients subsequently determined to have SLE were rheumatic fever, rheumatoid arthritis, and hemolytic anemia. Overall, about 50% of patients with lupus are initially suspected of having another disease. As noted above, the presence of four or more of the ACR criteria[34] give a 96% sensitivity and specificity when applied to a population of patients seen in rheumatology clinics. These criteria provide security in scientific studies that one is dealing with "typical" patients, but were not intended as diagnostic criteria. In the real world of the ward and clinic many patients fall outside this exclusive definition, but still need management and treatment.

Differentiation from rheumatic fever is relatively easy, but in a child or young adult with chorea it is not so easy. Nephritis has been reported in a minority of patients with mixed connective tissue disease (MCTD).[112] The differential diagnosis can be difficult clinically, as both disorders may be associated with positive ANA, anti-Ro and La antibodies and antiribonucleoprotein (anti-RNP). However, the presence of sclerodermatous features, high titer anti-RNP levels, and absence of anti-dsDNA antibodies should make the diagnosis clear. Systemic lupus erythematosus is often diagnosed initially as rheumatoid arthritis (RA), because arthritis is the most common presenting feature of SLE in up to 75% of cases, and the majority of lupus patients will have a positive rheumatoid factor. However, RA produces an erosive arthritis and does not affect the kidneys directly. Proteinuria may be induced by drugs used in its treatment, such as membranous nephropathy with nonsteroidal anti-inflammatory agents, or rapidly progressive glomerulonephritis (RPGN) with gold salts. The presence of apparently deforming arthritis makes SLE unlikely, but does not exclude it. Ligamentous laxity, seen in Jaccoud's arthropathy with lupus, may progress and appear similar to RA deformities. X-rays may reveal periarticular osteopenia or osteoarthritic changes similar to Charcot arthropathy. Some patients have a full clinical and immunological picture of SLE in addition to RA. These patients are overlap patients, meeting criteria fully for both disorders.

Henoch–Schönlein purpura (HSP) is far more common in children than lupus. Confusion may arise as lupus may produce a leukocytoclastic, purpuric rash, present only on lower limbs, and a few lupus patients may have predominant IgA in their renal biopsies with raised serum IgA concentrations. Lupus may manifest a small or medium vessel vasculitis, which causes difficulties of diagnosis with other forms of vasculitis. The presence of anti-dsDNA antibodies and a positive ANA remains crucial. But an ANA complicates the interpretation of antineutrophil cytoplasmic antibodies (ANCA) as the ANA may produce a positive perinuclear-staining ANCA (p-ANCA) on immunofluorescence.[113] In this case, the myeloperoxidase (MPO) or proteinase 3 (PR3) enzyme-linked immunosorbent assay (ELISA) may be positive, or more frequently is negative. On histology, however, the finding of multiple immunoglobulin deposits together with complement in the affected glomeruli, and a proliferative/membranous pattern rather than a necrotizing glomerulitis, should cause no difficulty.

In some older patients (>60 years of age) Sjögren's syndrome may be diagnosed as lupus, particularly on the basis of multi-system involvement and a positive ANA. Sjögren's may be associated with an interstitial nephritis leading to renal tubular acidosis and inability to concentrate the urine.[109] When patients have sicca symptoms in the setting of another rheumatic disease, approximately 70% will be seronegative for anti-Ro and La antibodies. In primary Sjögren's the converse is true. Seronegative patients may require salivary or parotid gland biopsy to confirm the diagnosis.

The clinical manifestations of lupus

Many attempts have been made to identify subgroups with particular disease manifestations, but these groupings have not been clinically useful. Fries and Holman[39] reported that patients with nephritis more frequently have alopecia and oral ulceration, and less commonly arthritis, facial rash, and Raynaud's phenomenon; Schaller[56] noted that childhood onset of lupus often is an acute process compared to adults. The Eurolupus project including 1000 patients, most seen in rheumatology clinics,[114] nearly all Caucasian, confirmed the greater incidence of nephritis in children compared to adults.

Table 1.2 illustrates the Eurolupus data,[114] a review by Wallace[115] of the literature up to 1993 on 1000 lupus patients, and the Carolina Lupus Study (CLU),[88] 265 lupus patients evaluated within a year of diagnosis of the disease. Note that in the predominantly Caucasian Eurolupus study, nephropathy was present in only 16% of patients at onset. In the CLU study, 31% of African American patients versus 13% of Caucasians had nephritis within 18 months of disease onset. Symptoms at onset of SLE are often nonspecific, many patients report a "flu-like illness," 75% of patients showed fever and malaise without weight loss.

Table 1.2 Organ involvement at presentation and during the course of the disease in patients with systemic lupus

Manifestations	Cervera et al.[114] At onset No. (%)	During evolution No. (%)	Wallace[115] 1956-1991 No. (%)	Cooper[88] CLU cohort No. (%)	African-Americans No. (%)	Caucasians No. (%)
Malar rash	40	58	10-61	38	35	44
Discoid	6	10	NA	15	21	3
Subacute cutaneous	3	6	NA	NA	NA	NA
Photosensitivity	29	45	11-48	39	30	53
Oral ulcers	11	24	7-36	17	12	22
Arthritis	69	84	53-95	75	75	74
Serositis	17	36	31-57	37	35	38
Pleuritis pericarditis				14	18	7
Renal	16	39	25-65	25	31	13
Neurologic	12	27	12-59	13	8	1
Seizures psychosis				6	3	1
Thrombo-cytopenia	9	22	7-30	11	10	12
Hemolytic anemia	4	8	2-18	11	14	7
Fever	36	52	41-86	NA	NA	NA
Raynaud's phenomenon	18	34	10-44	NA	NA	NA
Livedo reticularis	5	14	NA	NA	NA	NA
Thrombosis	4	14	NA	NA	NA	NA
Myositis	4	9	42-79*	NA	NA	NA
Lung involvement	3	7	1-22	NA	NA	NA
Chorea	1	2	NA	NA	NA	NA
Sicca syndrome	5	16	NA	NA	NA	NA
Lymphadenopathy	7	12	10-59	NA	NA	NA
Weight loss	NA	NA	31-71	NA	NA	NA
Hypertension	NA	NA	14-16	NA	NA	NA

NA, not available; *myalgia

Clinical presentations of lupus nephritis in childhood

The mean age at disease onset in patients with nephritis in the Wallace series was 4 years younger than in those with SLE without nephritis (27 versus 31 years of age and 230 versus 379 patients respectively). Most patients develop nephritis early in their disease; although as some investigators have noted the onset of renal disease can occur at any point in a patient's disease course. Table 1.3 compares data in children and older patients with those of more usual onset age.

An analysis of a subset of 208 from 770 children with lupus from our own experience and the literature[116] (Table 1.1) showed few differences from the data in adults.

The importance of achieving a remission of nephritis has recently been noted in adult patients by Chen et al.[117] Patient survival without ESRD is 92% for those achieving a complete remission, less than 50% at 10 years with partial remission, and 13% for those without response. In a pediatric lupus nephritis cohort (Table 1.4), Gibson et al.[118] report similar results. Children failing to reach complete or partial remission with immunosuppressive therapy had a significantly higher risk of ESRD within 6 years (Figure 1.1).

Renal lupus with "normal" urine

There is ample evidence that, in patients without obvious renal disease, renal biopsies will show immunological or structural abnormalities.[119–126] Most frequently these renal biopsy abnormalities take the form of mild mesangial expansion with immune aggregates visible on immunohistology and/or electron microscopy. In a smaller number of patients, the pattern is of a membranous nephropathy, but occasional patients with more severe diffuse patterns of nephritis can be found.[121]

Of course, the clinical diagnosis of these patients with "silent" lupus nephritis depends upon the zeal and skill with which the urine is examined, both chemically and by microscopy. Intermittent mild proteinuria, hematuria, and abnormalities of the urinary sediment may be missed unless the urine is examined repeatedly. If microalbuminuria is sought, it is usually present.[127]

Naturally, the presence of these histological abnormalities raises the question of whether patients with lupus and normal urine should have renal biopsies. If no action is contemplated in the light of the biopsy findings, then the answer must be "no". Some observers[125,126] have argued the opposite, in that even though renal function and urine are normal the occasional patient with more severe forms of nephritis

Table 1.3 Prevalence of nephritis in lupus of different age

	No.	Nephritis at onset (%)	Nephritis at any time (%)
Pediatric patients	76	28	46
Normal age patients	834	16	39
Older-onset patients*	90	3	22

* Onset over 50 years of age.
Data from Cervera et al.[114]

Table 1.4 Baseline characteristics of pediatric lupus nephritis cohort[118]

	All N=73	Complete responders N=15	Partial responders N=50	Nonresponders N=8	P-value[†]
Age	*15.6±3.4	15.4±3.7	15.5±3.4	16.4±4.1	0.76
BMI Z-score	0.72±1.42	0.25±1.75	0.78±1.31	1.3±1.25	0.30
Race					
White	22 (30%)	2 (13%)	20 (40%)		
Black	47 (64%)	11 (73%)	28 (56%)	8 (100%)	0.03
Hispanic	1 (2%)	1 (7%)	2 (4%)		
Native American	3 (4%)	1 (7%)			
Baseline GFR (ml/min/1.73m²)	81.3±43.9	98.4±36.5	84.3±42.0	34.3±35.6	0.003
Hypertension	47 (69%)	11 (73%)	28 (67%)	7 (87%)	0.49
Baseline proteinuria (mg/dl)	3740±3946	2848±3248	4159±4420	3777±3211	0.42
Histology class					
III	12 (16%)	5 (33%)	7 (14%)		
IV	54 (74%)	9 (60%)	38 (76%)	7 (88%)	0.29
V	7 (10%)	1 (7%)	5 (10%)	1 (12%)	
‡Relapse	24 (37%)	4 (27%)	19 (43%)		0.36
ESKD	17 (24%)	2 (13%)	8 (18%)	6 (75%)	0.004
Time to relapse (months)	44.6±32.2	52.5±44.9	46±30.3	NA	0.80
Time to ESKD (months)	57.8±47.3	105.5±77.1	67.8±41.4	26.7±36.1	0.12
Cytoxan	59 (80%)	14 (93%)	39 (78%)	6 (75%)	0.47
Mycophenolate mofetil	10 (14%)	1 (7%)	7 (14%)	2 (25%)	0.43
Hydroxychloroquine	32 (44%)	10 (67%)	21 (42%)	1 (13%)	0.05
ACE inhibitors	43 (59%)	11 (73%)	27 (54%)	5 (63%)	0.41

* Descriptive data represented as mean ± standard error or n (%).
† P-values calculated using Fisher's exact test for categorical data and Kruskal–Wallis for continuous variables due to independent variable with more than two levels.
‡ One patient in overall group who developed a partial response beyond first year and eventually relapsed. This patient excluded from analyses on relapse data. Denominator based on total number of responders.
ACE, angiotensin converting enzyme; BMI, body mass index; ESKD, end stage kidney disease; GFR, glomerular filtration rate.

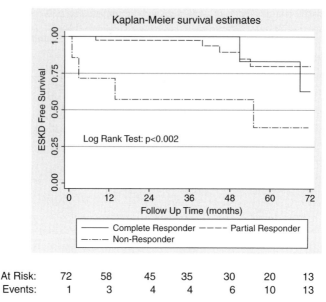

At Risk: 72 58 45 35 30 20 13
Events: 1   3   4   4   6   10 13

Fig. 1.1 Kidney survival by treatment response.[118] Reproduced from Gibson KL, Gipson DS, Massengill SA, Dooley MA, Primack WA, Ferris MA, Hogan SL. (2009). Predictors of Relapse and End Stage Kidney Disease in Proliferative Lupus Nephritis: Focus on Children, Adolescents and Young Adults. *Clin. J. Am. Soc. Nephrol.*, Dec **2009**; 4: 1962–1967, with permission from the American Society of Nephrology.

should be sought and treated. Does treating patients with corticosteroids at this point prevent or ameliorate evolution into more severe overt disease? This question has never been tested by a controlled trial, and is unlikely to be so. It seems likely that all forms of lupus nephritis must evolve through a symptomless phase before becoming overt, but the prognosis of "silent" nephritis has been little studied; occasionally such patients have evolved into renal failure.[121]

Lupus presenting as apparently idiopathic glomerulonephritis

Although multiple organ systems are involved from the onset in most patients with lupus, a minority of patients present initially with a single organ system affected. This is most commonly isolated arthritis, but patients with apparently idiopathic thrombocytopenia are seen who later develop other symptoms and signs consistent with SLE. Similarly, isolated glomerulonephritis may be seen, which evolves later into immunological and/or clinical lupus.[19,128] The renal biopsy appearance may be membranous or proliferative nephropathy.[129,130] Histological pointers to the diagnosis of lupus nephritis are the presence in the biopsy of a "full house" of all immunoglobulins and complement components studied (IgG, IgM, IgA, C3, C4, C1q), of mesangial deposits in otherwise epimembranous nephropathy, and the irregularity of the extracapillary aggregates in membranous disease. A mixed pattern of membranous and mesangiocapillary glomerulonephritis is highly suggestive of lupus (see Chapter 6). Care to exclude other etiologies of this immunohistological picture, such as hepatitis B or C, HIV, or syphilis, should be taken.

Renal manifestations of lupus

About 20–50% of unselected patients with lupus are reported to have abnormal urine tests or renal function early in their disease course,[130–132] and up to 60% of adults and 80% of children may go on to develop overt renal abnormalities. A recent study analyzed the annual incidence of nephritis in 384 lupus patients followed at the Johns Hopkins Medical Center between 1992 and 1994. The 1-year incidence of acute renal disease in established patients was 10%.[133]

Proteinuria

The mode of clinical onset is predominantly characterized by proteinuria. The dominant feature of renal lupus is proteinuria, which is often associated with some degree of edema[127,134] (Table 1.5).

Nephrotic syndrome

About 25% of all patients with lupus will show a nephrotic syndrome at some time in their disease course[39,134] (Tables 1.6 and 1.7). In series based on data from renal units, the proportion is, of course, higher, rising to 60% or more. As noted, Cameron's data show that a full nephrotic syndrome is more common in patients with WHO Class III and IV renal biopsy appearances, but the differences are not sufficiently great to be clinically useful. Other observers have noted the same: in Baldwin et al.,[134] only 2 of 24 patients judged to have mild focal nephritis or mesangial patterns were nephrotic, as compared to 16 of 24 with membranous nephropathy, and 41 of 44 with severe diffuse proliferative nephritis.

Looked at from the standpoint of the nephrotic syndrome, of 506 nephrotic adults seen in Cameron's unit during 1963–1986, 55 (10.8%) had lupus, but, of course, the proportion varies greatly with age, being highest in the twenties and almost negligible in the elderly. The clinical features of the nephrotic syndrome in patients with lupus do not differ from those with other renal biopsy appearances. Hypercholesterolemia is common in lupus patients with nephrotic syndrome.[137,138]

Table 1.5 Incidence of abnormal urinary findings in unselected patients with lupus

	Fries[39] (n=193)		Dubois[135] (n=520)
	First test % positive	Any test % positive	First test % positive
Glycosuria	2	2	—
Proteinuria*	48 (2.0 g)	57 (2.9 g)	46
Hematuria	51	51	33
Granular casts	26	35	32
Red cell casts	3	6	8
Fatty casts	—	—	6
Oval fat bodies	—	—	4.4
Waxy casts	—	—	1.7

* Mean daily excretion shown in parenthesis.

Table 1.6 Prevalence of nephrotic syndrome in patients with clinically overt lupus nephritis

Author	Reference no.	No. of patients	% with nephrotic syndrome	Type of clinic
Kellum and Haserick	131	173	29	Rheumatology
Estes and Christian	132	78	49	Rheumatology
Baldwin *et al.*	134	98	60	Nephrology
Adu and Cameron	127	102	59	Nephrology
Leaker *et al.*	136	135	34	Nephrology
Cameron	116*	179	59	Nephrology

* Collected pediatric series.

Renal tubular dysfunction

Both proximal and distal renal tubular dysfunction are present in many patients with lupus, which is not surprising in view of the presence of both tubular basement membrane immune aggregates and the interstitial infiltrate of monocytes and lymphocytes, these feature are more impressive and frequent in patients with Class III and IV biopsy appearances. However, it is rarely of any clinical significance. Urinary excretion of light chains and β32-microglobulin are both increased in a high proportion of patients.[139–143] Urinary concentration is "blunted"[142] and hyperkalemic renal tubular acidosis has been emphasized.[144–148] The hyperkalemia is common, affecting as many as 10% of patients with lupus nephritis[149] and may be a problem, requiring treatment with 9α-fluorhydrocortisone.[150]

Antinuclear antibodies are a sensitive screening test as more than 95% of lupus patients will be positive when the test is performed using a substrate containing human nuclei such as HEP-2 cells. A positive test for ANA is not specific for SLE, positive ANAs may occur in normal individuals, with increasing frequency with age such that

Table 1.7 Renal manifestations of adults with systemic lupus at presentation of renal disease

Renal presentation	All		WHO biopsy Class IV	
	No.	%	No.	%
Nephrotic syndrome	30	37	18	38
Asymptomatic urinary abnormality	30	37	11	23
Rapidly progressive renal failure	20*	24	17*	35
Acute nephrotic syndrome	2	2	2	4
Total	82	100	48	100

* Seven patients had proteinuria in the nephrotic range.
From S.O. McLigeyo and J.S. Cameron, unpublished data from patients presenting during 1980–1989 at Guy's Hospital.

15% above age 65 have been shown to have an ANA, usually at low titre. In 3–6% of cases, however, renal disease manifestations constitute the initial presentation of SLE.[39–42] This may occur before clinical symptoms of lupus are apparent. Cairns *et al.*[19] reported 11 ANA-negative patients whose onset of SLE began with clinical glomerulonephritis as the initial manifestation. All became ANA positive over a 6-year period. A similar group of 17 patients was described by Adu *et al.*[20] American College of Rheumatology criteria may not be fulfilled at first even if the ANA is positive.[46] The overwhelming majority of clinically relevant nephritis is evident within 5 years of the diagnosis of SLE.[47] Only 5 of Cameron's 230 patients with lupus nephritis who were seen between 1950 and 1980 had onset of renal disease after 10 years.[116] Others have confirmed this.[56]

A discussion of whether patients with lupus and nephrotic syndrome do worse in the long run than those with lesser degrees of proteinuria lies outside the scope of this chapter (but see Chapter 7). However, this is a source of controversy, with some researchers finding that they do worse,[151,152] whereas others see no difference in outcome. Proper studies correcting for age, histology, and renal function have not been performed, however, and the confounding effect of successful treatment on the prediction of outcome must be taken into account.

Complications of the nephrotic syndrome

The complications of the nephrotic syndrome differ in patients with lupus. First, the question of accelerated atherogenesis seems much more important, with young women or even children suffering myocardial infarcts. This is discussed further in Chapter 7. Second, patients with lupus, with or without APL, seem to suffer renal venous thrombosis more commonly than other nephrotics,[153] with the exception of those with membranous nephropathy, and it is often those lupus patients with a WHO Class V membranous pattern who show this complication.[154] It may be associated with thrombosis of the vena cava as described by Mintz *et al.*,[155] who found renal venous thrombosis in 3 of 11 patients; Cameron *et al.* diagnosed 4151 nephrotic lupus patients as having renal venous thrombosis in a systematic study, all had Class V nephropathy.[156] Coagulation in lupus is discussed in more detail in Chapter 9.

Hematuria

Although persistent microscopic hematuria is common, it is rarely found in isolation, whereas macroscopic hematuria is very rare although it may be seen in childhood lupus. Kincaid-Smith and her colleagues[136] have emphasized the prognostic value of quantifying hematuria, both in predicting the severity of renal biopsy appearances and the long-term outlook, a figure of more than 10 rbc/μl being associated with a poorer outlook. No other similar studies have been reported, however.

Casts

Casts are present in about one-third of unselected patients[39,135] (Table 1.5). The urinary sediment often contains granular casts and, sometimes, red cells, as well as red cells in excess of normal, depending upon the severity of the nephritis (Table 1.5).

Table 1.8 Prevalence of hypertension in systemic lupus

Author	Reference	No.	With hypertension (%)
General series			
Cervera *et al.*	114	1000	7
Wallace	115	520	25
Harvey *et al.*	130	105	14
Kellum and Haserick	131	275	43
Estes and Christian	132	150	46
Renal unit series			
Baldwin *et al.*	134	98	51
Adu and Cameron	127	82	27
Leaker *et al.*	136	135	36
Cameron*	116	79	41

* Collected pediatric series.

Hypertension

At presentation, 20–50% of patients were assessed as hypertensive (Table 1.8). Surprisingly, this was no more common in those with clinical nephritis than in those without. However, when the different histological grades of nephritis were examined, as expected from our own data (Table 1.6), it was seen that those with more severe nephritis were more commonly hypertensive (Class II, 17%; Class IV, 55%).[20,134] The hypertension is not often of great severity, retinopathy is usually mild, and accelerated hypertension rare, even in the presence of corticosteroid treatment. If retinopathy is present, however, distinguishing between features arising from the lupus and from the increased blood pressure may be difficult. Usually retinopathy is a marker for active lupus with involvement of the central nervous system, and carries a poor prognosis.[157]

Renal function–acute renal failure in lupus

More than half of patients reported by Cameron and colleagues had reduced renal function at diagnosis, as judged by a reduced glomerular filtration rate (GFR) or a raised plasma creatinine level (see further for details). Almost all studies report this as an adverse prognostic factor (see Chapter 7). Occasionally, patients with lupus glomerulonephritis present in acute renal failure.[158] There are several circumstances in which this may be seen. First, there may a diffuse, severe, crescentic nephritis, but, although smaller numbers of crescents frequently complicate Class III and IV nephritis (see Chapter 5), this finding is unusual in lupus.[159] Second, the glomeruli may show much more widespread capillary thrombi than usual.[160] A related group of patients are those who show an overlap with thrombotic thombocytopenic purpura (TTP).[161–164] Although the addition of plasmapheresis to steroids and cyclophosphamide therapy did not improve renal outcomes in the trial by Lewis *et al.*,[91] plasmapheresis is lifesaving in

TTP and renal recovery may be seen. Similarly, catastrophic APL syndrome with acute renal failure has been successfully treated with plasmapheresis.

Third, a pattern of intense, sometimes isolated, acute interstitial nephritis may be seen.[165–168] This does not seem to correlate with the presence of severe glomerular disease, nor with immune aggregates along the tubular basement membrane. Diagnosis can only be made by renal biopsy, as proteinuria may be trivial and the urine findings unimpressive. With dialysis and immunosuppression, the majority of patients recover at least some renal function, but some have died.

Finally, as previously discussed, renal venous, and much less commonly renal arterial, thrombosis occurs with some frequency in lupus nephritis, even in the absence of APL, and may be associated with acute deteriorations in renal function.

Although much diagnostic import is placed on glomerular findings, there is increasing recognition of tubulointerstitial injury in lupus nephritis. Rahman *et al.* have described proliferative lupus nephritis presenting with sterile pyuria alone.[169] Typically, the severity of interstitial damage parallels the degree of renal impairment. Tubular damage, fibrosis, and atrophy are linearly associated with long-term renal function and can be associated with hyperuricemia and renal tubular acidosis.

Clinical manifestations in other organ systems

Although this chapter focuses on lupus nephritis, nephrologists must remain aware that patients with lupus may have, or develop, involvement of other organ systems. In some patients these other manifestations may come to dominate the clinical picture and its management. Detailed accounts of these may be found in Wallace,[38] Wallace and Hahn,[168] and Boumpas *et al.*[170] The most common serious additional features are involvement of the central nervous system and of the heart.

Dermatological features

A rash is a common presentation[171] and was present in half the Eurolupus patients and three-quarters of the patients in the collected series, usually in the well-known "butterfly" distribution on the face. Livedo reticularis may be seen[172] in 5% of patients at onset, 15% later in the course. Occasionally the rash is purpuric, suggesting vasculitis, with alterations in the nailbed capillaries, and sometimes ulcerating lesions or vasculitic lesions, especially around the ankles. Photosensitivity is common in Caucasian patients with lupus nephritis. Alopecia is common, especially around the frontal and temple areas with broken hairs shafts or "lupus frizz." Patchy alopecia is rare; but is associated with more severe disease. Oral or nasal ulceration is a presenting feature in 10% of patients.

The activity score of the CLASI correlates with the improvement of global skin health, pain, and itch and is thus a useful tool to measure clinical response.

Musculoskeletal features

Joint pain in lupus is common, occurring in three-quarters of patients. The joint involvement may be arthralgia, in which pain is localized over the joints, although the external appearance is normal. Arthritis, observed as joint swelling or effusions accompanied by pain to palpation, is typically non-erosive and nondeforming, although this can occur with ligamentous laxity.[173,174] An initial diagnosis of "rheumatoid arthritis" is often made clinically. Usually several joints are affected at once, often in the hands or knees, and a symmetric pattern is common. The patient may also have myalgia at onset, typically involving the proximal muscles at the shoulders and hips. Myositis in lupus is rarely accompanied by significant proximal muscle weakness, but an overlap of lupus with dermatomyositis or polymyositis is not uncommon.

Cardiopulmonary features

Pleuritis and pericarditis[175–179] affect about 40% of patients, usually with pain, but occasionally symptomless effusions, most easily diagnosed on echocardiography. Cardiac tamponade is uncommon but may occur. Myocarditis with heart failure occurs but is rare. Endocarditis of the Libman–Sachs type recently has been associated more frequently with APL syndrome rather than SLE[180,181] (see Chapter 2). This may be difficult to diagnose except on echocardiography, which should be a routine investigation. Systolic murmurs are, of course, common in lupus patients in the presence of anemia, fever, and tachycardia; diastolic murmurs are more frequently sinister. Pulmonary hypertension in lupus[182] may be the result of the disease itself or due to multiple pulmonary emboli in association with APL, or vena caval thrombosis[155] associated clinically with Raynaud's phenomenon in about three-quarters of cases,[182] and may represent a similar phenomenon in the lung. Treatment with an intravenous, subcutaneous, or inhaled prostacyclin antagonist, or endothelin receptor blocker, has shown improved patient exercise tolerance and lifespan. In some institutions heart–lung transplantation is possible. In contrast to pulmonary arterial hypertension (PAH) associated with other connective tissue diseases (CTD), patients with SLE respond well to immunosuppressive agents (cyclophosphamide in conjunction with corticosteroids). Improvements or stabilization of PAH symptoms and quality of life have also been observed with the oral, dual endothelin receptor antagonists.

Acute pulmonary hemorrhage can be seen,[181] often presenting as a pulmonary–renal syndrome requiring distinction from ANCA vasculitis or antiglomerular basement membrane (anti-GBM) disease. This may also occur with infection and is associated with a high mortality rate. Early recognition and treatment with intravenous methylprednisolone plasmapheresis and activated factor VII preparations appear effective. Abramson and colleagues[182] have emphasized the frequency (27%) of acute reversible hypoxemia in young adults with acute lupus, which usually responds to treatment; its pathogenesis is, however, unclear. Chronic fibrosing alveolitis is a well-recognized feature of lupus, the treatment of which is unsatisfactory and the condition often progressive.[177,184]

Spleen and lymph node features

Splenomegaly and lymphadenopathy[184] are present in about one-quarter to one-third of patients with lupus. Care must be taken to distinguish lupus from lymphoma as the age at presentation and features may overlap significantly. In a large study involving nearly 10,000 lupus patients from cohorts followed around the world, the risk of lymphoma in lupus patients was elevated to 35-fold that of local age-matched controls.[185]

Neuropsychiatric features

Neuropsychiatric (NP) involvement[186–191] is a serious feature of systemic lupus, and is present at an obvious clinical level in about one-third of patients.[187,188] Neuropsychiatric lupus may be a presenting feature[188,189] in about 12% of patients, and can be an isolated feature at disease onset. Recently, the ACR established 16 categories of NP involvement with lupus. A recent inception cohort of nearly 1500 patients enrolled within 18 months of diagnosis suggests that all 16 syndromes are represented.[189,190] Neuropsychiatric involvement is an important source of morbidity and mortality, and is often present to some degree in patients with severe lupus nephritis.[191] Sensitive tests such as NP testing, cerebral blood flow,[192] position emission tomography (PET) scans,[193] and magnetic resonance imaging (MRI) scans[194] and angiography (MRA) may show abnormalities additional to those revealed even by computed axial tomography (CAT) scanning, but the significances of which are not yet clear.[195] In addition, extreme care should be taken to avoid gadolinium exposure in patients with nephritis at risk for renal impairment to avoid nephrogenic fibrosing dermopathy, a fatal illness associated with gadolinium in patients with renal impairment. Minor degrees of mood disorder and behavior are common, but difficult to interpret in the setting of an acute and disturbing illness. These, especially if associated with persistent headache (sometimes but not always of migrainous type), may be the prodrome of a serious overt NP disorder. The pathogenesis of NP lupus remains uncertain, but antineuronal antibodies and cerebral vascular lesions associated with an APL (see Chapter 2) may be responsible for the diffuse and focal infarctive patterns respectively.

Diagnosis of NP lupus can be difficult. Chorea may be seen, especially in children with neurological lupus,[195] sometimes associated with APL.[196,197] In addition, cranial nerve palsies,[133,138] for example ophthalmoplegias, seizures, and hemiparesis, as well as coma and frank psychosis,[198] or brainstem lesions[199] and transverse myelitis can be found. If the patient is already on immunosuppression therapy, infections may mimic NP lupus. Corticosteroids may be associated with psychosis, anxiety, and mood disorders. In practice this may occur even if the patient has tolerated higher doses of steroids previously without difficulty. Infection and illicit or mood-altering drugs must be excluded. If no other severe lupus features are present, the patient may be treated with appropriate psychiatric medications, and the dose of steroids decreased to confirm steroid-induced psychosis. The C-reactive protein (CRP) level may help to distinguish central nervous system (CNS) infections from active lupus,[200,201] cerebrospinal fluid investigations will exclude meningitis. Various immunological tests have been proposed, especially on the cerebrospinal fluid, but none has yet proven to be of clinical use.[201]

Hematopoietic features

Clinical hematological abnormalities are common. Many patients show a normochromic normocytic anemia from inflammation at presentation, and occasional patients present with purpura, not from associated vasculitis but from thrombocytopenia.[202] The classic anemia due to lupus is a Coombs positive hemolytic anemia. Some patients may be Coombs negative on testing, but have undetectable haptoglobin, elevated lactate dehydrogenase (LDH), or reticulocytosis indicating hemolysis. Bone marrow inflammation at presentation may be severe enough to produce marrow necrosis, but the typical bone marrow biopsy will show adequate precursors with peripheral consumption. Bone marrow dysplasia may be seen but the patient's blood count responds to corticosteroids. Overt thrombosis is rare at onset, but should it appear[85] it should, of course, prompt a search for APL (see Chapter 2).

Gastrointestinal and hepatic features

Gastrointestinal[203,204] and hepatic[205,206] abnormalities are relatively rare, although intestinal vasculitis is not infrequently seen in children or young adults with lupus, nausea is common, and at autopsy bowel infiltration with inflammatory cells is common.[206] Protein-losing enteropathy may be seen, or an inflammatory bowel disease overlap. Occasional patients suffer major vasculitic lesions in the bowel.[203]

Raynaud's phenomenon

This is common in adults with lupus, affecting 20–30% and often preceding the clinical onset of other manifestations of disease. In some patients it is very severe, with the loss of digital tissue, as in scleroderma. Patients with renal disease rarely have severe Raynaud's, however, and overall it is a favorable feature in terms of survival.[207]

Immunological abnormalities in lupus at presentation

This is dealt with in greater detail in Chapter 2, but it is of interest here to note how frequently the various immunological manifestations of lupus are seen at presentation. One would like to have these data for lupus nephritis alone, with an account of the evolution of the data, but surprisingly only a small body of data on few patients exists; the figures in Table 1.8 are derived, therefore, from a series of lupus patients with and without nephritis.

Clinicopathological correlations

Clinical features

A correlation of pathology with clinical features has been attempted by many authors. Although it is well known that the more severe histological forms of nephritis tend to have more severe clinical manifestations,[208] renal histology cannot be predicted with any certainty from the clinical picture (Figure 1.1). Table 1.5 shows the onset in relation to histology in the 1980–1989 cohort of our own series. Although there is a significant correlation between both the level of proteinuria and the presence of renal failure in predicting histology, the overlap is so great as to make this analysis useless in practice.

For example, although patients with Class IV biopsies are significantly more frequently nephrotic, hypertensive, with reduced renal function, these features do not predict the histology for an individual patient between Class I/II, IV, and V, whereas Class III is particularly variable in presentation.[208] Cameron observed a series of 82 patients with lupus nephritis and a full nephrotic syndrome during the period 1970–1989, 34 (42%) showed Class IV, 30 (37%) Class III, 10 (12%) Class V, and 8 (10%) Class II; 16 other Class IV patients were not nephrotic. Similarly 54 out of 109 were hypertensive, but only 39 of these showed Class IV biopsies, and 17 Class IV patients were normotensive. Renal function is perhaps the best clinical guide: GFR (measured by a single injection isotopic method) averaged 39±33 ml/min/1.73 m^2 in 51 Class IV patients, 91±35 ml/min/1.73/m^2 in 19 Class V, and 87±27 ml/min/1.73 m^2 in 30 patients showing Class II biopsies. Patients with Class V biopsies often show nephrotic range proteinuria, but normal renal function. Interstitial changes correlate well with GFR at the time of biopsy, both cells and interstitial volume, as well as with outcome (discussed in Chapter 7).

Serological studies

If a renal biopsy is performed after the patient has received immunosuppressive treatment for some time or the patient is flaring through a prior immunosuppressive regimen, the serological results may be negative. Titers of dsDNA antibody were noted to be higher in Class IV biopsies reported by Hill *et al.*[211] and Okamura *et al.*,[212] in adults, and Klein *et al.*[213] in children, not in all series. Those with Class IV biopsies tended to have lower C3 and C4 concentrations, as in Klein *et al.*'s study. In patients with no clinical renal disease, particularly noted in childhood onset lupus, extremely high dsDNA binding levels and very low complement concentrations have been seen.

Amyloidosis and systemic lupus

Amyloidosis is a rare finding in patients suffering from lupus, with or without nephritis; renal amyloid in lupus is extremely rare.[214,215] However, active lupus is not always associated with a rise in C-reactive protein or serum amyloid A protein in the plasma.

Summing up

Thus, systemic lupus with nephritis presents with features falling within the usual spectrum of renal syndromes, almost always with added features of a systemic disease. Today, with treatment graded to the severity of the disease (see Chapter 7), the prognostic value of the different clinical presentations has been all but eliminated, but this is another way of saying that the presence of, for example, a full nephrotic syndrome, renal dysfunction, and hypertension are indications for aggressive treatment. Nevertheless, each of these renal symptoms and signs needs to be dissected carefully, particularly in relation to histology (Chapter 8) if the most effective treatment, individualized for the particular patient under consideration, is to be achieved.

References

1 Walsh S.J., Algert C., Gregorio D.I., Reisine S.T., Rothfield N.F. (1995) Divergent racial trends in mortality from systemic lupus erythematosus. *J Rheumatol* **22**, 1663–68.

2 Ward M.M. (2009). Changes in the incidence of endstage renal disease due to lupus nephritis in the United States, 1996-2004. *J Rhemumatol* **36**, 63–7.

3 Alarcón G.S., McGwin G Jr., Roseman J.M., *et al.* (2004) Systemic lupus erythematosus in three ethnic groups. XIX. Natural history of the accrual of the American College of Rheumatology criteria prior to the occurrence of criteria diagnosis. *Arthritis Rheum* **51**, 609–15.

4 Bernatsky S. (2006) Mortality in systemic lupus erythematosus. *Arthritis Rheum* **54**, 2550–67.

5 Cameron J.S. (1999) Clinical Manifestations of lupus nephritis. In: *Lupus Nephritis* (ed. Lewis E.J., Schwartz M.M., Korbet S.M.), pp. 159–184. Oxford University Press, New York.

6 Virchow R. (1865) R. Historische notizzur lupus. *Arch Pathol Anat* **32**, 139–43.

7 Talbott J.H. (1993) Historical background of discoid and systemic lupus erythematosus. In: *Dubois' Lupus Erythematosus* (ed. Wallace D.J. and Hahn B.H.), pp. 3–10. Lea and Febiger, Philadelphia.

8 Kaposi M. (1872) Neue Beitrage zur Kentriss res Lupus Erythematosus. *Arch Dermatol Syph.*, **4**, 36–78. see also: Hebra, E and Kaposi, M. (1880) On diseases of the skin, including the exanthemata Vol. 4 (1875) (trans. W. Tay) (ed. Hilton Fagge C.), pp. 14–37. The New Sydenham Society, London.

9 Brooke H.G. (1895) Lupus erythematosus and tuberculosis. *Br J Dermatol* **7**, 73–77.

10 Osler W., Sir. (1904) On the visceral manifestations of the erythema group of skin diseases. *Am J Med Sci* **127**, 1–23.

11 Keith N.M. and Rowntree L.G. (1922) Study of renal complications of disseminated lupus erythematosus: report of four cases. *Trans Assoc Ain Physicians* **37**, 487–502.

12 Baehr G., Klemperer, P., and Schifrin, A. (1935) Diffuse disease of the peripheral circulation usually associated with lupus erythematosus. *Trans Assoc Am Physicians* **50**, 139–55.

13 Klemperer P., Pollack A.D., and Baehr G. (1941) Pathology and disseminated lupus erythematosus. *Arch Pathol* **32**, 569–631.

14 Muehrcke R.C., Kark R.M., Pirani C.L., and Pollak V.E. (1951) Lupus nephritis: a clinical and pathological study based on renal biopsies. *Medicine (Baltimore)* **36**, 1–146.

15 Friou G.J. (1958) The significance of the lupus globulin-nucleoprotein reaction. *Ann Intern Med* **49**, 866–74.

16 Seligmann M. (1957) Demonstration in the blood of patients with disseminated lupus erythematosus a substance determining a precipitation reaction with desoxyribonucleic acid. *C.R. Acad Sci (Paris)* **244**, 243–5.

17 Wallace D.J. (1993) Differential diagnosis and disease associations. In: *Dubois' lupus erythematosus* (ed. Wallace D.J. and Hahn B.H.), pp. 473–84. Lea and Febiger, Philadelphia.

18 Hargreaves M.M., Richmond H., and Morton R. (1948) Presentation of 2 bone marrow elements; the 'tart' cell and the 'LE' cell. *Proc Staff Meet Mayo Clinic* **23**, 25–8.

19 Cairns S.A., Acheson E.J., Corbett C.L. *et al.* (1979) The delayed appearance of an antinuclear factor and the diagnosis of systemic lupus erythematosus in glomerulonephritis. *Postgrad Med J* **55**, 723–7.

20 Adu D., Williams D.G., Taube D., *et al.* (1983) Late onset systemic lupus erythematosus and lupus-like disease in patients with apparent idiopathic glomerulonephritis. *Q J Med* **52**, 471–87.

21 Nissenson A.R., Port F.K. (1990) Outcome of end-stage renal disease in patients with rare causes of renal failure. *Q J Med* **74**, 63–74.

22 Mojcik C.F., Klippel J.H. (1996) End-stage renal disease and systemic lupus erythematosus. *Am J Med* **1011**, 100–7.

23 Ward M.M. (2000) Outcomes of remnalk transplantation among patients with end-satge renal disease caused by lupus nephroitis. *Kidney Int* **57**, 2136–2143.

24 Contreras G., Mattiazzi A., Guerra G., *et al.* (2010) Recurrence of lupus nephritis after kidney transplantation. *J Am Soc Nephrol* **21**, 1200–7.

25 Weening J.J., D'Agati V.D., Schwartz M.M., *et al.* International Society Of Nephrology Working Group On The Classification Of Lupus Nephritis; Renal Pathology Society Working Group On The Classification Of Lupus Nephritis (2004) The classification of glomerulonephritis in systemic lupus erythematosus revisited. *Kidney Int* **65**(2), 521–30.

26 Furness P.N., Taub N. (2006) Interobserver reproducibility and application of the ISN/RPS classification of lupus nephritis-a UK-wide study. *Am J Surg Pathol* **30**, 1030–5.

27 Markowitz G.S., D'Agati V.D., Weening J.J., D'Agati V.D. (2007) The ISN/RPS 2003 Classification Of Lupus Nephritis: An assessment at 3 years. *Kidney Int* **72**(7), 897–8.

28 Hiramatsu N., Kuroiwa H., Ikeuchi A., *et al.* (2008) Revised classification of lupus nephritis is valuable in predicting renal outcome with an indication of the proportion of glomeruli affected by chronic lesions. *Rheumatology* (Oxford) **47**(5), 702–7.

29 Gennerich W. (1922) [The present state of the lupus erythematosus question] (in German). *Arch Dermatol Syph* **138** 403–10.

30 Wallace D.J., and Hahn B.H. (ed). (1993) *Dubois' lupus erythematosus*. Section IV: Autoantibodies, pp. 181–276. Lea and Febiger, Phildelphia.

31 Le Worrall J., Snaith, M.L., Batchelor R., Isenberg D.A. (1990) SLE-a rheumatological view. *Q J Med* **275**, 319–30.

32 Fessel W.J. (1978). ANF negative systemic lupus erythematosus. *Am Med* **64**, 80–6.

33 Bielschowsky M., Helyer B.J., Howie J.B. (1959) Spontaneous haemolytic anaemia in mice of the NZB/ BI strain. *Proc Univ Otago Med School* (NZ), **37**, 9–11.

34 Tan E.M., Cohen A.S., Fries J.F., *et al.* (1982) The 1982 revised criteria for the classification of systemic lupus erythematosus. *Arthritis rheum* **25**,1271–7.

35 Hochberg M.C. (1997) Updating the American College of Rheumatology revised criteria for the classification of systemic lupus erythematosus. *Arthritis Rheum.* **40**, 1725(letter)

36 Bonilla-Martinez Z.L., Albrecht J., Troxel A.B., *et al.* (2008) The cutaneous lupus erythematosus disease area and severity index: a responsive instrument to measure activity and damage in patients with cutaneous lupus erythematosus. *Arch Dermatol* **144**, 173–80.

37 Lowenstein M.B., and Rothfield N.F. (1977) Family study of systemic lupus erythematosus. *Arthritis Rheum* **20**,1293–303.

38 Wallace D.J. (1993) The clinical presentation of SLE. In: *Dubois' lupus erythematosus* (ed. Wallace D.J. and Hahn B.H.), pp. 317–21. Lea and Febiger, Philadelphia.

39 Fries J.F., and Holman H.R. (1975) *Systemic lupus erythematosus: a clinical analysis.* Saunders, Philadelphia.

40 Arnett F.C., and Schulman L.E. (1976) Studies in familial systemic lupus erythematosus. *Medicine* **55**, 313–22.

41 Miles S., and Isenberg D. (1993) A review of serological abnormalities in relatives of SLE patients. *Lupus* **2**, 145–50.

42 de Horatius R.J., Rubin R.L., Messner R.P., *et al.* (1979) Lymphocytotoxic antibodies in laboratory personnel exposed to SLE sera. *Lancet* **2**, 1141 *(letter).*

43 Petri M., Perez-Gutthahn S., Longenecker C., Hochberg M. (1991) Morbidity of systemic lupus erythematosus: Role of race and socioeconomic status. *Am J Med* **91**, 345–53.

44 Dalle Vedove C., Del Giglio M., Schena D., Girolomoni G. (2009) Drug-induced lupus erythematosus. *Arch Dermatol Res* **301**, 99–105.

45 Steiman A.J., Gladman D.D., Ibañez D., Urowitz M.B. (2010) Prolonged serologically active clinically quiescent systemic lupus erythematosus: frequency and outcome. *Rheumatol.* **37**, 1822–7.

46 Scolari F., Savoldi S., and Costantino E. (1993) Antiphospholipid syndrome and glomerular thrombosis in the absence of overt lupus nephritis. *Nephrol Dialysis Transplant*, **8**, 1274–6.

47 Clemenceau S., Castellano F., de Oca M.M., Kaplan C., Danon F., and Levy M. (1990) C4 null alleles in childhood onset systemic lupus erythematosus. Is there any relationship with renal disease? *Pediatr Nephrol* **4**, 207–12.

48 Wilson J.G., and Fearon D.T. (1984) Altered expression of complement receptors as a pathogenetic factor in systemic lupus erythematosus. *Arthritis Rheum* **27**,1321–8.

49 Agnello V. (1978) Complement deficiency states. *Medicine* **57**,1–23.

50 Walport M., Ng Y.C., and Lachmann P.J. (1987) Erythrocytes transfused into patients with SLE and haemolytic anaemia lose complement receptor type 1 from their cell surface. *Clin Exp Immunol* **69**, 501–7.

51 Roberts J.L., Schwartz M.M., and Lewis E .J. (1978) Hereditary C2 deficiency and systemic lupus erythematosus associated with severe glomerulonephritis. *Clin Exp Immunol* **31**, 328–38.

52 Lewkonia R.M. (1992) The clinical genetics of lupus. *Lupus* **1**, 55–62.

53 Arnett F.C. (1993) The genetic basis of lupus erythematosus. In: *Dubois' lupus erythematosus* (ed. Wallace D.J. and Hahn B.H.), pp. 13–36. Lea and Febiger, Philadelphia.

54 Grossman J., Schwartz R.H., Callerame M.L., and Condemi 11. (1975) Systemic lupus erythematosus in a one year old child. *Am I Dis Child* **129**,123–5.

55 Lehman T.J.A., McCurdy D.K., Bernstein B.H., King K.K., and Hanson V. (1989) Systemic lupus erythematosus in the first decade of life. *Pediatrics* **83**, 235–9.

56 Schaller J. (1982) Lupus in childhood. *Clin Rheum Dis* **8**, 219–28.

57 Deapen D., Escalante A., Wienreb L., *et al.* (1992) A revised estimate of twin concordance in systemic lupus erythematosus. *Arthritis Rheum.*, **35**, 311–18.

58 Fronek Z., Timmerman L.A., Alper C.A., *et al.* (1988) Major histocompatibility complex associations with systemic lupus erythematosus. *Am J Med* **85** (Suppl. 6A), 42–4.

59 Reveille J.D., Schrohenloher R.E., Acton R.T., *et al.* (1989) DNA analysis of HLA-DR and DQ genes in American blacks with systemic lupus erythematosus. *Arthritis Rheum* **32**,1243–51.

60 Fielder A.H.L., Walport M.J., Batchelor J.R. *et al.* (1983) Family studies of the major histocompatibility complex in patients with systemic lupus erythematosus: importance of null alleles of C4A and C4B in determining disease susceptibility. *Br Med Y* **286**, 425–8.

61 Jacob C.O. (1992) Tumor necrosis factor alpha in autoimmunity: pretty girl or old witch? *Immunol. Today* **13**,122–5.

62 Lawley T.J., Hall R.P., Fauci A.S., Katz S.I., Hamberger, M.I., and Frank M.M. (1981) Defective Fc receptor functions associated with the haplotype HLA-AI-B8-DRw3 haplotype. *N Engl.J Med.*, **304**,185–92.

63 Flesher D.L., Sun X., Behrens T.W., Graham R.R., Criswell L.A. (2009) Recent advances in the genetics of systemic lupus erythematosus. Expert Rev Clin Immunol. 2010 May **6**(3), 461–79.

64 Fraser P.A., Ding W.Z., Mohseni M., *et al.* (2003) Glutathione S-transferase M null homozygosity and risk of systemic lupus erythematosus associated with sun exposure: a possible gene-environment interaction for autoimmunity. *J Rheumatol* **30**, 276–82

65 Iikuni N., Lourenço E.V., Hahn B.H., La Cava A. (2009) Cutting edge: Regulatory T cells directly suppress B cells in systemic lupus erythematosus. *J Immunol* **183**,1518–22.

66 Graham R.R., Hom G., Ortmann W., Behrens T.W. (2009) Review of recent genome-wide association scans in lupus. *J Intern Med* **265**, 680–8.

67 Citera G., and Wilson WA. (1993) Ethnic and geographic perspectives in SLE. *Lupus* **2**, 351–3.

68 Namjou B., Gray-McGuire C., Sestak A.L. *et al.* (2009) Evaluation of C1q genomic region in minority racial groups of lupus. *Genes Immun* **10**, 517–24.

69 Yewdall V., Cameron J.S., Nathan A.W., Neild G., Ogg C.S., and Williams D.G. (1983) Systemic lupus erythematosus and IgA deficiency. *3 Clin Lab Immunol* **10**,13–18.

70 Lawley T.J., Hall R.P., Fauci A.S., Katz S.I., Hamberger, M.I., and Frank, M.M. (1981) Defective Fc receptor functions associated with the haplotype HLA-AI-B8-DRw3 haplotype. *N Engl J Med* **304**, 185–92.

71 James J.A., Harley J.B., Scofield R.H. (2006) Epstein-Barr virus and systemic lupus erythematosus. *Curr Opin Rheumatol*, 18462–7.

72 Cooper G.S., Dooley M.A., Treadwell E.L., St Clair E.W., Gilkeson G.S. (2002) Risk factors for development of systemic lupus erythematosus: allergies, infections, and family history. *J Clin Epidemiol* **55**, 982–9.

73 Batchelor J.R., Welsh K.I., Mansilla R., *et al.* (1983) Hydralazine-induced systemic lupus erythematosus: influence of HLA-DR and sex on susceptibility. *Lancet* **1**,1107–9.

74 Mongey, A.-B. and Hess, EV (1993) The potential role of environmental agents in systemic lupus erythematosus and associated disorders. In: *Dubois' lupus erythematosus* (ed. Wallace D.J. and Hahn B.H.), pp. 37–48. Lea and Febiger, Philadelphia.

75 Cooper G.S., Treadwell E.L., Dooley M.A., St. Clair E.W., Gilkeson G.S., Taylor J.A. (2004) N-Acetyl Transferase Genotypes in Relation to Risk of Developing Systemic Lupus Erythematosus. *J Rheum* **30**, 276–82.

76 Cooper G.S., Wither J, Bernatsky S, Claudio J.O., Clarke A, Rioux JD; CaNIOS GenES Investigators, Fortin P.R. (2010) Occupational and environmental exposures and risk of systemic lupus erythematosus: silica, sunlight, solvents. *Rheumatology (Oxford)*. [Epub ahead of print]

77 Kiyohara C., Washio M., Horiuchi T., *et al.* Sapporo SLE (KYSS) Study Group. Collaborators. (2009) Cigarette smoking, N-acetyltransferase 2 polymorphisms and systemic lupus erythematosus in a Japanese population. Lupus**18**, 575–80.

78 Li X., Sundquist J., Sundquist K. (2009) Risks of rheumatic diseases in first- and second-generation immigrants in Sweden: a nationwide follow up study. *Arthritis Rheum* **60**, 1588–96.

79 Hochberg M.C. (1993) The epidemiology of systemic lupus erythematosus. In: *Dubois' lupus erythematosus* (ed. Wallace D.J. and Hahn B.H.), pp49–57. Lea and Febiger, Philadelphia.

80 Citeras G., and Wilson W.A. (1993) Ethnic and geographic perspectives in SLE. *Lupus* **2**, 351–3.

81 Siegel M. and Lee S.L. (1973) The epidemiology of systemic lupus erythematosus. *Semin Arthritis Rheum* **3**, 1–54.

82 Fessel W.J. (1974) Systemic lupus erythematosus in the community Incidence, prevalence, outcome, and first symptoms; the high prevalence in African ancestry women. *Arch Intern Med* **134**, 1027–35.

83 Johnson A.E., Gordon C., Palmer R.G., and Bacon P.A. (1995) The prevalence and incidence of systemic lupus erythematosus in Birmingham, England. *Arth Rheum* **38**, 551–8.

84 Nived O., Sturfelt G., and Wollheim F. (1985) Systemic lupus erythematosus in an adult population in Southern Sweden: incidence, prevalence, and validity of the ARA revised classification criteria. *Br J Rheumatol* **24**, 147–54.

85 Symmons D.P.M. (1995) Lupus around the world. *Frequency of lupus in people of African origin. Lupus* **4**, 176–8.

86 Serdula M.K., and Rhoads G.G. (1979) Frequency of systemic lupus erythematosus in different ethnic groups in Hawaii. *Arthritis Rheum* **22**, 328–33.

87 Maskarinec G., and Katz A.R. (1995) Prevalence of systemic lupus erythematosus in Hawaii: is there a difference between ethnic groups? *Hawaii Med J* **54**, 406–9.

88 Cooper G.S., Parks C.G., Treadwell E.L., *et al.* (2002) Differences by race, sex and age in the clinical and immunologic features of recently diagnosed systemic lupus erythematosus patients in the southeastern United States. *Lupus* **11**, 161–167.

89 Dooley M.A., Hogan S., Jennette C., Falk R. (1997) Cyclophosphamide therapy for lupus nephritis: poor renal survival in black Americans. *Kidney Int* 1997 **51**,1188–95.

90 Bastian H.M., Alarcón G.S., Roseman J.M., *et al.* LUMINA Study Group. (2007) Systemic lupus erythematosus in a multiethnic US cohort (LUMINA) XL II: factors predictive of new or worsening proteinuria. *Rheumatology* **46**, 683–9

91 Lewis E.J., Hunsicker L.G., Lan S.P., Rohde R.D., Lachin J.M. (1992) A controlled trial of plasmapheresis therapy in severe lupus nephritis. The Lupus Nephritis Collaborative Study Group. *N Engl J Med* **326**,1373–9.

92 Johnson S.R., Urowitz M.B., Ibañez D., Gladman D.D. (2006) Ethnic variation in disease patterns and health outcomes in systemic lupus erythematosus. *Rheumatol* **33**,1990–5.

93 Sutcliffe N., Clarke A.E., Gordon C., Farewell V., Isenberg D.A. (1999) The association of socio-economic status, race, psychosocial factors and outcome in patients with systemic lupus erythematosus. *Rheumatology* **38**,1130–7.

94 Freedman B.I., Wilson C.H., Spray B.J., Tuttle A.B., Olorenshaw I.M., Kammer G.M. (1997) Familial clustering of end-stage renal disease in blacks with lupus nephritis. *Am J Kidney Dis* **29**, 729–32.

95 Mok C.C., Ho C.T., Chan K.W., Lau C.S., Wong R.W. (2004) Outcome and prognostic indicators of diffuse proliferative lupus glomerulonephritis treated with sequential oral cyclophosphamide and azathioprine. *Arthritis Rheum* **46**, 1003–13.

96 Mok C.C., Ying K.Y., Lau C.S., *et al.* (2004) Treatment of pure membranous lupus nephropathy with prednisone and azathioprine: an open-label trial. *Am J Kidney Dis* **43**, 197–208.

97 Chan T.M., Li F.K., Tang C.S., *et al.* (2000) Efficacy of mycophenolate mofetil in patients with diffuse proliferative lupus nephritis. Hong Kong-Guangzhou Nephrology Study Group. *N Engl J Med* **343**, 1156–1162.

98 Hu W., Liu Z., Chen H., Tang Z., Wang Q., Shen K., *et al.* Mycophenolate mofetil vs cyclophosphamide therapy for patients with diffuse proliferative lupus nephritis. *Chin Med J* 2002 **115**, 705–9.

99 Ong L.M., Hooi L.S., Lim T.O., *et al.* (2005) Randomized controlled trial of pulse intravenous cyclophosphamide versus mycophenolate mofetil in the induction therapy of proliferative lupus nephritis. *Nephrology* **10**, 504–10.

100 Lopez-Acuna D., Hochberg M.C., and Gittelsohn A.M. (1982) Mortality from discoid and systemic lupus erythematosus in the United States 1968–78. *Arthritis Rheum* **25** (Suppl), S80.

101 Kaslow R.A. (1982) High rate of death caused by systemic lupus erythematosus among US residents of Asian descent. *Arthritis Rheum* **25**, 414–16.

102 Levy M., Montes de Oca M., and Babron M.C. (1989) Lupus erythematux dissemine chez l'enfant. Etude collaborative en region parisienne. *Journées Parisiennes de Pediatric.* p. 52–8 Flammarion, Paris.

103 Costenbader K.H., Feskanich D., Stampfer M.J., Karlson E.W. (2004) Reproductive and menopausal factors and risk of systemic lupus erythematosus in women. *Arthritis Rheum* **56**, 1251–62.

104 Petri M., Kim M.Y., Kalunian K.C., Grossman J., Hahn B.H., Sammaritano L.R. *et al.* (2005) OC-SELENA Trial Combined oral contraceptives in women with systemic lupus erythematosus. *N Engl J Med* **353**, 2550–8.

105 Sánchez-Guerrero J., Uribe A.G., Jiménez-Santana L., *et al.* (2005) A trial of contraceptive methods in women with systemic lupus erythematosus. *N Engl J Med* **353**, 2539–49.

106 Buyon J.P., Petri M.A., Kim M.Y., *et al.* (2005) The effect of combined estrogen and progesterone hormone replacement therapy on disease activity in systemic lupus erythematosus: a randomized trial. *Ann Intern Med* **142**, 953–62.

107 Sánchez-Guerrero J., González-Pérez M., Durand-Carbajal M., *et al.* (2007) Menopause hormonal therapy in women with systemic lupus erythematosus. *Arthritis Rheum* **56**, 3070–9.

108 Lu Q., Wu A., Tesmer L., Ray D., Yousif N., Richardson B. (2007) Demethylation of CD40LG on the inactive X in T cells from women with lupus. *J Immunol* **179**, 6352–8.

109 Ward M.M., Studenski S. Age associated clinical manifestations of systemic lupus erythematosus: a multivariate regression analysis. (1990) *J Rheumatol* **17**, 476–81.

110 Maddison P., Farewell V., Isenberg D., *et al.* Systemic Lupus International Collaborating Clinics. (2002) The rate and pattern of organ damage in late onset systemic lupus erythematosus. *J Rheumatol* **29**(5),913–7.

111 Cohen I.M., Swerdlin A.H.R., Steinberg S.M., and Stone R.A. (1980) Mesangial proliferative glomerulonephritis in mixed connective tissue disease. *Clin Nephrol* **13**, 93–6.

112 Schnabel A., Csernok E., Isenberg D.A., Mrowka C., and Gross W.L. (1995) Antineutrophil cytoplasmic antibodies in systemic lupus erythematosus. *Arthritis Rheum* **38**, 633–7.

113 Bridoux F, Kyndt X, Abou-Ayache R., *et al.* (2004) Proximal tubular dysfunction in primary Sjögren's syndrome: a clinicopathological study of 2 cases. *Clin Nephrol* **61**, 434–9.

114 Cervera R., Khamashta M., Font J. *et al.* (1993) Systemic lupus erythematosus: clinical and immunologic patterns of disease expression in a cohort of 1000 patients. *Medicine* **72**,113–24.

115 Wallace D.J. (1993) The clinical presentation of SLE. In: *Dubois' lupus erythematosus* (ed. DJ Wallace and B.H. Hahn) pp.317–21. Lea and Febiger, Philadelphia.

116 Cameron J.S. (1994) Lupus nephritis in childhood and adolescence. *Pediatr Nephrol* **8**, 230–49.

117 Chen Y.E., Korbet S.M., Katz R.S., Schwartz M.M., Lewis E.J., Collaborative Study Group. (2008): Value of a complete or partial remission in severe lupus nephritis. *Clin J Am Soc Nephrol* **3**(1): 46–53.

118 Gibson K.L., Gipson D.S., Massengill S.A., *et al* (2009) Predictors of Relapse and End Stage Kidney Disease in Proliferative Lupus Nephritis: Focus on Children, Adolescents and Young Adults. *Clin J Am Soc Nephrol* **4**, 1962–7.

119 Hollcraft R.M., Dubois E.L., Lundberg G.D., *et al* (1976) Renal change in systemic lupus erythematosus with normal renal function. *J Rheumatol* **3**, 251–61.

120 Mahajan S.K., Ordóñez N.G., Feitelson P.J., Lim V.S., Spargo B.H., and Katz A.I. (1977) Lupus nephropathy without clicical renal involvement. *Medicine (Baltimore)* **56**, 493–501.

121 Cavallo T., Cameron W.R., and Lapenas, D., (1977) Immunopathology of early and clinically silent lupus nephropathy. *Am J Pathol* **87**,1–15.

122 Leehey D.J., Katz A.I., Azaran A.H., Aronson A.J., and Spargo, B.H. (1982) Silent diffuse lupus nephritis: long term follow-up. *Am J Kidney Dis* **2** (Suppl. 1), 188–96.

123 O'Dell J.R., Hays R.C., Guggenheim S.J., and Steigerwald J.C. (1985) Systemic lupus erythematosus without clinical renal abnormalities: renal biopsy findings and clinical course. *Ann Rheum Dis* **44**, 415–19.

124 Stamenkovic I., Favre H., Donath A., Assimacopoulos A., and Chatelanat F. (1986) Renal biopsy in SLE irrespective of clinical findings: long term follow-up. *Clin Nephrol* **26**, 109–15.

125 Font J., Torras A., Cerevera R., Darnell A., Revert L., and Ingelmo M. (1987) Silent renal disease in systemic lupus erythematosus. *Clin Nephrol* **27**, 283–8.

126 Terai C., Nojima Y., Takano K., Yamada A., and Takaku F. (1987) Determination of urinary albumin excretion by radioimmunoassay in patients with subclinical lupus nephritis. *Clin Nephrol* **27**, 79–83.

127 Adu D., and Cameron J.S. (1982) Lupus nephritis. *Clin Rheum Dis* **8**, pp. 153–63.

128 Simenhoff M.L., and Merrill J.P. (1964) The spectrum of lupus nephritis. *Nephron* **1**, 3480–74.

129 Shearn M.A., Hopper J., and Biava C.G. (1980) Membranous lupus nephropathy initially seen as idiopathic membranous nephropathy. *Arch Intern Med* **140**, 1521–3.

130 Harvey A.M., Schulman L.E., Tumulty A., Lockard Conley C., and Schonrich E.H. (1954) Systemic lupus erythematosus. Review of the literature and clinical analysis of 138 cases. *Medicine (Baltimore)* **33**, 2914–37.

131 Kellum R.E., and Haserick J.R. (1964) Systemic lupus erythematosus. A statistical evaluation of mortality based upon a consecutive series of 299 patients. *Arch Intern Med* **113**, 200–7.

132 Estes D., and Christian C.L. (1971) The natural history of systemic lupus erythematosus by prospective analysis. *Medicine* **50**, 85–95.

133 Petri M., Singh S., Tesfasyone H., Malik A. (2009) Prevalence of flare and influence of demographic and serologic factors on flare risk in systemic lupus erythematosus: a prospective study. *J Rheumatol* **36**, 2476–80.

134 Baldwin D.S., Gluck M.C., Lowenstein J., and Gallo G.R. (1977) Clinical course as related to the morphologic forms and their transitions. *Am J Med* **62** 12–30.

135 Dubois (1976). *Systemic lupus erythematosus* 2nd edn (revised) Lea and Febiger, Philadelphia.

136 Leaker B., Fairley K.F., Dowling J., and Kincaid-Smith P. (1987) Lupus nephritis: clinical and pathological correlation. *Q Med* **62**,163–79.

137 Shearn M.A. (1964) Normocholesterolemic nephrotic syndrome of systemic lupus erythematosus. *Am J Med* **36**, 250–61.

138 Groggel G.C., Cheung A.K., Ellis-Benigni K., and Wilson D.E. (1989) Treatment of nephrotic hyperlipoproteinemia with gemfibrozil. *Kidney Int* **36**, 266–71.

139 Tu W.H., and Shearn M.A. (1967) Systemic lupus erythematosus and latent renal tubular dysfunction. *Ann Intern Med* **67**, 100–9.

140 Spriggs B., and Epstein W.V. (1974) Clinical and laboratory correlates of L-chain proteinuria in systemic lupus erythematosus. *J Rheumatol* **1**, 287–92.

141 Parving H-H., Sorensen F., Mogensen C.E., and Helin P. (1980) Urinary albumin and β2-microglobulin excretion rates in patients with systemic lupus erythematosus. *Scand J Rheumatol* **9**, 49–51.

142 Yeung C.K., Wong K.L., Ng R.P., and Ng W.L. (1984) Tubular dysfunction in systemic lupus erythematosus. *Nephron*, **36**, 84–8.

143 Kozeny G.A., Barr W., Bansal VK. *et al.* (1987) Occurrence of renal tubular dysfunction in lupus nephritis. *Arch. Intern. Med* **147**, 891–5.

144 Cryer P.E., and Kissane J.M. (1980) Washington University case conference. Interstitial nephritis in a patient with systemic lupus erythematosus. *Am J Med* **69**, 775–81.

145 Gur H., Kopolovic Y., and Gross D.J. (1987) Chronic predominant interstitial nephritis in patients with systemic lupus erythematosus. A follow-up of three years and review of the literature. *Ann Rheum Dis* **46**, 617–23.

146 De Fronzo R.A., Cooke C.R., Goldberg M., Cox M., Myers A.R., and Agus Z.S. (1977) Impaired renal potassium secretion in systemic lupus erythematosus. *Arch Intern Med* **86**, 268–71.

147 Herrera Acosta J., Gurrero J., Erkesod M.L., *et al.* (1978) Normotensive hyperreninemia in systemic lupus erythematosus. An indicator of tubular dysfunction. *Nephron* **22**, 128–37.

148 Kiley J., and Zager P. (1984). Hyporeninemic hypoaldosternism in two patients with systemic lupus erythematosus. *Am J Kidney Dis* **4**, 439–43.

149 Lee F.O., Quismorio F.P., Troum O.M., Anderson P.W., Do Y.S., and Hsueh W.A. (1989) Mechanisms of hyperkalemia in systemic lupus erythematosus. *Arch Intern Med* **148**, 397–401.

150 Dreyling K.W., Wanner C., and Schollmeyer P. (1980) Control of hyperkalemia with fluorocortisone in a patient with systemic lupus erythematosus. *Clin Nephrol* **33**, 179–83.

151 Gruppo Italiano per lo Studio della Nefrite del Lupus (GISNEL). (1992) Lupus nephritis: prognostic factors and probability of sustaining life-supporting renal function 10 years after diagnosis. *Am J Kidney Dis* **19**, 473–9

152 Donadio J.V., Jr. Hart G.M., Bergstralh E.J., and Holley K.E. (1995) Prognostic determinants in lupus nephritis: a long term clinicopathologic study. *Lupus* **4**, 109–15.

153 Hasselaar P., Derksen R.H.W.M., Blokzijl L., *et al.* (1989) Risk factors for thrombosis in lupus patients. *Ann Rheum Dis* **48**, 933–40.

154 Appel G.B., Williams G.S., Melzer J.I., and Pirani C.L. (1976) Renal vein thrombosis, nephrotic syndrome and systemic lupus erythematosus. *Ann Intern Med* **85**, 310–17.

155 Mintz G., Acevedo Vasquez E., Guterriez-Espinosa G., and Avelar-Garnica F. (1984) Renal vein thrombosis and inferior vena cava thrombosis in systemic lupus erythematosus. *Arthritis Rheum* **27**, 539–44.

156 Cameron J.S., Ogg C.S., and Wass C.S. (1988) Complications of the nephrotic syndrome. In: *The nephrotic syndrome* (ed. Cameron J.S. and Glassock R.J.), pp. 849–920. Marcel Dekker, New York.

157 Stafford-Brady F.J., Urowitz M.B., Gladman D.D., and Easterbrook M. (1988) Lupus retinopathy: patterns, associations and prognosis. *Arthritis Rheum* **31**, 1105–10.

158 Phadke K., Trachtman H., Nicastri A., Chen C.K., and Tejani A. (1984) Acute renal failure as the initial manifestation of systemic lupus erythematosus in children. *J Pediatr* **105**, 38–41.

159 Ywung C.K., Wong K.L., Wong W.S., Ng M.T., Chan K.W., and Ng W.L. Crescentic lupus glomerulonpehritis. *Clin Nephrol* **21**, 251–8.

160 Ponticelli C., Imbasciati E., Brancaccio D., Tarantino A., and Rivolta E. (1979) Acute renal failure in systemic lupus ervthematosus. *Br Med J* **3**, 716–19.

161 Cecere E.A., Yishinoya S., and Pope R.M. (1981) Fatal thrombotic thrombocytopenic purpura in a patient with systemic lupus erythematosus. Relationship to circulating immune complexes. *Arthritis Rheum* **24**, 550–3.

162 Finkelstein R., Carter A., Marel A., and Brook J.G. (1982) Plasma infusions in thrombotic thrombocytopenic purpura complicating systemic lupus erythematosus. *Postgrad Med J* **58**, 577–9.

163 Gelfand J., Truong L., Stern L., Pirani C.L., and Appel G.B. (1985) Thrombotic thrombocytopenic purpura syndrome in systemic lupus erythematosus: treatment with plasma exchange. *Am J Kidney Dis* **6**, 154–60.

164 Fox D.A., Faix J.D., Coblvn J., Fraser J., Smith B., and Weinblatt M.E. (1986) Thrombotic thrombocytopenic purpura and systemic lupus erythematosus. *Ann Rheum Dis* **45**, 319–22.

165 Case records of the Massachusetts General Hospital. (1976) Case no 2-1976. Principal discussant: Epstein, F.H. *N Engl J Med* **294**, 100–5.

166 Cunningham E., Prevost J., Bretjens J., Reichlin M., and Venuto C. (1978) Acute renal failure secondary to interstitial lupus nephritis. *Arch Intern Med* **138**, 1560–1.

167 Tron F., Ganeval D., and Droz D. (1979) Immunologically-mediated acute renal failure of non-glomerular origin in the course of systemic lupus erythematosus (SLE). Report of two cases. *Am J Med* **67**, 529–32.

168 Wallace D.J., and Hahn B.M. (1993). *Dubois' lupus erythematosus* 4th edn. Lea and Febiger, Philadelphia.

169 Rahman P., Gladman D.D., Ibanez D., Urowitz M.B. (2001) Significance of isolated hematuria and isolated pyuria in systemic lupus erythematosus. *Lupus* **10**, 418–23.

170 Boumpas D.T., Austin H.A., III Fessler B.J., *et al* (1995) Systemic lupus erythematosus: emerging concepts. Part 1: Renal, neuropsychiatric, cardiovascular, pulmonary and hematologic disease. *Ann Intern Med* **122**, 940–50.

171 Sontheimer R.D. (ed.) (1997) Special issue: Skin disease in lupus erythematosus. *Lupus* **6**, 75–217.

172 Dessar K.B., Sartiano G.P., and Cooper, J.L. (1969) Lupus livedo and cutaneous infarction. *Angiology* **20**, 261.

173 Wallace D.J. (1993) The musculoskeletal system. In: *Dubois' lupus erythematosus* (ed. Wallace D.J. and Hahn B.H.), pp. 322–31. Lea and Febiger, Philadelphia.

174 Bywaters E.G.L. (1975) Jaccoud's syndrome. A sequel to the joint involvement of systemic lupus erythematosus. *Clin Rheum. Dis.*, **1**, 125–48.

175 Quismorio F.P. (1993) Cardiac abnormalities in systemic lupus erythematosus. In: *Dubois' lupus erythematosus* (ed. Wallace D.J. and Hahn B.H.), pp. 332–42. Lea and Febiger, Philadelphia.

176 Nihoyannopoulos P., Gomez P.M., Joshi J., Loizou S., Walport M.J., and Oakley C. (1990) Cardiac abnormalities in systemic lupus erythematosus. *Circulation* **82**, 369–75.

177 Quismorio F.P. (1993) Pulmonary manifestations. In: *Dubois' lupus erythematosus* (ed. Wallace D.J. and Hahn B.H.), pp. 343–355. Lea and Febiger, Philadelphia.

178 Galve E., Candell-Riera J., Pigrau C., *et al.* (1988) Prevalence, morphological types, and evolution of cardiac valvular disease in systemic lupus erythematosus. *N Eng J Med* **319**, 817–23.

179 Leung W-H., Wing K.-L., Lau C.-P., Wong C.-K., and Liu H.-W. (1988) Association between antiphospholipid antibodies and cardiac abnormalities in patients with systemic lupus erythematosus. *Am J Med* **89**, 411–19.

180 Asherson R.A., and Oakley C. (1986) Pulmonary hypertension and systemic lupus erythematosus. *J Rheumatol* **13**, 1–5.

181 Schwab E.P., Schumacher H.R., Jr, Freundlich B., and Callegari P.E. (1993) Pulmonary hemorrhage in systemic lupus erythematosus. *Semin Arthritis Rheum* **23**, 8–15.

182 Abramson S.B., Dobro J., Eeberle M., *et al.* (1991) Acute reversible hypoxemia in systemic lupus erythematosus. *Ann Intern Med* **114,** 941–7.

183 Weinreb L., Sharma O.P., and Quismorio F.P., Jr. (1990) A long-term study of interstitial lung disease in systemic lupus erythematosus. *Semin Arthritis Rheum* **20,** 48–56.

184 Quismorio F.P. (1993) Hemic and lymphatic abnormalities in SLE. In: *Dubois' lupus erythematosus* (ed. Wallace D.J. and Hahn B.H.), pp. 418–30. Lea and Febiger, Philadelphia.

185 Bernatsky S., Boivin J.F., Joseph L., *et al.*(2005) An international cohort study of cancer in systemic lupus erythematosus. *Arthritis Rheum* **52**, 1481–90.

186 Lim L., Ron M.A., Ormerod I.E.C., *et al.* (1988) Psychiatric and neurological manifestations in systemic lupus erythematosus. *Q J Med* **66**, 27–38.

187 Van Dam A.P. (1991) Diagnosis and pathogenesis of CNS lupus. *Rheumatol Int.,* **11,** 1–11.

188 West S.G. (1994). Neuropsychiatric lupus. *Rheum Clin N Am* **20**, 129–58.

189 Wallace D.J., and Metzger A.L. (1993) Systemic lupus erythematosus and the nervous system. In: *Dubois' lupus erythematosus* (ed. Wallace D.J. and Hahn B.H.), pp. 370–85. Lea and Febiger, Philadelphia.

190 Hanly J.G., Urowitz M.B., Su L., *et al*; Systemic Lupus International Collaborating Clinics (2008); Short-term outcome of neuropsychiatric events in systemic lupus erythematosus upon enrollment into an international inception cohort study. *Arthritis Rheum* **59**, 721–9.

191 Hanly J.G., Urowitz M.B., Siannis F., *et al.* Systemic Lupus International Collaborating Clinics (2008). Autoantibodies and neuropsychiatric events at the time of systemic lupus erythematosus diagnosis: results from an international inception cohort study. *Arthritis Rheum* **58**, 843–53

192 Rubbert A., Miarienhagen J., Pirner K., *et al.* (1993) Single-photon emission computed tomography analysis of cerebral bloodflow in the evaluation of central nervous system involvement in systemic lupus erythematosus. *Arthritis Rheum* **36**, 1253–62.

193 Holman B.L. (1993) Functional imaging in systemic lupus erythematosus: an accurate indicator of central nervous system involvement? *Arthritis Rheum* **36**, 1193–5.

194 Kent D.L., Haynor D.R., Longstreth W.T., Jr, and Larson E.B. (1994) The clinical efficacy of magnetic resonance imaging in neuroimaging. *Ann Intern Med* **120**, 856–71.

195 Herd J.K., Mehdi M., Uzendoski D.M., and Saldivar V.A. (1978) Chorea associated with systemic lupus erythematosus: report of 2 cases and review of the literature. *Pediatrics* **61**, 308–13.

196 Khamashta M.A., Gil A., Anciones B., *et al* (1988) Chorea in systemic lupus erythematosus: association with antiphospholipid antibodies. *Ann Rheum Dis* **47**, 681–3.

197 Frampton G., Hicks J., and Cameron J.S. (1991) Significance of anti-phospholipid antibodies in patients with lupus nephritis. *Kidney Int* **39**, 1225–31.

198 Ginsburg K.S., Wright E.A., Larson M.G., *et al.* (1992) A controlled study of the prevalence of cognitive dysfunction in randomly selected patients with systemic lupus erythematosus. *Arthritis Rheum* **35**, 776–82.

199 McAbee G.N., and Barasch E.S. (1990) Resolving MRI lesions in lupus erythematosus selectively involving the brainstem. *Pediatr Neurol* **61**, 186–9.

200 Becker G.J., Waldburger M., Hughes G.R.V., and Pepys, M. (1980) Value of serum C-reactive protein measurement in the investigation of fever in systemic lupus erythematosus. *Ann Rheum Dis* **39**, 50–2.

201 Honig S., Gorevic P., and Weissmann G. (1977) C-reactive protein in systemic lupus erythematosus. *Arthritis Rheum* **20**, 1065–70.

202 Itoh Y., Sekine H., Hosono O., *et al.* (1990) Thrombotic thrombocytopenic purpura in two patients with systemic lupus erythematosus: clinical significance of anti-platelet antibodies. *Clin Immunol* **57**, 125–36.

203 Nadorra R.L., Nakazato Y., and Landing B.H. (1987) Pathologic features of gastrointestinal tract lesions in childhood onset systemic lupus erythematosus: study of 26 patients with review of the literature. *Pediatr Pathol* **7**, 245–59.

204 Laing T.J. (1988) Gastrointestinal vasculitis and pneumatosis intestinalis due to systemic lupus erythematosus: successful treatment with pulse intravenous cyclophosphamide. *Am J Med* **85**, 555–8.

205 Runyon B.A., La Brecque D.R., and Anuras S. (1980) The spectrum of liver disease in systemic lupus erythematosus. Report of 33 histologically-proved cases and review of the literature. *Am J Med* **60**, 187–94.

206 Miller M.H., Urowitz M.B., Gladman D.D., and Blendis L.M. (1984) The liver in systemic lupus erythematosus. *Q J Med* **53**, 401–9.

207 Dimant J., Gonzler E., Slesinger M., *et al.* (1979) The clinical significance of Raynaud's phenomenon in systemic lupus erythematosus. *Arthritis Rheum* **28**, 815–19.

208 Schwartz M.M., Kawala K.S., Corwin H.L., and Lewis E.J. (1987) The prognosis of segmental glomerulonephritis in systemic lupus erythematosus. *Kidney Int* **52**, 274–9.

209 Alexopoulos E., Cameron J.S., and Hartley B.H. (1990) Lupus nephritis: correlation of interstitial cells with glomerular function. *Kidney Int* **37**, 100–9.

210 Magil A.B., Ballon H.S., Chan V., Lirenman D.S., Rae A., and Sutton R.A.L. (1984) Parognotic factors in diffuse proliferative glomerulonephritis. *Kidney Int* **34**, 511–17.

211 Hill G.S., Hinglais N., Tron F., and Bach J.-E (1978) Systemic lupus erythematosus. Morphologic correlations with immunologic and clinical data at the time of biopsy. *Am J Med* **64**, 61–79.

212 Okamura M., Kanayama Y., Amatsu K., *et al.* (1993) Significance of enzyme-linked immunosorbent assay (ELISA) for antibodies to double stranded and single stranded DNA in patients with lupus nephritis: correlation with severity of renal histology. *Ann Rheum Dis* **52**,14–20.

213 Klein M.H.,Thorner P.S., Yoon S.-J., Poucell S., and Baumal R. (1984) Determination of circulating immune complexes, C3 and C4 complement components and anti-DNA antibody in different classes of lupus nephritis. *Int J Pediatr* Nephrol **5**, 75–82.

214 Huston D.P., McAdam K.P.W.J., Balow J.E. *et al.* (1981) Amyloidosis in systemic lupus erythematosus. *Am J Med* **70**, 320–3.

215 Orellana C., Collado A., Hernandez M.V., Font J., Del Olmo J.A., and Munoz-Gomez J. (1995) When does amyloidosis complicate systemic lupus erythematosus? *Lupus* **4**, 415–17.

Chapter 2

Autoantibodies and lupus nephritis

Anisur Rahman, Jessica J. Manson and
David A. Isenberg

Introduction

Systemic lupus erythematosus (SLE) is an autoimmune rheumatic disease with an incidence of approximately four cases per 10^5 people per year in the UK.[1] The peak age of onset is between the ages of 20 and 40, and women are affected approximately 10 times more often than men. The condition is more common in some racial groups than others. In Birmingham (UK), the prevalence of SLE in women is 206 per 10^5 in Afro-Caribbeans, 91 per 10^5 in Asians, and 36 per 10^5 in Caucasians. For men the corresponding figures were 9.3 per 10^5, 2.6 per 10^5, and 3.4 per 10^5 for these three ethnic groups respectively.[1]

The clinical manifestations of the disease are protean and it is often characterized by a relapsing and remitting pattern in which the frequency of flares varies between patients. The disease can affect practically any organ or system, for example causing pleurisy, psychosis, anemia, miscarriage, and fetal cardiac abnormalities, arthritis, skin rash, and/or glomerulonephritis.[2,3] Estimates of the frequency of renal involvement in this disease usually vary between 25 and 65% (reviewed in[4]) but will obviously be closer to 100% in those patients seen in a nephrology department.

Lupus nephritis is recognized as one of the most severe forms of organ involvement, both in terms of direct mortality and of the degree of immunosuppression required to treat it. The mortality rate due to all causes in SLE has remained relatively stable in the past 50 years (see Table 2.1). Before 1950, a high percentage of these deaths were due to renal failure. More recently, the proportion of deaths due to renal failure has fallen as therapy has improved. Cardiovascular disease and infection are increasingly important causes of death in patients with SLE. Infection can often occur in patients who are taking high-dose immunosuppression, for example due to renal disease. Thus, it is clear that the development of nephritis in a patient with SLE has serious prognostic implications, which makes it imperative to gain a greater understanding of the role played by autoantibodies in causing this renal damage.

Just as the clinical features of SLE are manifold, so serological studies of patients with the disease indicate that many different autoantibodies can be found in these patients.[7–9] The majority of these are directed against antigens found in the cell nucleus. However, many of these antibody specificities only occur in a minority of patients with SLE. Furthermore, significant evidence for a link to the pathogenesis of the

Table 2.1 Trends in the causes of death in systemic lupus erythematosus

	Dubois et al.[5,6] 1950–1955	Dubois et al.[5,6] 1956–1962	Dubois et al.[5,6] 1963–1973	Reveille et al.[7] 1973–1987	Centre for Rheumatology UCH 1978–2008
Patients studied	491	491	491	389	500
Deaths (all causes) (%)	12	20	19	22	15
Percentage of deaths due to nephritis	26	36	14	4	8
Percentage of deaths due to infection	16	12	18	39	25

UCH, Rheumatology Unit (unpublished data).
Superscript numbers are reference numbers.

disease has only been obtained for a few autoantibodies, as discussed in a recent review.[10] Thus, in discussing the role of autoantibodies in the pathogenesis of lupus nephritis, we will concentrate primarily on these specificities. In a large European study of 1000 patients, 96% had antinuclear antibodies, and in particular 78% had raised titres of antibodies against double-stranded DNA (anti-dsDNA).[3] In contrast to antibodies against single-stranded DNA (anti-ssDNA), anti-dsDNA antibodies are very infrequently found in any disease other than SLE.[11–12] Table 2.2 shows the percentages of patients with antibodies to various nuclear antigens, both in the European study and in a cohort of 500 patients in our unit, followed for 1 year or until death.

However, there is a striking restriction amongst the autoantigenic targets in lupus. Using two-dimensional gel electrophoresis of HeLa cell extracts, it has been estimated that a typical mammalian cell contains physiologically significant quantities of 1500–2000 different proteins.[13] However, Gharavi et al.[14] showed that only a small minority of these bind to sera from patients with SLE. Thus, they deduced that the presence of autoantibodies to intracellular proteins in SLE could not be explained simply by postulating a polyclonal activation of B cells. This conclusion was underlined by their finding that SLE sera bound fewer bacterial proteins but more mammalian proteins than sera from healthy subjects.

Because so few of the possible autoantibody specificities are represented in patients with lupus, the question arises whether these particular antibodies are important in causing the tissue damage of the disease. In their review of the role of autoantibodies in autoimmune disease, Naparstek and Plotz[15] reiterated the important difference between demonstrating that an antibody is associated with a particular clinical effect and showing that it plays a role in causing that effect. To prove the former, it is only necessary to show that the antibody is present at higher frequency or in higher titers in patients who develop the clinical complication in question than in those who do not. Serological evidence of this kind has been obtained linking several of the antibodies

Table 2.2 Prevalence of different autoantibodies in patients with systemic lupus erythematosus

Antibody	% Prevalence in 500 patients seen at the Centre for Rheumatology UCH	% Prevalence in 1000 European patients[3]
Antinuclear	95	96
Anti-dsDNA	64	78
Anti-Ro	32	25
Anti-La	13	19
Anti-Sm	13	10
Anti-U$_1$RNP	27	13
Anticardiolipin IgG	21	24
Anticardiolipin IgM	9	13
Lupus anticoagulant	14	15
Rheumatoid factor	25	18

listed in Table 2.2 to the occurrence of lupus nephritis, and each of these antibodies will be considered in turn in this chapter.

To show that an autoantibody is involved in the pathogenesis of lupus nephritis, however, one must also show that both it and a suitable target antigen are present in damaged glomerular tissue, that the introduction of the antigen and antibody to a suitable experimental system leads to the development of such damage, and, ideally, that reduction of antibody levels in the glomerulus leads to amelioration of disease. Proof of this kind has been much more difficult to obtain, and most of the experimental data published so far pertains to dsDNA and its physically associated antigens.

Anti-DNA antibodies in lupus nephritis

Antibodies with the ability to bind DNA were isolated from sera of patients with SLE by four different research groups in 1957.[16–19] Using immunoprecipitation in gel-diffusion studies, Tan et al.[20] demonstrated that the amount of antibody to dsDNA varied during the course of the disease. In one patient, in particular, they showed that on four separate occasions the level rose just prior to disease exacerbation, which included proteinuria. A very similar relationship between disease activity and presence of anti-dsDNA antibodies in serum was described by Schur and Sandson (1968).[21] They looked at serum samples taken from 96 patients with SLE (44 with nephritis) over a 2-year period. Antibodies to both native (double-stranded) and heat-denatured (single-stranded) DNA were found in more than 60% of patients with active nephritis but in only 10–15% of those with inactive disease. Characteristically, exacerbations of nephritis in these patients were preceded by the appearance of anti-DNA antibodies and a fall in serum complement. These changes were reversed as the nephritis resolved. Using a different assay, Schur and colleagues then showed that serum samples from patients with SLE had significantly higher levels of DNA-binding activity than those from healthy subjects or people with other rheumatic diseases.[22] When immunoglobulin (Ig)G was isolated from these sera, most of the DNA-binding activity was retained in the IgG fraction, suggesting that this binding was mediated by antigen–antibody interaction. Among 140 samples, 38 of the 45 sera with the highest binding affinity were derived from patients with active lupus nephritis.

Koffler et al.[23] used immunofluorescent staining to demonstrate that the kidneys of patients who had died from lupus nephritis contained plentiful glomerular deposits of IgG and complement, but less IgM compared to IgG. Elution of this glomerular antibody showed that it had a higher content of antinuclear binding activity per unit of IgG than serum from the same patient in each case. Eluates from kidneys of patients without SLE did not show antinuclear reactivity. Though a specific test for anti-DNA binding was not carried out, antinuclear binding of the eluates could be partially inhibited by adding dsDNA. These results suggested that high serum anti-dsDNA antibody levels might be associated with lupus nephritis due to the concentration of a proportion of these antibodies (particularly those of the IgG isotype) in the glomeruli followed by the activation of complement. This group then used hemagglutination of antigen-coated erythrocytes to look more specifically at serum antibodies to different polynucleotides during the course of the disease.[10] They found that antibodies to dsDNA were in 60% of 25 patients with SLE, were almost never found in other rheumatic conditions, and that levels were often raised during periods of disease activity. Although anti-ssDNA antibodies were found in 87% of these patients, they were also found in a number of other conditions, for example rheumatoid arthritis and chronic active hepatitis, and levels in patients with SLE did not reflect disease activity closely.

In studying the activity of serum antibodies to dsDNA in patients with SLE, Winfield et al.[24] found that although this was usually higher when the disease was active, avidity was reduced if this activity took the form of glomerulonephritis. The explanation appeared to be that the highest avidity antibodies were being removed from serum by their deposition in the glomeruli, as glomerular eluates from autopsy specimens of patients who had died from lupus nephritis showed much higher avidity for dsDNA than serum from the same patients. There were no similar changes in avidity when anti-ssDNA antibodies were studied. Although this again suggests that it is anti-dsDNA antibodies that are of critical importance in lupus nephritis, it is important to recognize that a role for ssDNA is not excluded by these results. Some patients with lupus nephritis have anti-ssDNA but no detectable anti-dsDNA antibodies.[25–26] A Japanese study in patients with untreated renal lupus, although emphasizing that most patients with severe nephritis had high IgG anti-dsDNA titres, also identified a small number with high levels of anti-ssDNA but lower levels of anti-dsDNA.[27]

Hahn[28] has noted that native dsDNA may contain single-stranded regions, whereas ssDNA contains sequences capable of forming helical areas of secondary structure that may react with anti-dsDNA antibodies. Thus, the populations of anti-ssDNA and anti-dsDNA antibodies in an individual patient are not totally distinct, and monoclonal antibodies that react with both antigens are well recognized (reviewed in[29]). The variety of histopathological patterns seen in SLE (see Chapter 5) emphasizes the fact that lupus nephritis is a heterogeneous condition and that different autoantibodies may be important in different patients.

Nevertheless, large cohort studies confirm that, in the majority of cases, anti-dsDNA levels are linked most closely to the occurrence and severity of renal involvement. Swaak et al.[30] compared 51 lupus patients with 660 patients who had other auto-immune conditions, and found that 50 of the SLE sera contained anti-dsDNA antibodies, in contrast to only one of the control sera. In most patients with renal exacerbations of the disease, there was a sharp fall in the anti-dsDNA titre, usually preceded by a rise. This result could be explained either by postulating that blood samples had been taken too late to show the rise in some patients, or that the fall was due to serum anti-dsDNA antibodies having become sequestered in the kidney. Subsequent studies suggest that the former explanation is more likely. Lloyd and Schur[31] studied renal and nonrenal exacerbations of SLE in 27 patients and found that complement depletion and raised anti-dsDNA levels were associated more closely with renal exacerbations. Both Ter Borg et al.[32] in a prospective study of 72 patients and Cervera et al.[3] in a multi-center study of 1000 patients showed that active lupus nephritis was usually associated with a higher titer of anti-dsDNA antibody. Echoing the original work of Koffler et al.,[23] a Japanese group carried out renal biopsies on 40 untreated patients with SLE, and found a close correlation between the degree of nephritis and the titer of IgG, but not IgM, anti-dsDNA antibodies (Okamura et al. 1993).[27]

The particular connection between anti-dsDNA (as opposed to other autoantibodies commonly found in lupus patients' sera) and renal lupus was shown in a long-term follow-up study.[33] Fourteen patients bled up to seven times over a 3–15-year period were tested for binding to antibodies to dsDNA, Ro, La, Sm, RNP, and ribosomal P. Their clinical activity was assessed using the British Isles Lupus Assessment Group (BILAG) system, which divides activity into eight organs/systems. The connection between anti-dsDNA and renal involvement was very strong ($P < 0.00006$) but no other antibody was linked to renal activity. However, in a study of kidney biopsies taken from patients with end stage renal disease/post-mortem, antibodies of varying specificity (e.g. anti-Ro, anti-La, and anti-Sm) were noted.[34]

On balance, it seems highly likely that anti-DNA antibodies are involved in lupus nephritis and that their precise contribution is influenced by isotype, specificity, and avidity. Immunoglobulin G antibodies that bind to dsDNA with high affinity seem particularly closely associated with nephritis. Might these properties be important in enabling such antibodies to damage the glomerulus?

Anti-DNA antibodies and mechanisms of glomerular damage

Are DNA/anti-DNA complexes present in the bloodstream of patients with lupus?

Following the original demonstrations that anti-DNA antibodies were associated with lupus nephritis, the favored explanation was that of immune complex deposition.[35] This hypothesis held that DNA/anti-DNA complexes, formed in the circulation, could be deposited in the glomeruli, leading to complement fixation and glomerulonephritis. This would explain the immunofluorescence evidence showing IgG and complement deposition,[23] but implied that it should be possible to demonstrate such complexes in the blood of patients with SLE.

Early attempts to quantify circulating DNA gave inconsistent results. The confusion arose partly because DNA can be released from leukocytes during the clotting process, so that serum DNA levels may be artifactually high.[36] Other difficulties include that of excluding contamination by bacterial DNA, especially in stored serum samples.[37] Once measurement in plasma rather than serum became accepted practice, a number of authors reported that there was very little circulating DNA in the blood of healthy people, Using four different methods, Steinman concluded that any level of plasma DNA greater than 100 ng/ml could be considered pathogenic. Raptis and Menard[38] subsequently employed a more accurate method in which the DNA chain could be uniformly labeled by nick translation. They were able to demonstrate levels of DNA 10–20 times higher in the plasma of patients with active SLE than in normal subjects. In one such patient, the level fell from 4000 ng/ml to 350 ng/ml over a period of 6 months as the disease responded to treatment. This method also allowed the length of circulating DNA molecules to be estimated. It appeared that most of these were of low molecular weight (up to 500 base pairs (bp) long). The immune-complex deposition hypothesis would predict that much of this DNA might be found complexed to anti-DNA antibodies. Early attempts to identify such complexes were largely unsuccessful. Izui et al.[39] attempted to radiolabel either the DNA or the antibody component of immune complexes and then precipitate the label by a method that relied on the binding properties of the nonlabeled component. These methods were shown to be capable of detecting DNA/anti-DNA complexes formed in vitro in a wide range of antibody to antigen ratios. There was no significant difference in precipitable radioactivity between plasma samples from patients with active SLE and healthy controls. One possible explanation might be that these complexes are cleared from the circulation,[40] a phenomenon that has been demonstrated in mice.[41] Clearance in the mouse occurs mainly in the liver and the rate of clearance depends on the size and DNA content of the complexes. Emlen and Burdick[41] suggested that complexes were trimmed by the action of plasma deoxyribonuclease (Dnase), a mechanism that they were able to replicate both in vivo and in vitro. The products of such digestion were low molecular weight DNA molecules of 40–200 bp. It was postulated that this represented the length protected from Dnase by binding to IgG. Such protection could explain the preponderance of low molecular weight DNA extracted from the gamma globulin fraction of blood taken from patients with active SLE by Sano and Morimoto.[42] No DNA was present in the corresponding fraction from healthy people or from a patient with inactive SLE. Further studies by this group showed that the DNA was of human origin and was present in two fractions of 30–40 bp and 150 bp, respectively.[43] This DNA also had a higher content of guanine and cytosine than most human DNA.[44]

Fournie[45] noted that raised plasma DNA levels were also seen in some other conditions, particularly those characterized by cytolysis. In each case a DNA fraction 120–200 bp in length was a characteristic finding, and this might be explained by postulating that it is a breakdown product of chromatin. The base unit of chromatin is the nucleosome, in which a length of 120–200 bp is associated with an octamer comprising two molecules each of histones H2A, H2B, H3, and H4 (reviewed in[46]). The whole DNA/octamer complex is stabilized by binding to a single molecule of histone 1 (H1). Evidence that circulating DNA in patients with SLE occurs predominantly in the form of oligonucleosomes came from the experiments of Rumore and Steinman.[47] DNA purified from the plasma of such patients (but not specifically from the gamma globulin fraction) was radiolabeled, and shown by electrophoresis to occur in fractions of 150–2200, 400, 600, and 800 bp lengths. This pattern of bands was exactly like that of DNA extracted from oligonucleosomes. Furthermore, the radiolabeled DNA could be precipitated by binding to anti-histone antibodies, showing that it was associated with histones in the plasma.

Experimental evidence suggests, therefore, that circulating DNA exists in patients with SLE, some in nucleosomes and some complexed to antibody. High titers of antinucleosome antibodies have been found in 56–286% of patients with SLE (reviewed in[46]). At least part of this variability is dependent on the purity of the antigen used in the test assays. It has also been shown that antinucleosome antibodies might be a better predictor of a flare than anti-dsDNA antibodies in patients who are clinically quiescent but with evidence of serological activity.[48] There is no evidence to suggest that the immune complexes, whether dsDNA/anti-dsDNA or nucleosome/antinucleosome, migrate preferentially to the kidney. For this reason, alternative mechanisms have been proposed to explain how anti-dsDNA antibodies bind to the glomerulus. These will be discussed in the following sections to show how the original focus on binding to dsDNA itself has been widened to include cross-reactivity with tissue proteins and chromatin components. A fuller consideration follows in subsequent chapters.

Could circulating autoantibodies bind exposed DNA in the glomerulus?

If anti-dsDNA antibodies are not already bound to DNA when they migrate to the kidney, perhaps they might bind to DNA exposed in the glomerulus. Koffler *et al.*[23] and Andres *et al.*[49] used polyclonal anti-DNA antibodies to label renal tissue from patients with lupus nephritis. Both groups reported staining of glomeruli and concluded that DNA was present at this site. It is now clear, however, that such polyclonal sera may bind to other tissue components, and attempts to demonstrate glomerular DNA by more specific methods have been less convincing.[40] For example, Stockl *et al.*[50] used the fluorescence of intercalated dyes to test for ssDNA and dsDNA in renal biopsy specimens from 48 patients with SLE. Despite intense staining of cell nuclei in the same specimens (a positive control), there was no staining of glomerular deposits in any of the biopsies. It has been argued that DNA is unlikely to be deposited in the glomerular basement membrane (GBM) due to repulsion by similarly charged molecules.[40,42] The sugar–phosphate backbone of DNA is negatively charged. The GBM also carries a strong negative charge due to the presence of glycosaminoglycan side chains, particularly heparan sulfate (HS).[51] DNA may, however, be present in the mesangium where it could bind to collagen. Gay *et al.*[52] showed that dsDNA binds type V collagen immobilized on a column or in solution. Type V collagen is characteristically found in the mesangial matrix, which is interesting in view of evidence that the perfusion of isolated rat kidneys with DNA followed by monoclonal mouse anti-dsDNA antibody led to the deposition of the antibody in the mesangium.[53]

Could circulating autoantibodies bind the glomerulus by cross-reaction with intrinsic renal antigens?

The capacity of an autoantibody to cause renal damage may be determined by its ability to cross-react with particular glomerular epitopes. A number of candidates have emerged. These include constituents of the GBM and the podocyte, the glomerular parietal epithelial cell. Varying capacity to cross-react with different targets may ultimately explain why some patients, notably those with diffuse proliferative glomerulonephritis, have subendothelial antibody deposits, in contrast to others who have membranous glomerulonephritis where the deposition is subepithelial.[54]

Alpha-actinin is an actin-associated protein, which has been the subject of great interest in the study of lupus nephritis in recent years. There are several different types of alpha-actinin, but alpha-actinin 4 is the major type expressed in the renal glomerulus, where it localizes predominantly in the podocyte. Point mutations in the gene for alpha-actinin 4 are responsible for some forms of familial focal segmental glomerosclerosis,[55] although these diseases are not characterized by autoantibody production or deposition. Two separate research groups, in New York and Israel, showed independently that the ability of some murine monoclonal antinuclear antibodies to cause glomerulonephritis after passive transfer to recipient mice correlated with their ability to bind alpha-actinin but not with their ability to bind dsDNA.[56,57] The New York group subsequently showed that a human monoclonal antibody that cross-reacted with dsDNA and alpha-actinin also caused glomerulonephritis in these mice.[58] These results suggested the possibility that some anti-dsDNA antibodies in lupus cause renal dysfunction by interacting with alpha-actinin to cause changes in the cytoskeletal structure of podocytes. However, clinical studies did not support a close association between anti-alpha-actinin antibodies and lupus nephritis. In a small study, Mason *et al.* showed that purified anti-dsDNA antibodies from patients with SLE were more likely to bind alpha-actinin if the patients had nephritis than if they did not have nephritis.[59] However, two subsequent studies showed that anti-alpha-actinin antibodies were present both in patients with and without lupus nephritis and that these antibodies were not specific for lupus.[60] One group did suggest that anti-alpha-actinin positivity distinguished nephritis from non-nephritis patients with SLE more clearly than anti-dsDNA positivity, but the number of patients studied was small and fewer than half the patients with lupus nephritis were positive for anti-alpha actinin.[61]

Heparan sulfate and laminin are two other possible glomerular targets for autoantibody binding. Binding to HS has been reported to be higher in patients with lupus nephritis than in other forms of lupus.[62–63] Intriguingly, it has been shown in a murine model of lupus that treatment with peptides derived from laminin reduced renal antibody deposition and caused some reduction in kidney disease.[64]

Several groups have shown that monoclonal anti-dsDNA antibodies bind to proteins in glomerular cells. Such binding is not dependent on anti-DNA affinity of the molecules as it is characteristically unaffected by Dnase treatment. Madaio *et al.*[65] showed that two monoclonal murine anti-DNA antibodies bound to mouse glomeruli *in vitro*. One also bound when infused intravenously into BALB/c mice or when hybridoma cells secreting the monoclonal antibody (mAb) were introduced intraperitoneally. Electron-dense deposits were seen in the glomeruli of these mice by electron microscopy. Raz et al.[66] produced similar results by perfusing isolated rat kidneys with monoclonal murine anti-dsDNA antibodies or polyclonal human IgG from patients with SLE. Proteinuria and reduced inulin clearance developed and deposition of foreign antibodies was demonstrated by immunofluorescence. No deposits were seen on electron microscopy. Importantly, only IgG from SLE patients with active nephritis gave these results. Antibodies from SLE patients without nephritis did not affect the rat kidneys, even though their content of anti-DNA activity was similar. Perfusion with DNA/anti-DNA complexes under the same conditions did not lead to proteinuria. Therefore, it appeared that these results were due to direct binding of the antibodies to the glomerulus. The molecular binding site was explored in a subsequent study, which showed that murine monoclonal anti-DNA antibodies, but not anti-RNA or anti-histones, could bind to five cell-surface proteins present in various tissues, including renal epithelium.[67] These proteins were isolated by immunoblotting and were found to be distinct from histones. This was in contrast to the work of Jacob et al.,[68] which demonstrated binding of the murine monoclonal antibody PME77 to five proteins present in many cell types, including glomerular cells. Sequence analysis later revealed that these proteins were histones.[69]

Ehrenstein et al.[70] investigated the ability of five human monoclonal IgG anti-dsDNA antibodies to cause glomerular damage in severe combined immunodeficiency (SCID) mice. Hybridomas secreting the antibodies were administered intraperitoneally to these mice. Examination of their kidneys by immunofluorescence showed that only one such antibody was deposited in the glomeruli. This antibody (33.C9) had originated from a patient with active lupus nephritis. Another two antibodies bound to the kidney and other tissues, but this binding was confined to cell nuclei. Proteinuria was seen only in mice given the three kidney-binding antibodies, but there were no visible deposits observed on light microscopy. Applying the same protocol, we demonstrated that a sixth monoclonal IgG, RH 14, was deposited in the glomeruli of SCID mice and that the appearance of these subendothelial deposits on electron microscopy, with fusion of the foot processes, was very similar to that seen in human lupus nephritis.[71]

A common thread in the work of these three groups was that not all anti-DNA antibodies tested bound to the glomerulus. This implies that only some anti-dsDNA antibodies are nephritogenic, which accords with clinical studies showing that the presence of high anti-dsDNA titers is not always associated with nephritis.[21,30–32,37,72]

By staining renal biopsies with anti-idiotype antibodies, it has been shown that antibodies carrying certain idiotypic determinants are found at higher frequency in glomeruli damaged by lupus nephritis than by other forms of nephritis.[73–76] Perhaps such public idiotypes are markers of pathogenic subpopulations of anti-dsDNA antibodies. Hahn[28] and others have attempted to define the characteristics of such subpopulations. As indicated above, positive charge, IgG isotype, and specific, high-affinity binding to dsDNA may all be important. Sequence studies of monoclonal murine and human antibodies that possess these attributes show that they tend to accumulate somatic mutations in the complementarity determining regions (CDRs) of the variable domains (reviewed in[77]). The distribution of these mutations suggests that they have been selected by an antigen-driven process, and the net effect is often to increase the positive charge in the CDRs. As these form the antigen-binding site of the immunoglobulin molecule, it is easy to see that this might enhance binding to negatively charged DNA. The critical test of the hypothesis that specific somatic mutations play a dominant role in allowing pathogenic monoclonal antibodies to bind antigens and to cause nephritis is to use expression systems to create variants of these antibodies in which these mutations have been reverted back to the germline sequence. Several groups have done this for both murine[78] and human monoclonal autoantibodies.[79,80] The results show consistently that reverting somatic mutations does reduce binding to dsDNA, but the type of mutation that is important varies from one study to another. Thus, although both Wellman[79] and Mason[80] found that mutations to arginine were especially important in enhancing binding to dsDNA, Katz[78] found the opposite. Furthermore, binding to dsDNA does not always correlate well with ability to cause glomerulonephritis. In the series of mutated variants of the murine monoclonal antibody R4A studied by Katz and colleagues,[78] the highest binding to dsDNA was seen in an antibody that had lost two arginines from heavy chain framework region 3 (FR3), but this antibody did not cause glomerulonephritis. Nephritogenic properties of anti-DNA antibodies are considered in greater detail elsewhere.[81,82]

The importance of DNA–histone complexes

As described above there is now considerable evidence that circulating DNA exists primarily in the form of DNA–histone complexes derived from chromatin, possibly as a product of cell apoptosis.[29] The idea that these complexes play a major role in the pathogenesis of lupus nephritis is attractive both because it provides a possible explanation for the development of high-affinity anti-DNA antibodies and because it suggests a mechanism for binding to the negatively charged GBM.

As already mentioned, the sequences of IgG anti-DNA antibodies show evidence that antigen-driven clonal expansion leads to the accumulation of mutations. Although DNA itself is not a potent antigen, DNA–protein complexes might play this immunogenic role. Krishnan and Marion[83] have induced a lupus-like syndrome in healthy strain mice by immunizing them with just such a complex. In other mouse models it has been possible to identify monoclonal antibodies that bind intact nucleosomes but not their components.[51,84] This suggests that some immunogenic epitopes are present only in the three-dimensional structure of chromatin itself. If chromatin derivatives are also important immunogens in SLE, one would expect the serum of patients to contain antibodies to histones and the nonhistone chromatin proteins, as well as anti-dsDNA. Such antibodies are considered in the next section.

DNA–histone complexes also provide a possible mechanism for the binding of anti-dsDNA to HS glycosaminoglycan in the GBM. Cross-reactivity of anti-DNA antibodies from serum and glomerular eluates of patients with SLE with HS was demonstrated more than 20 years ago.[85] Schmiedeke[86] suggested a mechanism for the binding of anti-DNA antibodies to HS by showing that various histone fractions were capable of binding similar glycosaminoglycans in vitro, and also to the GBM when introduced to rat kidneys by the intravascular route. These bound histones could act as a site of deposition for subsequently injected DNA. The concept that anti-DNA bound HS through a DNA–histone complex was consistent with the finding that purified mono-clonal anti-dsDNA could only bind HS if both these components were added.[87] van den Born et al.[88] showed that binding of a monoclonal anti-HS glycosaminoglycan antibody was reduced in renal biopsies from lupus nephritis and that binding of this antibody to rat kidney was competitively inhibited by histones. Termaat et al.[53] then produced large subendothelial glomerular deposits of murine monoclonal anti-dsDNA antibody by perfusing rat kidneys, sequentially with histones, DNA, and anti-body. Similar results were obtained by perfusing the kidneys with the same components in the more physiologically relevant form of nucleosome/antinucleosome complexes, but deposition was much reduced by prior perfusion with heparatinase.[51] Morioka et al.[89] have shown that when radiolabeled complexes of low-molecular weight DNA with anti-DNA antibody are introduced into rat kidney via the aorta, the deposition of radioactivity in glomeruli increases almost 100-fold if histones are injected into the same kidney first. Thus, there is a considerable body of evidence in support of the idea that this is one mechanism whereby anti-DNA antibodies cause nephritis. It is clearly not the only mechanism as some patients with renal lupus have no detectable anti-HS activity at all.

More recently, Rekvig's group have carried out elegant electron microscopy studies showing co-localization of autoantibodies in both human and murine lupus nephritis with chromatin in electron-dense deposits.[90,91] The chromatin is believed to arise from apoptotic glomerular cells. The antibodies did not co-localize with alpha-actinin or other intraglomerular proteins.

Antibodies to protein components of chromatin

Anti-histone reactivity was first demonstrated in SLE sera by Robbins[18] and Kunkel et al.[92] Although found in virtually all drug-induced lupus syndromes in which nephri-tis is not a common feature,[7] anti-histone antibodies also occur in patients with 'idiopathic' SLE. Using an enzyme-linked immunosorbent assay (ELISA) in which the substrate consisted of glass beads coated with histone, Gioud et al.[93] found levels of activity significantly greater than those of a healthy control population in 32 of 62 SLE patients. However, only one of 70 patients with other rheumatic conditions had raised anti-histone levels. It may be argued that at least part of the activity in such assays is due to the presence of DNA/anti-DNA complexes, which bind histones through their DNA component. Viard et al.[94] showed that purified anti-dsDNA antibodies from SLE patients would only bind histones if pre-incubated with DNA, and conversely that partially purified anti-dsDNA would lose the ability to bind histones if treated with Dnase. The total serum anti-histone activity in these patients was associated with disease activity but not correlated with nephritis. In the earlier report[87] there was only a weak correlation between levels of anti-dsDNA and anti-histone activity, suggesting that little of the anti-histone activity measured was due to DNA/anti-DNA complexes. Again, although patients with active disease were more likely to have raised anti-histone levels, these were not related to the occurrence of nephritis.

Antibodies to nonhistone constituents of chromatin, such as high-mobility group protein 17 (HMG-17) and ubiquitin, are also found in SLE. Anti-HMG-17 antibodies were found in 16 of 46 parents with SLE, and levels correlated with disease activity and with those of anti-dsDNA.[95] Levels were higher in those with active rather than inactive nephritis. Ubiquitin is a highly conserved 77-amino acid protein, present in all mammalian cells, which binds to histones H2A and H2B, particularly in areas of active chromatin. Antibodies in ubiquitin seem to be very common in SLE. Of 161 patients studied by Muller et al.,[96] 79% possessed such antibodies (as opposed to only 55% with anti-dsDNA). Only 16% of patients with other autoimmune diseases showed anti-ubiquitin antibodies. Using rabbit antisera raised against ubiquitin or N-terminal peptides of histones H2A and H3, Stockl et al.[50] showed the presence of at least one of these antigens in glomeruli of renal biopsy specimens from 36 of 48 patients with lupus nephritis but in only two of 70 with other forms of nephritis. Serum samples were available for 15 of these patients: 13 of these contained antibodies to the histone N-terminal peptides, seven anti-ubiquitin, and 11 anti-ubiquitinated H2A. Thus, not only do antibodies to protein components of chromatin exist in patients with SLE, but there is also evidence that these antigens may be present in glomeruli of the same patients.

Antibodies to other nuclear antigens

The Ro and La antigens were first described as components present in a human spleen extract, which would react with sera from SLE patients.[97] They were later found to be identified with SS-A and SS-B, two nuclear antigens that reacted with sera from patients with Sjögren's syndrome.[98,99] It is now clear that anti-Ro/SS-A antibodies bind at least two separate protein components with molecular weights of 60 and 52 kDa.

The Sm antigen was first defined by Tan and Kunkel[100] as a nuclear antigen resistant to Dnase or Rnase, which reacted with sera from patients with SLE. Further studies showed that this antigen was associated with a complex of RNA and protein found in the nucleus.[8] Lerner and Steitz[101] then showed that the Sm autoantigen was a subcellular particle containing small uridine-rich RNA and a number of proteins. At least four Sm proteins (B, B', D and E) exist, and the complex is thought to play an important role in splicing of mRNA (reviewed in[8]). Antibodies to the Sm antigen are almost never seen in diseases other than SLE. The occurrence of lupus nephritis in anti-Sm positive patients is not uncommon. Winn et al.[102] described 135 patients with SLE, of whom 103 carried anti-Sm, and 47% of these showed clinical or histological evidence of renal involvement. Biopsies suggested that the nephritis in patients with anti-Sm, but not anti-dsDNA, was less severe than in anti-dsDNA positive patients. However, this large percentage of anti-Sm positive patients with SLE is most unusual. Approximately 30% of black patients with SLE but only 10% of white patients have anti-Sm antibodies (discussed in[2]). In large studies anti-Sm antibodies do not appear to be associated with nephritis.[2,3]

Up to 5% of patients with SLE persistently show no antinuclear antibodies (ANA) in their serum in standard tests.[2,3,26] Anti-Ro antibodies are thought to be associated with nephritis in some such patients. Provost et al.[103] described seven ANA negative, anti-Ro positive patients with membranoproliferative glomerulonephritis on biopsy. Subsequently, the same group published details of a larger group of 66 ANA negative patients with SLE: eight had proteinuria, although biopsies showed mild cellular proliferation only.[26] These eight patients had no anti-dsDNA antibodies, but four had anti-Ro and seven anti-ssDNA. A pathogenic role for anti-Ro was postulated in two patients who died of lupus nephritis.[25] Both were anti-Ro positive and serum titers of this antibody fell during the development of rapidly progressing renal failure. Glomerular eluates from autopsy specimens of both patients showed higher titers of IgG anti-Ro than the final serum samples, indicating that anti-Ro was concentrated in the glomerular lesions. It was impossible, however, to demonstrate Ro antigen in the eluates. In a much larger and more recent prospective study of 100 anti-Ro positive patients over 10 years, Simmons-O'Brien et al.[104] showed that 18 of 50 patients with SLE suffered glomerulonephritis and in eight of these patients there were no antibodies to ss- or dsDNA. A subpopulation of nine patients with antibodies to Ro, Sm, and U_1ribonucleoprotein (U1RNP) was identified. Of these patients, five developed glomerulonephritis, a finding in keeping with the earlier report of McCarthy et al.[72] showing that black women with all three of these antibodies were particularly likely to develop renal lupus.

Antibodies to cytoplasmic antigens

Antineutrophil cytoplasmic antibodies (ANCA)

Antineutrophil cytoplasmic antibodies are a group of autoantibodies directed against proteins found in the cytoplasm of neutrophils and monocytes.[105,106] Their presence is most closely associated with vasculitic illness such as Wegener's granulomatosis, in which raised ANCA titers may be seen during nephritis. Antibodies to different antigens give two distinct patterns on immunofluorescence. Antibodies to lysosomal protease 3 (PR3) are found in 80% of cases where the cytoplasm is stained diffusely (c-ANCA pattern). Perinuclear staining (p-ANCA) results from the presence of antibodies to any of a number of antigens, including myeloperoxidase, lactoferrin, and lysozyme.[105]

Whereas c-ANCA are not found in SLE, p-ANCA may be found in up to 25% of SLE patients.[106] The clinical relevance of these antibodies is uncertain. In a group of 79 consecutive patients attending an SLE clinic in Hong Kong, 31 had antibodies to lactoferrin.[107] Although there was no significant correlation between antilactoferrin positivity and the incidence of nephritis, the occurrence of crescents in 12 patients with the most severe degree of nephritis was statistically more likely to occur if these antibodies were present. However, other authors have not found an association between ANCA and lupus nephritis.[108] In a study of 157 sera from 120 patients with SLE, Schnabel et al.[106] reported that although 40 had antibodies to lactoferrin, elastase, or lysozyme, there was no correlation of either p-ANCA or any of these specificities with renal involvement. Thus, at present, there is no conclusive evidence to link ANCA to lupus nephritis but their links to lupus have been reviewed or detailed elsewhere.[109]

Antibodies to complement component C1q

Clq is the first component in the classical pathway of complement activation. It is characteristically activated by binding to immune complexes. Serum from patients with SLE shows reactivity with C1q in binding assays. At least a part of this activity may be due to circulating immune complexes. However, Uwatoko and Mannik[110] demonstrated that these patients also possess monomeric IgG molecules that bind C1q even after treatment with Dnase. $F(ab)_2$ fragments of these antibodies also bound C1q, showing that this was a true antigen–antibody reaction. Antibodies to C1q are found in healthy people and increased levels are found more frequently in older age groups.[111] In patients with SLE, however, the highest levels of IgG anti-C1q are found in young patients (aged 20–49), and these patients are significantly more likely to have raised levels than age-matched individuals from the general population. This may be explained partially by the presence of raised anti-C1q titers in young patients with highly active disease. Siegert *et al.*[112] showed that 30 of 88 patients with SLE had raised levels of anti-C1q antibodies: 20% of these patients had clinical evidence of nephritis and there was a strong correlation between the presence of nephritis and raised titer of anti-C1q. Renal biopsies were carried out in 13 patients, 10 of whom showed membranoproliferative glomerulonephritis. Of these 10 patients, nine had raised levels of anti-C1q. Raised anti-C1q levels were also positively correlated with raised anti-dsDNA and reduced complement levels. Thus, it remains unclear whether high levels of anti-C1q in the absence of anti-dsDNA antibodies are related to nephritis.

Antiphospholipid (APL) antibodies

Antiphospholipid antibodies occur in 1.5–5% of the population,[113] but are present at much higher frequency (up to 25–40%) in patients with SLE (reviewed in[114]). APL antibodies can occur in patients with a variety of infectious or neoplastic conditions, but under these circumstances they appear to bind cardiolipin without the need for a cofactor and are not associated with an increased risk of thrombosis.[115] Antiphospholipid antibodies found in patients with autoimmune disorders appear to recognize the antigen in association with a serum cofactor known as β_2 glycoprotein I (β2GPI),[116] and are, in some cases, associated with an increased risk of thrombosis leading to the clinical features of antiphospholipid syndrome (APS).[115,117] These features include venous thromboses, increased prevalence of stroke, skin rash, thrombocytopenia, and recurrent spontaneous miscarriages.[114–119] Where these clinical and serological abnormalities occur in the absence of a known autoimmune disorder, patients are said to have primary antiphospholipid syndrome (PAPS).[119]

There are three types of test in routine clinical use for detection of APL. The anticardiolipin ELISA detects the presence of antibodies that can bind to cardiolipin on a plate. The strength of binding is normally expressed in standardized international units (GPL or MPL depending on whether IgG or IgM antibodies are being measured). According to the most recent international classification criteria,[120] APL levels above 40 GPL or 40 MPL must be detected on at least two occasions at least 12 weeks apart to allow APS to be diagnosed. This is an important criterion because the levels found in healthy people and in patients with SLE are often much lower than this. The second test commonly used is the lupus anticoagulant test. This is not a binding assay but an assay of the ability of blood to clot under differing conditions. Prolonged clotting in this assay is known to be due to the presence of APL. The assay is confusingly known as the lupus *anticoagulant* test, even though the effect of aPL *in vivo* is to *promote* coagulation. This confusing terminology arises because in this *in vitro* assay the aPL delay clotting, whereas *in vivo* they have the opposite effect. As in the case of the anticardiolipin test described above, the lupus anticoagulant assay must be positive on at least two occasions 12 weeks apart for APS to be diagnosed. Some patients are positive for both anticardiolipin and lupus anticoagulant, but many are positive in only one of these assays. Both should be done in patients with SLE. A third (less widely used) assay is a specific ELISA for anti-β2GPI antibodies, which has been introduced because binding to this antigen shows more specificity for APS than binding to cardiolipin.

A number of authors have reported cases in which deteriorating renal function in patients with SLE and APL antibodies is associated with histological changes, suggesting thrombosis and intimal proliferation in the small vessels.[121–124] These are not a common feature in lupus nephritis occurring in the absence of APL antibodies, and the conclusion that APL antibodies are responsible for their presence is supported by the report of a similar clinical and histological picture in a patient with PAPS.[118] Patients typically suffer an insidious loss of renal function with falling creatinine clearance, but with little proteinuria and benign urinary sediment.[125]

These cases in which APL antibodies actually cause renal problems in SLE are rare, but it is nevertheless important to know the APL status of a patient with lupus nephritis. This is particularly true in cases where very low serum protein levels, occurring as a result of nephrotic syndrome, can also promote thrombosis, and a patient with both low albumin and high serum APL may warrant treatment with anticoagulants until the protein level improves.

The origin of pathogenic autoantibodies in SLE

For many years, one of the great mysteries surrounding SLE was the conundrum of why autoantibodies were formed to its nuclear and cytoplasmic structures 'hidden' with the cell. Although, as discussed earlier in this chapter, the possibility of autoantibodies penetrating living cells may occur, this is relatively uncommon. The seminal paper by Casciola-Rosen and colleagues demonstrates how human keratinocytes under the influence of ultraviolet radiation undergo apoptosis, in normal physiological process, leading to formation on the surface of dead and dying cells of smaller and larger blebs, which contain many of the autoantigens against which autoantibodies are found in patients with lupus.[126] It has become evident from the work of Hermann *et al.* and other groups,[127,128] that efficient removal of apoptotic material is delayed in lupus and this led to the notion that lupus is a disease of "waste disposal." This topic is discussed in more detail by us elsewhere,[10] but, in brief, the inappropriate collection of apoptotic material is thought to lead to a persisting presence of autoantigens and a loss of peripheral tolerance. The persisting nuclear (and cytoplasmic) fragments are, it is now believed, collected and presented by "professional" antigen presenting cells to T cells and subsequently to B cells, leading to the formation of antibodies against these inciting antigens. This could explain why patients with lupus characteristically develop autoantibodies against antigens such as nucleosomes, anionic phospholipids, and Ro, which are present on the surface of this apoptotic debris, and/or antigens such as β2GPI and C1q that may become attached to the debris.

Conclusions

Lupus nephritis is a strikingly heterogeneous condition. This heterogeneity is exemplified in the role played by autoantibodies. Serological studies provide evidence that a number of different antibodies may be linked to the occurrence of renal involvement in patients with SLE, but some are only important in a small subset of patients. Anti-dsDNA antibodies are the most commonly seen antibodies in lupus nephritis, and those for which evidence of a pathogenic role is strongest.[129] However, some anti-dsDNA negative patients have nephritis in association with anti-ssDNA or anti-Ro. Conversely, not all patients with high titers of anti-dsDNA develop nephritis. This shows that only a subset of anti-dsDNA antibodies are nephritogenic, and factors important in defining this subset are likely to include affinity, specificity, isotype, idiotype, and an ability to cross-react with cell-surface antigens. These nephritogenic antibodies can exert their effects on the glomeruli by different mechanisms. These include binding to DNA attached to collagen, binding to cell-surface proteins, and binding of anti-DNA/DNA/histone complexes to HS in the GBM. In any one patient, a number of different mechanisms may be operating and their relative importance is likely to vary from case to case. Thus, the task of finding a specific form of therapy directed against autoantibodies is a challenging one.

References

1. Johnson, A.E., Gordon, C., Palmer, R.G., and Bacon, P.A. (1995) The prevalence and incidence of systemic lupus erythematosus in Birmingham, England; relationship to ethnicity and country of birth. *Arthritis Rheum* **38**, 551–8.

2. Moss, K., Ioannou, Y., Sultan, S.M., May, I, and Isenberg, D.A. (2002) Outcome of a cohort of 300 patients with systemic lupus erythematosus attending a dedicated clinic for over two decades. *Am Rheum Dis* **61**, 409–13.

3. Cervera, R., Khamashta, M.A., Font, J., Sebastiani, G.D., Gil, A., Lavilla, P., *et al.* (1993) Systemic lupus erythematosus: clinical and immunologic patterns of disease expression in a cohort of 1000 patients. *Medicine (Baltimore)* **72**, 113–24.

4. Cameron, J.S. (2001) Clinical manifestations of lupus nephritis. In: *Rheumatology and the Kidney* (Adu, D., Emery, P., Madaio, M. eds), pp. 17–32. Oxford University Press, Oxford.

5. Dubois, E.L., and Tuffanelli, D.L. (1964) Clinical manifestations of systemic lupus erythematosus. Computer analysis of 530 cases. *J Am Med Assoc* **190**, 104–11.

6. Dubois, E.L., Wierzchowiecki, M., Cox, M.B., and Weiner, J.M. (1974) Duration and death in systemic lupus erythematosus. An analysis of 249 cases. *J Am Med Assoc* **227**, 1399–402.

7. Ravirajan, C.T., Rahman, M.A., Papadaki, L., Griffiths, M.H., Kalsi, J., Martin, A.C., *et al.* (1998) Genetic, structural and functional properties of an IgG DNA-binding monoclonal antibody from a lupus patient with nephritis. *Eur J Immunol* **28**, 339–50.

8. Reveille, J.D., Barolucci, A., and Alarcon, G.S. (1990) Prognosis in systemic lupus erythematosus. Negative impact of increasing age at onset, Black race and thrombocytopenia as well as causes of death. *Arthritis Rheum* **33**, 37–48.

9. Tan, E.M. (1989) Antinuclear antibodies: diagnostic markers for autoimmune diseases and probes for cell biology. *Adv Immunol* **44**, 93–138.

10. Rahman, A., and Isenberg, D.A. (2008) Mechanisms of Disease, Systemic Lupus Erythematosus. *N Engl J Med* **358**, 53–63.

11. Koffler, D., Carr, R., Agnello, Thoburn, R., and Kundel H.G. (1971) Antibodies to polynucleotides in human sera: antigenic specificity and relation to disease. *J Exp Med* **134**, 294–312.

12. Isenberg, D.A., Shoenfeld, Y., Walport, M., Mackworth-Young, C., Dudeney, C., Todd-Pokropek, A., *et al.* (1985) Detection of cross-reactive anti-DNA idiotypes in the serum of systemic lupus erythematosus patients and of their relatives. *Arthritis Rheum* **28**, 999–1007.

13. Duncan, R., and McConkey, E.H. (1982) How many proteins are there in a typical mammalian cell? *Clin Chem* **28**, 749–55.

14. Gharavi, A.E., Chu, J.-L., and Elkon, K.B. (1988) Autoantibodies to intracellular proteins in human systemic lupus erythematosus are not due to random polyclonal B cell activation. *Arthritis Rheum* **11**, 1337–45.

15. Naparstek, Y., and Plotz, P.H. (1993) The role of autoantibodies in autoimmune disease. *Annu Rev Immunol* **11**, 79–104.

16. Cepellini, R., Polli, E., and Celada, F. (1957) A DNA-reacting factor in serum of a patient with lupus erythematosus diffuses. *Proc Soc Exp Biol Med* **96**, 572–4.

17. Meischer, P., and Strassle, R. (1957) New serological methods for the detection of the LE factor. *Vox Sang* **2**, 283.

18. Robbins, W.C., Holman, H.R., Deicher, H., and Kunkel, H.G. (1957) Complement fixation with cell nuclei and DNA in lupus erythematosus. *Proc Soc Biol Med* **96**, 575–9.

19. Seligmann, M. (1957) Mise en evidence dans le serum des maladies atteints de lupus erythemateux dissemine de precipitation avec l'acide desoxyribonucleique. *Comptes Rendu l'Acad Sci (Paris)* **245**, 243–5.

20. Tan, E.M., Schur, P.H., Carr, R.I., and Kunkel, H.G. (1966) Deoxyribonucleic acid (DNA) and antibodies to DNA in the serum of patients with systemic lupus erythematosus. *J Clin Invest* **45**, 1732–7.

21. Schur, P.H. and Sandson, J. (1968) Immunologic factors and clinical activity in systemic lupus erythematosus. *N Engl J Med* **278**, 533–8.

22. Pincus, T., Schur, P.H., Ross, J.A., Decker, J.L., and Talal, N. (1969) Measurement of serum DNA-binding activity in systemic lupus erythematosus. *N Engl J Med* **281**, 533–8.

23. Koffler, D., Schur, P.H., and Kunkel, H.G. (1967) Immunological studies concerning the nephritis of systemic lupus erythematosus. *J Exp Med* **126**, 607–24.

24. Winfield, J.B., Faiferman, L., and Koffler, D. (1977) Avidity of anti-DNA antibodies in serum and IgG glomerular eluates from patients with systemic lupus erythematosus. Association of high avidity anti-native DNA antibody with glomerulonephritis. *J Clin Invest* **59**, 90–6.

25. Maddison, P.J., and Reichlin, M. (1979) Deposition of antibodies to a soluble cytoplasmic antigen in the kidneys of patients with systemic lupus erythematosus. *Arthritis Rheum* **22**, 858–63.

26. Maddison, P.J., Provost, T.T., and Reichlin, M.M. (1981) Serologic findings in patients with 'ANA-negative' SLE. *Medicine (Baltimore)* **60**, 87–94.

27. Okamura, M., Kanayama, Y., Amastu, K., Negoro, N., Kohda, S., Takeda, T., *et al.* (1993). Significance of enzyme linked immunosorbent assay (ELISA) for antibodies to double stranded and single stranded DNA in patients with lupus nephritis: correlation with severity of renal histology. *Ann Rheum Dis* **52**, 14–20.

28. Hahn, B.H. (1982) Characteristics of pathogenic subpopulations of antibodies to DNA. *Arthritis Rheum* **25**, 747–52.

29. Isenberg, D.A., Ehrenstein, M.R., Longhurst, C., and Kalsi, J.K. (1994) The origin, sequence, structure, and consequences of developing anti-DNA antibodies: a human perspective. *Arthritis Rheum* **37**, 169–80.

30. Swaak, A.J.G., Aarden, L.A., Statius van Eps, L.W., and Feltkamp, T.E.W. (1979) Anti dsDNA and complement profiles as prognostic guides in systemic lupus erythematosus. *Arthritis Rheum* **22**, 226–35.

31. Lloyd, W., and Schur, P.H. (1981) Immune complexes, complement, and anti-DNA in exacerbations of systemic lupus erythematosus (SLE). *Medicine (Baltimore)* **60**, 208–17.

32. Ter Borg, E.J., Horst, G., Hummel, E.J., Limburg, P.L., and Kallenberg, C.G.M. (1990) Measurement of increases in anti-double-stranded DNA antibody levels as a predictor of disease exacerbation in systemic lupus erythematosus. *Arthritis Rheum* **33**, 634–43.

33. Isenberg, D.A., Garton, M., Reichlin, M.W., and Reichlin, M. (1997) Long term follow up of autoantibody profiles in black female lupus patients and clinical comparison with Caucasian and Asian patients. *Brit J Rheum* **36**, 229–233.

34. Mannik, M., Merrill, C.E., Stamps, L.D., and Wener, M.H. (2003) Multiple autoantibodies form the glomerular immune deposits in patients with systemic lupus erythematosus. *J Rheumatol* **30**, 1495–1504.

35. Koffler, D., Agnello, V., Thoburn, R., and Kunkel, H.G. (1971) Systemic lupus erythematosus: prototype of immune complex nephritis in man. *J Exp Med* **134**, 1695–705.

36. Steinman, C.R. (1975) Free DNA in serum and plasma from normal adults. *J Clin Invest* **56**, 512–5.

37. McCoubrey-Hoyer, A., Okarma, J.B., and Holman, H.R. (1984) Partial purification and characterization of plasma DNA and its relation to disease activity in systemic lupus erythematosus. *Am J Med* **77**, 23–34.

38. Raptis, L. and Menard, H.A. (1980) Quantitation and characterization of plasma DNA in normals and patients with systemic lupus erythematosus. *J Clin Invest* **66**, 1391–9.

39. Izui, S., Lambert, P.H., and Miescher, P.A. (1977) Failure to detect circulating DNA anti-DNA complexes by four radioimmunological methods in patients with systemic lupus erythematosus. *Clin Exp Immunol* **30**, 384–92.

40. Eilat, D. (1985) Cross-reactions of anti-DNA antibodies and the central dogma of lupus nephritis. *Immunol Today* **6**, 123–7.

41. Emlen, W., and Burdick, G. (1988) Clearance and organ localization of small DNA-antiDNA immune complexes in mice. *J Immunol* **140**, 1816–22.

42. Sano, H., and Morimoto C. (1981) Isolation of DNA from DNA/anti-DNA antibody immune complexes in systemic lupus erythematosus. *J Immunol* **126**, 538–9.

43. Sano, H., and Morimoto, C. (1982) DNA isolated from DNA/anti-DNA antibody immune complexes in systemic lupus erythematosus is rich in guanine-cytosine content. *J Immunol* **128**, 1341–5.

44. Sano, H., Imokawa, M., Steinberg, A.D., and Morimoto, C. (1983) Accumulation of guanosine-cytosine enriched low M.W. DNA fragments in lymphocytes of patients with systemic lupus erythematosus. *J Immunol* **130**, 186–90.

45. Fournie, G.J. (1988) Circulating DNA and lupus nephritis. *Kidney Int* **33**, 487–97.

46. Manson J.J., and Isenberg D.A. (2006) The origin and pathogenic consequences of anti-dsDNA antibodies in systemic lupus erythematosus. *Expert Rev Clin Immunol* **2**, 377–85.

47. Rumore, P.M., and Steinman, C.R. (1990) Endogenous circulating DNA in systemic lupus erythematosus. *J Clin Invest* **86**, 69–74.

48. Ng KP, Manson J.J., Rahman A., and Isenberg D.A. (2006) Association of antinucleosome antibodies with disease flare in serologically active clinically quiescent patients with systemic lupus erythematosus. *Arthritis Care Res* **55**, 900–904.

49. Andres, G.A., Accini, L., Beiser, S.M., Christian, G.A., Cinotti, B.F., Hsu, K.C., *et al.* (1970) Localisation of fluorescein-labeled antinucleoside antibodies in glomeruli of patients with active systemic lupus erythematosus. *J Clin Invest* **49**, 2106–18.

50. Stockl, F., Muller, S., Batsford, S., Schmiedeke, T., Waldherr, R., Andrassy K., *et al.* (1994) A role for histones and ubiquitin in lupus nephritis? *Clin Nephrol* **41**, 10–17.

51. Kramers, C., Hylkema, M.N., van Bruggen, M.C.J., van de Lagemaat, R., Dijkman, H.B.P.M., Assmann, K.J.M., *et al.* (1994) Anti-nucleosome antibodies complexed to nucleosomal antigen show anti-DNA reactivity and bind to rat glomerular basement membrane in vivo. *J Clin Invest* **94**, 568–77.

52. Gay, S., Losman, M.J., Koopman, W.J., and Miler, E.J. (1985) Interaction of DNA with connective tissue matrix proteins reveals preferential binding to type V collagen. *J Immunol* **135**, 1097–100.

53. Termaat, R.M., Assmann, K.J.M., Dijkman, H.P.B.M., van Gompel, F., Smeenk, R.T.J., and Berden J.H.M. (1992) Anti-DNA antibodies can bind to the glomerulus via two distinct mechanisms. *Kidney Int* **42**, 1363–71.

54. Weening, J.J., D'Agati, V.D., Schwartz, M.M., *et al.* (2004) The classification of glomerulonephritis in systemic lupus erythematosus revisited. *J Am Soc Nephrol* **15**, 241–50.

55. Kaplan, J.M., Kim, S.H., North, K.N. *et al.* (2000) Mutations in ACTN4 encoding α – actinin-4 cause familial focal segmental glomerulodosis. *Nat Gen* **24**, 251–6.

56. Mostoslavsky, G., Fischel, R., Yachimonich, N., *et al.* (2001) Lupus anti-DNA auto antibodies cross-react with glomerular structural protein: a case for tissue injury by molecular mimicry. *Eur J Immunol* **31**, 1221–7.

57. Deocharan, B., Qing, X., Lichauco, J., and Putterman, C. (2002) α actinin is a cross-reactive renal target for pathogenic anti-DNA antibodies. *J Immunol* **168**, 3072–8.

58. Zhao, Z., Weinstein, E., Tuzova, M., *et al.* (2005) Cross-reactivity of human lupus anti-dsDNA antibodies with α actinin and nephrogenic potential. *Arthritis Rheum* **52**, 522–530.

59. Mason, L.J., Ravirajan, C.T., Rahman, A., Putterman, C., and Isenberg, D.A. (2004) Is α actinin a target for pathogenic anti-DNA antibodies in lupus nephritis? *Arthritis Rheum* **50**, 866–870.

60. Renaudineau, Y., Croquefer, S., Jousse., S, Renaudineau, E., Devauchelle, V., Guegen, P., *et al.* (2006) Association of anti-alpha-actinin binding anti-double-stranded DNA antibodies with lupus nephritis. *Arthritis Rheum* **54**, 2523–32.

61. Becker-Merok, A., Kalaaji, M., Haugbro, K., Nikolaisen, C., Kilsen, K., Rekvig, O.P., *et al.* (2006) Alpha-actinin-binding antibodies in relation to systemic lupus erythematosus and lupus nephritis. *Arthritis Res Ther* **8**, R162.

62. Ravirajan C.T., Rowse L., MacGowan, J.R., and Isenberg, D.A. (2001) An analysis of clinical disease activity and nephritis associated serum autoantibody profiles in patients with systemic lupus erythematosus: a cross sectional study. *Rheumatology* **40**, 1405–12.

63. Kramers, C., Termaat, R.M. ter Borg, E.J., *et al.* (1993) Higher anti-heparan sulphate reactivity during systemic lupus erythematosus (SLE) disease exacerbations with renal manifestations: a long term prospective analysis. *Clin Exp Immunol* **93**, 34–8.

64. Amital, H., Heilweil, M., Ulmansky, R., *et al.* (2005) Treatment with laminin derived peptide suppresses lupus nephritis. *J Immunol* **175**, 5516–23.

65. Madaio, M.P., Carlson, J., Cataldo, J., Ucci, A., Migliorini, P., and Pankewycz, O. (1987) Murine monoclonal anti-DNA antibodies bind directly to glomerular antigens and form immune deposits. *J Immunol* **138**, 2883–9.

66. Raz, E., Breziz, Rosemann, E., and Eilat, D. (1989) Anti-DNA antibodies bind directly to renal antigens and induce kidney dysfunction in the isolated perfused rat kidney. *J Immunol* **42**, 3076–82.

67. Raz, E., Ben-Basset, H., Davidi, T., Shlomai, Z., and Eilat, D. (1993) Cross-reactions of anti-DNA autoantibodies with cell surface proteins. *Eur J Immunol* **23**, 383–90.

68. Jacob, L., Lety, M.A., Louvard, D., and Bach, J-F. (1985) Binding of a monoclonal anti-DNA autoantibody to identical protein(s) present at the surface of several human cell types involved in lupus pathogenesis. *J Clin Invest* **75**, 315–17.

69. Jacob, L., Viard, J-P., Allenet, B., Anin, M.-F., Slama, F.B.H., Vandekerckhove, J., *et al.* (1989) A monoclonal anti-dsDNA autoantibody binds to a 94 kDa cell surface protein on various cell types via nucleosomes or a DNA-histone complex. *Proc Natl Acad Sci USA* **86**, 4669–73.

70. Ehrenstein, M.R., Katz, D.R., Griffiths, M.H., Papadaki, L., Winkler, T.H., Kalden, J.R., *et al.* (1995) Human IgG anti-DNA antibodies deposit in kidneys and induce proteinuria in SCID mice. *Kidney Int* **48**, 705–11.

71. Ravirajan, C.T., Rahman M.A., Papadaki L., Griffiths, M.H., Kalsi, J., Martin, A.C., *et al.* (1998) Genetic, structural and functional properties of an IgG DNA-binding monoclonal antibody from a lupus patient with nephritis. *Eur J Immunol* **28**, 339–50.

72. McCarthy, G.A., Harley, J.B., and Reichlin, M. (1993) A distinctive autoantibody profile in black female patients with lupus nephritis. *Arthritis Rheum* **36**, 1560–5.

73. Bernstein, K.A., Kahl, L.E., Balow, J.E., and Lefkowith, J.B. (1994) Serologic markers of lupus nephritis in patients: use of a tissue-based ELISA and evidence of immunopathogenic heterogeneity. *Clin Exp Immunol* **98**, 60–5.

74. Isenberg, D.A., and Collins, C. (1985) Detection of cross-reactive anti-DNA antibody idiotypes on renal tissue-bound immunoglobulins from lupus patients. *J Clin Invest* **76**, 287–94.

75. Kalunian, K.C., Panosian-Sahakian, N., Ebling, F.M., Cohen, A.H., Louie, J.S., Kaine, J., *et al.* (1989) Idiopathic characteristics of immunoglobulins associated with systemic lupus erythematosus: studies of antibodies deposited in glomeruli of humans. *Arthritis Rheum* **32**, 513–22.

76. Isenberg, D.A., Spellerberg, M., Williams, W., Griffiths, M., and Stevenson, F. (1993) Identification of a role for the 9G4 idiotope in systemic lupus erythematosus. *Br J Rheumatol* **32**, 876–82.

77. Rahman, A., Giles, I., Haley, J., and Isenberg, D.A. (2002) Systemic analysis of sequences of anti-DNA antibodies-relevance to theories of origin and pathogenicity. *Lupus* **11**, 807–823.

78. Katz, J.B., Limpansithikul, W., and Diamond, B. (1994) Mutational analysis of an autoantibody: differential binding and pathogenicity. *J Exp Med* **180**, 925–32.

79. Wellman, U., Letz, M., Herrmann, M., Angermuller, S., Kalden, J.R., and Winkler, T.H. (2005) The evolution of human anti-double-stranded DNA autoantibodies. *Proc Natl Acad Sci USA* **102**, 9258–63.

80. Mason, L.J., Lambrianides A., Haley, J.D., Manson, J.J., Latchman, D.S., Isenberg, D.A., and Rahman, A. (2005) Stable expression of a recombinant human antinucleosome antibody to investigate relationships between antibody sequence, binding properties and pathogenicity. *Arthritis Res Ther* **7**, R971–83.

81. Van Bavel, C.C., Fenton, K.A. Rekvig, U.P., van der Vlag, J., and Berden, J.H. (2008) Glomerular targets of nephritogenic autoantibodies in systemic lupus erythematosus. *Arthritis Rheum* **58**, 1892–1899.

82. Van Bavel, C.C., van der Vlag J., and Berden J.H. (2007) Glomerular-binding of anti-dsDNA autoantibodies: the dispute resolved? *Kidney Int* **71**, 1–3.

83. Krishnan, M.R., and Marion, T.N. (1993) Structural similarity of antibody variable regions from immune and autoimmune anti-DNA antibodies. *J Immunol* **150**, 4948–57.

84. Losman, J.A., Fasy, T.M., Novick, K.E., Massa, M., and Monestier, M. (1993) Nucleosome-specific antibody from an autoimmune MRL/Mp-*lpr/lpr* mouse. *Arthritis Rheum* **36**, 552–60.

85. Faaber, P., Rijek, T.P.M., van de Putte, L.B.A., Capel, P.J.A., and Berden, H.H.M. (1986) Cross reactivity of human and murine antiDNA antibodies with heparan sulfate: the major glycosaminoglycan in glomerular basement membranes. *J Clin Invest* **77**, 1824–30.

86. Schmiedeke, T.M.J, Stockl, F.W., Weber, R., Sugisaki, Y., Batsford, S.R., and Vogt, A. (1989) Histones have high affinity for the glomerular basement membrane: relevance for immune complex formation in lupus nephritis. *J Exp Med* **169**, 1879–94.

87. Brinkman, K., Termaat, R.M., Berden, J.H.M., and Smeenk, R.J.T. (1990) Anti-DNA antibodies and lupus nephritis: the complexity of cross-reaction. *Immunol Today* **11**, 232–4.

88. van den Born, J., Kramers, C., Bakker, M.A.H., van Bruggen, M.C.J., Assmann, K.J.M., and Berden, J.H.M. (1992) Decreased anti-heparan sulfate staining of the glomerular basement membrane in lupus nephritis. Possible role of histones. *Lupus* **1** (Suppl 1), 10.

89. Morioka, T., Woitas, R., Fujiaki, Y., Batsford, S.R., and Vogt, A. (1994) Histone mediates glomerular desposition of small size DNA anti-DNA complex. *Kidney Int* **43**, 991–7.

90. Kalaaji, M. Mortensen, E., Jorgensen, L., Olsen, R., and Rekvig, O.P. (2006) Nephritogenic lupus antibodies recognise glomerular basement membrane-associated chromatin fragments released from apoptotic intraglomerular cells. *Am J Path* **168**, 1779–92.

91. Kalaaji, M., Fenton, K.A., Mortensen, E.S., Olsen, R., Sturfelt, G., Alm, P., *et al.* (2007) Glomerular apoptotic nucleosomes are central targets for nephritogenic antibodies in human SLE nephritis. *Kidney Int* **71**, 664–72.

92. Kunkel, H.G., Holman, H.R., and Deicher, H.R.G. (1960) Multiple 'autoantibodies' in cell constituents in systemic lupus erythematosus. *Ciba Found Symp* **8**, 429–37.

93. Gioud, M., Ait Kaci, M., and Monier, J.C. (1982) Histone antibodies in systemic lupus erythematosus: a possible diagnostic tool. *Arthritis Rheum* **25**, 407–13.

94. Viard, J.P., Choquette, D., Chabre, H., Slama, F.B.H., Primo, J., Letrait, M., *et al.* (1992) Anti-histone reactivity in systemic lupus erythematosus sera: a disease activity index linked to the presence of DNA: anti-DNA immune complexes. *Autoimmunity* **12**, 61–8.

95. Tzioufas, A.G., Boumba, V.A., Seferiadis, K., Tsolas, O., and Moutsopoulos, M. (1993) Autoantibodies to HMG-17 nucleosomal protein in autoimmune rheumatic diseases: correlation with systemic lupus erythematosus clinical activity and with antibodies to double-stranded DNA. *Arthritis Rheum* **36**, 955–61.

96. Muller, S., Briand, J.-P, and Van Regenmortel, M.H.V. (1988) Presence of antibodies to ubiquitin during the autoimmune response associated with systemic lupus erythematosus. *Proc Natl Acad Sci USA* **85**, 8176–80.

97. Clark, G., Reichlin, M., and Tomasi, T.B. (1969) Characterization of a soluble cytoplasmic antigen reactive with sera from patients with systemic lupus erythematosus. *J Immunol* **102**, 117–24.

98. Alspaugh, M.A., and Tan, E.M. (1975) Antibodies to cellular antigen in Sjogren's syndrome. *J Clin Invest* **55**, 1067–73.

99. Alspaugh, M.A., and Maddison, P. (1979) Resolution of the identity of certain antigen-antibody systems in systemic lupus erythematosus and Sjogren's syndrome: an inter-laboratory collaboration. *Arthritis Rheum* **22**, 796–8.

100. Tan, E.M., and Kunkel, H.G. (1966) Characteristics of a soluble nuclear antigen precipitating with sera of patients with systemic lupus erythematosus. *J Immunol* **96**, 464–71.

101. Lerner, M.R., and Steitz, J.A. (1979) Antibodies to small nuclear RNAs complexed with proteins are produced by patients with systemic lupus erythematosus. *Proc Natl Acad Sci USA* **76**, 5495–7.

102. Winn, D.A., Wolfe, F., Lindberg, D.A., Fristoe, F.H., Kingland, I., and Sharp, G.C. (1979) Identification of a clinical subset of systemic lupus erythematosus by antibodies to the Sm antigen. *Arthritis Rheum* **22**, 1334–7.

103. Provost, T.T., Ahmed, A.R., Maddison, P.L., and Reichlin, M. (1977) Antibodies to cytoplasmic antigens in systemic lupus erythematosus: serologic marker for systemic disease. *Arthritis Rheum* **20**, 1457–63.

104. Simmons-O'Brien, E., Chen, S., Watson, R., Antoni, C., Petri, M., Hochberg, M., *et al.* (1995) One hundred anti-Ro (SS-A) antibody positive patients: a 10-year follow-up. *Medicine (Baltimore)* **74**, 109–30.

105. Gross, W.L., and Casernock, E. (1995) Antineutrophil cytoplasmic antibodies (ANCA): immunodiagnostic and pathophysiological aspects in vasculitis. *Curr Opin Rheumatol* **7**, 1–19.

106. Schnabel, A., Csernok, E., Isenberg, D.A., Mrowka, C., and Gross, W.L. (1995) Antineutrophil cytoplasmic antibodies in systemic lupus erythematosus: prevalence, specificities, and clinical significance. *Arthritis Rheum* **38**, 633–7.

107. Lee, S.S., Lawton, J.W.M., Chan, C.E., Li, C.S., Kwan, T.H. and Gross, W.I. (1995) Anti-actoferrin antibody in systemic lupus erythematosus. *Br J Rheumatol* **31**, 660–73.

108. Cambridge, G., Wallace, H., Bernstein, R.M., and Leaker, B. (1994) Autoantibodies to myeloperoxidase in idiopathic and drug-induced systemic lupus erythematosus and vasculitis. *Br J Rheumatol* **33**, 109–14.

109. Sen, D., and Isenberg, D.A. (2002) Anti neutrophil cytoplasmic antibodies in systemic lupus erythematosus. *Lupus* **12**, 651–8.

110. Uwatoko, S., and Mannik, M. (1988) Low molecular weight C1q binding immunoglobulin G in patients with systemic lupus erythematosus consists of autoantibodies to the collagen-like region of C1q. *J Clin Invest* **82**, 816–24.

111. Siegert, C.E.H., Daha, M.R., Swaak, A.J.G., van der Voort, E.A.M, and Breedveld, F.C. (1993) The relationship between serum titers of autoantibodies to C1q and age in the general population and in patients with systemic lupus erythematosus. *Clin Immunol Immunopathol* **67**, 204–9.

112. Siegert, C.E.H., Daha, M.R., Westedt, M.L., van der Voort, E.A.M, and Breedveld, F.C. (1991) IgG autoantibodies against C1q are correlated with nephritis, hypocomplementaemia, and dsDNA antibodies in systemic lupus erythematosus. *J Rheumatol* **18**, 230–4.

113. Petri, M. (2000) Epidemiology of the anti-phospholipid antibody syndrome. *J Autoimmun* **15**, 145–51.

114. Levine, J.S., Ware Branch, D., and Rarch, J. (2002) The anti-phospholipid antibody syndrome. *N Engl J Med* **346**, 752–63.

115. Hunt, J.E., McNeil, H.P., Morgan, G.J., Crameri, R.M., and Krillis, S.A. (1992) A phospholipid-β2-glycoprotein I complex is an antigen for anticardiolipin antibodies occurring in autoimmune disease but not with infection. *Lupus* **1**, 75–81.

116. Galli, M., Confurius, P., Maasen, C., Hemker, H.C., de Baets, M.M., van Brieda-Vriesman, P.J.L., *et al.* (1990) Anticardiolipin antibodies directed not to cardiolipin but to a plasma cofactor. *Lancet* **335**, 1544–7.

117. Ordi, J., Selva, A., Monegal, F., Porcel, J.M., Martinez-Costa, X., and Villardel, M. (1993) Anticardiolipin antibodies and dependence on a serum cofactor. A mechanism of thrombosis. *J Rheumatol* **20**, 1321–4.

118. Alarcon-Segovia, D., Deleze, M., Oria, C.V., Sanchez-Guerro, J., Gomez-Pacheco, L., Cabiedes, J., *et al.* (1989) Antiphospholipid antibodies and the antiphospholipid syndrome in systemic lupus erythematosus. *Medicine (Baltimore)* **68**, 353–65.

119. Asherson, R.A., Khamashta, M.A., Ordi-Ros, J., Derksen, R.H.W.M., Machin, S.J., Barquinero, J., *et al.* (1989) The 'primary' antiphospholipid syndrome: major clinical and serological features. *Medicine (Baltimore)* **68**, 366–75.

120. Miyakis, S. Lockshin, M.D., Atsumi, T., Branch, D.W., Brey, R.L., Cervera, R., *et al.* (2006) International consensus statement on an update on the classification criteria for definite antiphospholipid syndrome (APS). *J Thromb Haemost* **2**, 295–306.

121. Kleinknecht, D., Bobrie, G., Meyer, O., Noel, L.H., Callard, P., and Ramdane, M. (1989) Recurrent thrombosis and renal vascular disease in patients with a lupus anticoagulant. *Nephrol Dial Transplant* **4**, 854–8.

122. Leaker, B., MacGregor, A., Griffiths, M., Snaith, M., Neild, G.H., and Isenberg, D.A. (1991) Insidious loss of renal function in patients with anticardiolipin and antibodies and absence of overt nephritis. *Br Rheumatol* **30**, 422–5.

123. Asherson, R.A., and Kant, K.S. (1993) Antiphospholipid antibodies and the kidney. *J Rheumatol* **20**, 1268–72.

124. Rankin, E.C.C., Neild, G.H., and Isenberg, D.A. (1994) Deterioration of renal function in a patient with lupus. *Ann Rheum Dis* **53**, 67–71.

125. Isenberg, D.A., Griffiths, M., and Neild, G.H. (1995) Woman with livedo reticularis, renal failure, and benign urinary sediment. *Nephrol Dial Transplant* **10**, 295–7.

126. Casciola-Rosen, L.A., Anhalt, G., and Rosen, A. (1994) Autoantigens targeted in systemic lupus erythematosus are clustered in two populations of surface structures. *J Exp Med* **179**, 1317–30.

127. Herrmann, M., Voll, R.E., Zoller, O.M. *et al.* (1998) Impaired phagocytosis of apoptotic cell material by monocyte-derived macrophages from patients with systemic lupus erythematosus. *Arthritis Rheum* **41**, 1241–50.

128. Licht, R., Dicker, J.W., Jacobs, C.W., Tex, W.J., and Berden, J.H. (2004) Diseased phagocytosis of apoptotic cells in diseased SLE mice. *J Autoimm* **22**, 139–145.

129. Isenberg, D.A., Manson, J.J., Ehrenstein, M.R., and Rahman, A. (2007) Fifty years of anti-dsDNA antibodies: are we approaching 'journey's end'? *Rheumatology* **46**, 1052–6.

Chapter 3

T cells and B cells in lupus nephritis

Mary H. Foster

Introduction

The immune system plays a central role in the pathogenesis of systemic lupus erythematosus (SLE) and lupus nephritis, the most common serious complication. Disease manifestations result from effector pathways set in motion by activated and tissue-infiltrating lymphocytes and mononuclear cells, secreted cytokines, and circulating and deposited autoantibodies. These effectors are, in turn, the product of an autoimmune response unleashed from normal controls by the interaction of complex genetic and environmental factors. T and B lymphocytes lie at the heart of autoimmunity, defining antigen specificity and modulating each step in pathogenesis: initiation, regulation, amplification, tissue infiltration, organ destruction, and disease resolution. This chapter will review the role of adaptive immunity and its dysregulation in lupus nephritis, with emphasis on recent insights and promising new targets for immune intervention.

Initiation of nephritogenic autoimmune responses

Tolerance and lupus susceptibility

Systemic lupus erythematosus results from failed immune tolerance to self. In healthy individuals, self-reactive T and B cells are produced routinely as a by-product of the gene recombination and somatic processes that generate a vast repertoire of receptors capable of binding an infinite variety of foreign antigens. It is estimated that as many as 75% of newly formed and 40% of mature germinal center B cells recognize self.[1,2] Self-reactivity in the T cell repertoire is similarly ensured by the dependence of T cell selection and activation on recognition of peptide within the context of self-major histocompatibility complex (MHC) molecules. Nonetheless, autoreactive disease is uncommon because self-reactivity is normally held in check by any one of a series of mechanisms acting on developing and mature lymphocytes (Table 3.1).[3]

Antigen-specific tolerance results from lymphocyte receptor engagement of self-antigen within a permissive, noninflammatory microenvironment (Figure 3.1). In this setting, an antigen-induced "signal 1" will trigger lymphocyte deletion, receptor replacement, also known as editing, or nonresponsiveness, termed anergy, depending in part on the net strength of the receptor–antigen interaction. These mechanisms are highly effective at controlling autoreactivity but can be bypassed in an inflammatory environment. Co-delivery of both signal 1 and a co-stimulatory second signal leads to

Table 3.1 Mechanisms regulating autoimmunity*

Deletion
Anergy
Receptor editing
Clonal ignorance
Peritoneal homing
Follicular exclusion
Competition for survival factors
Regulatory B and T cell subsets[†]
Th1, Th2, and Th17 skewing
Immune suppressive cytokines (TGFβ, IL-10)
Receptor and co-receptor modulation
Idiotypic networks
Antigen sequestration

[†] IL-10 or TGFβ-producing B cells; prototypic CD4+CD25+foxp3+ Treg, TGFβ-producing T-helper-3 (Th3) T cells, T regulatory type 1 (Tr1) T cells, and inhibitory CD8+, TCRγ/δ or NK T cells.

* Adapted from Foster, M.H. (2007). T cells and B cells in lupus nephritis. *Semin Nephrol* **27**(1), 47–58, with permission from Elsevier.

cell activation. Signal 2 is typically delivered by a cognate member of a co-stimulatory pair, such as CD40/CD40L, B7(CD80)/CD28, or inducible co-stimulator ligand (ICOSL)/ICOS, expressed on an antigen presenting cell (APC).[4] Alternatively, potent mitogen or microbial products such as lipopolysaccharide, dsRNA, or unmethylated CpG DNA can transmit a "danger" signal to self-reactive B cells by engaging toll-like receptors (TLRs).[5] These situations nonetheless fail to induce disease in healthy individuals because a variety of additional downstream regulatory mechanisms are in place to block progression of autoimmune responses and to prevent or limit tissue infiltration and immune damage (Table 3.1).

Thus, development of lupus nephritis requires concomitant multi-focal breakdown in immune regulation: activation of autoreactive B and T cells, failure of multiple serial immune regulatory checkpoints, local antigen exposure, renal recruitment of immune mediators, and a renal microenvironment that promotes effector activity and organ destruction (Table 3.2). This breakdown, in turn, results from interactions of as yet poorly defined environmental triggers with a polygenic inherited autoimmune susceptibility.[6,7]

Animal models have revealed a variety of environmental antigens or microbial products that precipitate or exacerbate lupus-like disease in genetically predisposed hosts. Growing evidence suggests that a subset of environmental toxins acts through epigenetic mechanisms. Procainamide and hydralazine interfere with methyltransferase Dnmt1 to alter lymphocyte chromatin structure.[8,9] T cell DNA hypomethylation leads to overexpression of methylation-sensitive genes, such as leukocyte function-associated antigen-1 (LFA-1) and loss of tolerance. Adoptive transfer of

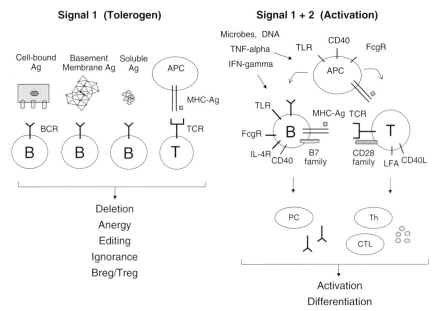

Fig. 3.1 Antigen regulation of autoimmunity. Self-antigen contact with the T or B cell receptor (TCR, BCR) can induce specific tolerance or activation in the responding lymphocyte. Antigen is presented either in native conformation for recognition by B cells or as peptide antigen presented by cell-bound MHC molecules for recognition by TCR-alpha/beta-expressing T cells. The outcome of the interaction depends on the microenvironment and whether an inflammatory milieu upregulates costimulatory signals. Ag, antigen; Breg, regulatory B cell; Treg, regulatory T cell; PC, plasma cell; CTL, cytotoxic T lymphocyte. Reproduced from Foster, M. H. (2007). T cells and B cells in lupus nephritis. *Semin Nephrol* **27**(1):47–58, with permission from Elsevier.

drug-treated T cells induces lupus-like disease in syngeneic mice.[10] Procainamide also alters T cell thymic selection and signaling thresholds.[11] In contrast, hydrocarbon oil (pristane) appears to induce experimental lupus indirectly by augmenting production of type I interferon (IFN) and inflammatory responses to TLR7.[12] The molecular mechanisms by which mercuric chloride, gold, and allogeneic reactions induce Th2-type autoreactive CD4+ T cells, interleukin (IL)-4, and IFNγ have yet to be elucidated.[13,14]

Genetic mapping in the major models of spontaneous lupus and in SLE patients recruited through multi-center consortia has revealed over 40 genes or genetic loci that predispose to lupus.[15,16] Key allelic variants or mutations linked to SLE in patients to date include: MHC Class II alleles encoding molecules critical to antigen presentation; B-lymphoid tyrosine kinase (BLK) involved in B cell signaling; interferon regulatory factor 5; programmed death 1 (PD-1); genes encoding immunoglobulin (Ig)G Fc receptors and complement components that regulate B cell activation, tolerance, and effector cell functions; signal transducer and activator of transcription 4 (STAT4), engaged in T cell differentiation and cytokine signaling; and protein

Table 3.2 Initiation and amplification of nephritogenic autoimmune responses in lupus

Altered DNA methylation or histone acetylation*
Dendritic cell activation[†]
Antigenic mimicry due to foreign/self homology
Exposure of cryptic or neo- (modified) self-antigen
Expression of dormant self-antigen (heat shock protein)
Imbalance or defect in T or B cell regulatory subsets
Bystander activation
Polyclonal activation (mitogens, superantigens, lectins)
Biased T helper subset expansion (Th1/Th2/Th17 shift)
Defective, abnormal, or excessive apoptosis[‡]
Altered antigen receptor signaling (BCR, TCR)
Decreased inhibitory receptor signaling (FcγRIIB, CD21, CD22, CD5)
Enhanced accessory receptor signaling (TLR, co-stimulators, activating FcγR, adhesion molecules)
Enhanced lymphocyte survival (elevated BLyS/BAFF, mutated Fas)
Epitope spreading

* A given type of environmental challenge (infectious agents, chemicals, drugs, pharmacological agents, ultraviolet light) may induce acquired defects by multiple mechanisms shown here.
† Activation of IFNα/β-producing dendritic cells by viruses, nucleic acid-IgG immune complexes, or microbial products may be a major cause of loss of peripheral tolerance.
‡ Apoptosis defects may contribute to autoimmunity at multiple levels. Apoptosis is crucial for autoreactive B and T cell deletion, and apoptotic cells expose a variety of lupus self-antigens that can either tolerize or immunize, depending on context.
Reproduced from Foster, M.H. (2007) T cells and B cells in lupus nephritis. *Semin Nephrol* **27**(1), 47–58, with permission from Elsevier.

tyrosine phosphatase, nonreceptor type 22 (Ptpn22), which encodes a known negative regulator of lymphocyte signaling. The Ptpn22 C1858T (R620W) allelic variant, recently implicated in multiple human autoimmune disorders, is a gain-of-function variant that appears to raise lymphocyte signaling thresholds.[17] Gene profiling in murine lupus suggests a role for Ptpn22 in modulating B cell anergy.[18] In lupus-prone mouse strains, genetically determined defects in central and peripheral B and T cell tolerance were confirmed by introduction of autoreactive B and T cell receptor transgenes.[19,20] The list of potential SLE susceptibility genes continues to grow as experimental manipulations in normal mouse strains induce unexpected lupus-like phenotypes; lupus nephritis has been induced by overexpression or gene-targeted disruption of immune-related molecules involved in B and T cell signaling, selection, activation, and survival.[21–24] Interpreted in light of the clinical heterogeneity of human SLE, it is clear that multiple different combinations of regulatory defects lead to lupus.

It was recently recognized that immune networks are themselves regulated by clusters of small noncoding RNAs, termed microRNAs or miRNAs. These 19–25 nucleotide

RNAs act as post-transcriptional repressors by annealing to the 3' untranslated region of specific target mRNAs, with profound effects on protein synthesis and cell function. To date, miR-155, miR-181, and miR-150 have emerged as key orchestrators of lymphocyte activation and selection.[25] Aberrant lymphocyte expression and function of miR-101 and the miR-17-92 cluster were recently implicated in lupus pathogenesis.[26,27]

T and B cell abnormalities in lupus

Multiple abnormalities are reported in lupus B and T cells, many of which are potential targets for therapeutic intervention.[28–30] Defects central to SLE T cell dysfunction are deficiency and replacement of the TCR/CD3 ζ chain by the Fc receptor γ chain, constitutive clustering of lipid rafts, and unusual raft composition (reviewed in[31]). These anomalies lead to enhanced but aberrant early TCR signaling, with heightened calcium responses, lowered activation threshold, and upregulated expression of multiple molecules, including CD40L, ICOS, β2 integrins CD11a/CD18 (LFA-1), CD11c/CD18 (Mac-1), CD70, CD44, phosphorylated ERM (esrin, radixin, and moesin), Syk, focal adhesion kinase, pp125FAK, protein phosphatase 2A (PP2A), calcium/calmodulin-dependent protein kinase (CaMKIV), COX-2, agrin proteoglycan, and perforin. T cell DNA is hypomethylated and other responses are blunted or dysfunctional: NFκB signaling, IL-2 production, mitogen activated protein (MAP) kinase responses, Ras activation, transcriptional regulator expression and activation, activation-induced death, mitochondrial function, negative regulator cbl-b, and extracellular signal-related kinase (ERK) pathways.[31–34] Imbalanced signaling yields a lupus T cell phenotype with features of activation and anergy manifest as impaired regulatory and effector functions, paradoxical spontaneous hyperexcitability, depressed Ag-specific responsiveness, enhanced B cell help, and deficient cytotoxicity. It is notable that genetic dampening of ERK signaling in T cells *in vivo* by inducible overexpression of dominant-negative MEK induces a lupus biochemical phenotype.[35]

Lupus B cells are also intrinsically abnormal and hyperactive, demonstrating widespread upregulation of multiple signaling axes.[36,37] Reported abnormalities include enhanced phosphorylation of JAK2, STAT5, mTOR, retinoblastoma protein, and the MAPK and AKT pathways; upregulation of NFκB, cyclin dependent kinases, CD40L, and antiapoptotic pathways; and downregulation of PKCα and Lyn kinase.[38–41] A similar pattern of signal activation was recently observed among B cells from genetically distinct murine lupus strains (B6.Sle1z, B6.Sle1z.Sle3z, BXSB, Fas-deficient MRL/LpJ-Tnfrsf6lpr, hereafter MRL/lpr),[41] fueling optimism that therapy targeted to a shared core signaling pathway may be universally effective in a genetically diverse patient population.

Local immune responses in lupus kidneys

CD4+ and CD8+ T cells, B cells, macrophages, and dendritic cells infiltrate the renal interstitium and glomerulus in lupus nephritis. The biology of local immune regulation, lymphocyte trafficking and expansion, and lymphocyte-mediated tissue destruction remains poorly understood and is an area of intense interest. Lupus kidneys are rich in chemokines known to recruit lymphocytes.[42] Renal infiltration in SLE is also dependent on IFNγ, a key cytokine in lupus pathogenesis; infiltrates are almost completely abolished in IFNγ- or IFNγ-receptor-deficient MRL/lpr or (NZBxNZW)F1 (BWF1) mice.[43–48] Interferon γ also facilitates cognate interactions between T cells and renal parenchymal cells, in particular proximal tubular epithelial cells (PTEC) (reviewed in[49]). Interferon γ upregulates parenchymal cell accessory molecules, including MHC Class II proteins, ICOSL, and PD-1 ligand (PDL-1), a negative regulator that mediates T cell tolerance to peripheral tissues.[46,50–52] Co-stimulators B7-1 and B7-2 (CD80 and CD86 respectively), in contrast, are not expressed on intrinsic kidney cells.[53] Inducible MHC Class II expression permits antigen presentation to CD4+ T cells, an interaction that can either activate or anergize the responding T cell depending on accompanying co-stimulation. Collective findings suggest that in healthy individuals PTEC–T cell interactions primarily function to maintain tolerance to self-antigen.[54,55]

The primary role of parenchymal–T cell interactions in the course of lupus nephritis is less clear, and not resolved by murine studies based on genetic elimination of co-stimulators. In MRL/lpr mice, global loss of PD-L1 leads to early death from autoimmune myocarditis and pneumonitis, before the development of nephritis and classic systemic lupus.[56] Conversely, ICOS deficiency depresses IgG autoantibody titers but has little effect on renal pathology or function, with the exception of conflicting reports on the fate of renal infiltrating ICOS+ T cells.[42,57] In human lupus nephritis, tumor necrosis factor apoptosis-inducing ligand (TRAIL), a pleiotropic member of the tumor necrosis factor (TNF) family with recently recognized co-stimulator actions, is implicated in local nephritogenic responses. Tumor necrosis factor apoptosis-inducing ligand and two TRAIL agonistic receptors, TRAIL-R1/DR4 and TRAIL-R2/DR5, are upregulated in renal tubules in proliferative nephritis and in human PTEC co-cultured with TNFα, and exogenous TRAIL induces human PTEC to proliferate and produce intercellular adhesion molecule (ICAM)-1 and IL-8.[58]

T cells and cellular immunity in lupus nephritis

Pivotal role for T cells in lupus

T cells play a central but complex role in pathogenesis of lupus nephritis (Figure 3.2).[29,59] Autoreactive T cells are expanded and activated by defects in thymic and peripheral T cell tolerance and by deficiency of regulatory T cells (Treg). Activated effector T cells provide help for B cell production of mutated, high-affinity, IgG isotype-switched nephritogenic autoantibodies, regulate B cell responses, modulate differentiation and function of other T cell subsets, and mediate effector functions. T cells infiltrate the kidney in lupus to interact with renal parenchymal cells, modulate local immunity, and injure kidney cells via cytokine secretion, recruitment of macrophages or natural killer (NK) cells, or direct cytotoxicity. A key role in kidney injury is suggested by correlation of renal interstitial inflammation with the degree of kidney damage and progression to end stage renal failure.[60] It is notable, however, that Treg are critical to limit nephritogenic responses and renal immune injury in lupus, and their deficiency can initiate or exacerbate disease. Because Treg share phenotypic markers and activation pathways with T effectors, manipulations that delete major

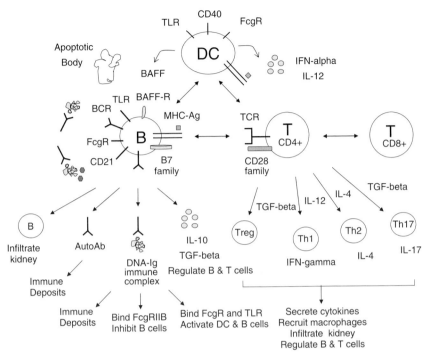

Fig. 3.2 Diverse roles for B cells, T cells, and dendritic cells (DC) in the control of autoimmunity and pathogenesis of lupus nephritis. Reproduced from Foster, M. H. (2007). T cells and B cells in lupus nephritis. *Semin Nephrol* **27**(1):47–58, with permission from Elsevier.

T cell populations or interrupt common pathways may have unpredictable outcomes on disease.

Autoreactive CD4+, CD8+, and CD4-CD8- (double-negative, DN) TCRα/β and TCRγ/δ T cells can be isolated from the blood of lupus patients and from blood, lymphoid organs, kidney, and extrarenal tissue of lupus mice.[54,61–66] Abnormalities in T cell subset absolute numbers, frequencies, and functions are reported, including an increase in the CD4+/CD8+ ratio, increased frequency of double-negative CD4-CD8- T cells, increased IFNγ production, and altered Th1 and Th2 ratios and cytokine production.[67]

A critical role of T cells in mediating disease in murine lupus was confirmed by demonstration of disease amelioration through depletion of select T cell subsets or interference with several major T cell co-stimulatory pathways. In general, murine lupus nephritis is ameliorated by genetic or antibody depletion of CD4+ and α/β T cells or antagonism of CD28/B7, CD40/CD40L, and ICAM-1/LFA-1 co-stimulatory pathways.[50,53,68–71] These manipulations variably decrease proteinuria, renal histopathological injury, and lymphocytic infiltration, improve urea and creatinine clearances, and lower autoantibody titers. The predominant effect of these maneuvers presumably is elimination of pathogenic effector T cells. The ICOS/ICOSL pathway appears less critical to kidney injury; whereas anti-ICOS antibody administration improves nephritis in BWF1 mice, targeted deletion of ICOS has little or no effect on renal function or pathology in MRL/lpr mice.[42,57,72] A key role for T cells is likewise revealed by interference in a normally nonautoimmune strain with a major T cell negative regulatory pathway. Targeted deletion of CD152 (CTLA-4), a molecule critical to limiting T cell activation in the periphery, leads to global T cell dysregulation, early onset humoral autoimmunity, glomerular immune deposition, and interstitial nephritis in C57BL/6 mice, even in the absence of B cell activating factor (BAFF).[73]

In contrast, targeted deletion of β2-microglobulin, which eliminates both classical and nonclassical (CD1) MHC Class I expression and thus eliminates CD8+ and NK1 T cells, accelerates disease in BWF1 mice.[74] β2-Microglobulin deletion alleviates kidney injury but accelerates dermatitis in MRL/lpr mice.[75,76] The renal effect in MRL/lpr mice is attributed to deletion of effector CD8+ T cells, because isolated CD1-deletion does not alter nephritis in this strain. However, prolonged administration of anti-CD8 monoclonal antibody fails to alter disease in either MRL/lpr or (NZWxBXSB) F1 mice.[77] Genetic manipulations reveal activity of both effector and regulatory TCRγ/δ T cell subsets in MRL/lpr lupus nephritis: deletion of TCRγ/δ T cells accelerates nephritis and mortality and expands CD4+ T cell populations, whereas deletion of TCRα/β cells partially ameliorates nephritis, and TCRγ/δ–TCRα/β-double-deficient MRL/lpr mice are free of autoantibodies and disease.[78]

The role of natural killer T (NKT) cells in SLE is similarly complex (reviewed in[79]). Natural killer T cells express an invariant TCRα chain rearrangement and NK cell receptor NK1.1, and recognize glycolipid presented by the nonpolymorphic, nonclassical MHC Class I molecule CD1d expressed on APC, including subsets of B cells. When activated, particularly by the potent agonist α-galactosylceramide (α-GalCer), NKT cells produce large amounts of IFNγ, IL-4, and other cytokines that activate dendritic cells (DC), NK cells, B cells, and conventional T cells. Natural killer T cells generally have been considered negative immune regulators and their deficiency and dysfunction have been considered risk factors for autoimmunity. However, BWF1 NKT cells are expanded and activated *in vivo* and promote CD1- and CD40L-dependent IgG autoantibody production by B-1 and marginal zone, but not conventional follicular, B cells.[80–82] Glycolipid therapy is nonefficacious in diseased MRL/lpr and detrimental in BWF1 lupus strains.[79]

Regulatory T cells in lupus

Regulatory T cells control immune hyperactivity and are key in preventing peripheral activation of autoreactive cells that escape central tolerance. Major Treg subsets include CD4+CD25highFoxp3+CD127low thymus-committed natural and peripherally induced adaptive Treg cells, as well as CD4+CD25-, CD8+CD25+, CD8+CD28-Tregs and subsets of TCRγ/δ and NKT cells. Regulatory T cells exert both Ag-specific and bystander suppressor activities, via either cognate interactions with effector cells or via secreted cytokines (IL10, TGFβ) or other soluble mediators.[83,84] Decreased peripheral Treg cell numbers or functionally anomalous Tregs are implicated in the pathogenesis of murine lupus,[84–87] whereas the status of Tregs in human lupus is inconclusive (reviewed in[84,88]). Many, but not all, investigators report abnormalities in SLE patient Treg numbers or function. These discrepancies are due in part to overlap in phenotypic markers that limits accurate discrimination between Treg and other

T cell subsets; activated T cells express CD25+ and transiently low levels of Foxp3, and small populations of CD4+ CD25-foxp3+ T cells have regulator activities. Some effects attributed to defective regulatory function may, in fact, be due to effector T cell resistance to suppression.[89,90] Additionally, Treg numbers and function are influenced by disease activity and immunosuppressive therapy; urinary FOXP3 mRNA levels were recently correlated with disease activity in lupus nephritis.[91] Enhancement of Treg numbers or activity is a promising approach to therapy in SLE.[84,92]

Contrary to initial expectations, evidence suggests that cytotoxic T cells in lupus are also predominantly regulatory, directed toward controlling pathogenic B and T cells, not primarily pathogenic themselves.[93,94] T cell cytotoxic responses are mediated primarily through Fas, perforin, and the cytokine TNF. Genetic ablation of any of these pathways in lupus-prone mice leads to acceleration, not improvement, of lupus and nephritis.[95–97] This also may explain in part the association of drug-induced lupus with anti-TNFα therapy.

Expansion of a normally rare population of IL-10-, TGFβ-, and FasL-producing autoreactive regulatory CD4+ T cells that express NKG2D, a marker typically restricted to CD8+ and NK effector cells, and circulating soluble NKG2D ligands were recently described in human juvenile-onset SLE.[98] NKG2D+ CD4+ T cell frequency inversely correlated with SLE disease activity. Notably, these cells are distinct from pathogenic IFNγ producing autoreactive NKG2D+ CD4+ T cell effectors described in rheumatoid arthritis, celiac disease, and recently in SLE.[99]

T cell effector mechanisms in lupus

Differentiated T cell effector subsets active in SLE include TCRα/β CD4+ helper subsets, Th1, Th2, and Th17, distinguished in part by their distinct transcription factors and signature cytokine patterns (Figure 3.2), TCRα/β CD4+ T follicular helper cells (Tfh), differentiated TCRα/β CD8+ cells, TCRγ/δ, and NKT cells. T cell effectors exert their functions through cognate interactions with other cells, including B cells, other T cells, macrophages, dendritic cells, NK cells, and parenchymal cells, or through secretion of immunomodulatory cytokines.

A subset of lupus autoreactive CD4+ T cells responds to major epitopes in nucleosomal histones to provide help to antinucleosome and anti-DNA B cells.[100–102] In addition to supporting humoral autoimmunity, CD4+ T helpers promote lupus nephritis by generating proinflammatory cytokines that upregulate adhesion and MHC Class II molecules on APC and kidney parenchymal cells and by infiltrating the kidney to recruit macrophages, activate parenchymal cells, and promote fibrosis.[54,61,102] Renal parenchymal cells, in turn, produce nephritogenic cytokines, macrophage growth factors, and chemokines that amplify T cell responses and perpetuate local injury.[103–105]

Activated CD4+ and CD8+ T cells are present in glomerular lesions and renal interstitium in murine and human lupus,[64,65] and autoreactive CD4+ DN and cytotoxic T cells can be isolated from murine lupus kidneys.[54,66] MRL/lpr kidney-derived CD4+ DN T cell clones induce MHC Class II and ICAM-1 expression on cultured renal PTEC, and proliferate *ex vivo* in response to renal PTEC.[54] CD4+ TCRα/β T cell effectors isolated from nephritic kidneys of mice with chronic graft-versus-host-disease (GVHD) induce glomerular crescents and mononuclear infiltrates in histocompatible recipients when transferred under the renal capsule.[66] Whereas the contribution of T cell direct cytotoxicity to kidney cells is not fully established in lupus nephritis, it is notable that in nonlupus model systems, nephritogenic CD4+ and CD8+ T cell clones can mediate MHC-restricted, perforin- and granzyme-mediated cytotoxicity toward cultured PTEC.[106]

Kidney infiltrates in MRL/lpr mice include the unique population of B220+ Class I-restricted DN CD4-CD8- TCRα/β T cells that are expanded in this strain due to the lpr gene associated defective CD95/Fas antigen. Crispin et al. recently determined that kidneys of patients with lupus nephritis are also infiltrated by DN CD4-CD8- TCRα/β and IL-17-producing T cells,[107] presumably derived from the population of IL-17-producing DN T cells expanded in the blood of SLE patients.[61,107]

All major subsets of CD4+ T helper cells contribute to lupus pathogenesis, via complex cellular and cytokine interactions. Initial studies focused on Th1 and Th2 cells, the first characterized subsets, and identified no dominant pathogenic subset (reviewed in[108,109]). Both Th1 (IFNγ, IL-12, TNFα/β) and Th2 (IL-4, IL-10) cytokines are elevated in murine lupus. Therapeutic administration of histone deacetylase inhibitors in MRL/lpr lupus downregulates transcription of cytokines (IL-12, IFNγ, IL-6, and IL-10) from both Th subsets.[110] Genetic and biological manipulations that modulate cytokine production or actions in vivo show inconsistent results in altering disease in lupus-prone mice. Administration of either IL-10 or IFNγ accelerates nephritis in BWF1 mice, whereas antibody blockade of either cytokine delays disease. Targeted disruption of either IFNγ or IL-4 reduces nephritis in MRL/lpr mice, whereas administration of IL-12 to MRL/lpr mice accelerates kidney injury and promotes intrarenal accumulation of IFNγ-secreting T cells.

Recent investigations confirm involvement of Th17 and additional Th subsets and related cytokines in SLE. Reverse transcriptase polymerase chain reaction (RT-PCR) of laser microdissected renal T cells detected predominantly IFNγ, IL-13, and IL-17 production in nephritic MRL/lpr mouse kidneys.[111] Interleukin-10 was present but primarily limited to perivascular T cells. Serum IL-17 levels are elevated in SLE patients and correlate with disease severity; Th17 cell populations are expanded in murine and human SLE.[112–114] T follicular helper cells express ICOS and the chemokine CXCR5 that facilitates their migration to B cell follicles, where they are critical for germinal center selection of mutated high-affinity antigen-specific B cells. Mice with a mutated roquin gene develop enhanced ICOS expression, high numbers of Tfh cells and germinal centers, and lupus-like disease with immune complex glomerulonephritis (ICGN).[115] Interleukin-21, a multifunctional CD4+ Th cell cytokine, promotes T and B cell effector functions and autoimmunity; genetic elimination of the IL-21 receptor alleviates BXSB-Yaa murine lupus.[116]

Interleukin-27, a pleiotropic member of the IL-6/IL-12 family, modulates differentiation and survival of Th1 and Th17 cells. Interference with IL-27 signaling alters the murine lupus nephritis phenotype. In MRL/lpr mice, deficiency of WSX-1, a component of the IL-27 receptor, reduces CD4+ T cell IFNγ production and converts diffuse proliferative glomerulonephritis to a disease resembling membranous nephropathy.[117] Conversely, WSX-1 overexpression reduces MRL/lpr production of IFNγ, IL-4, and autoantibodies, and ameliorates kidney injury.[118]

B cells and humoral immunity in lupus nephritis

Multi-functional B cells

B cells have a profound impact in shaping immune, autoimmune, and inflammatory responses (reviewed in[119–123]). B cells modulate cellular immunity via direct interactions with T cells and DC and through generation of regulatory and effector antibodies and cytokines (IL-10, TGFβ, IL-4, IL-6, IFNγ, IL-2, and TNFα) (Figure 3.2 and Table 3.3).[122,124] Antigen specificity is imparted by cell membrane-bound Ig, which transduces antigen-triggered signals and is capable of internalizing and processing bound antigen for highly efficient peptide–MHC presentation to T cells.[125] Diverse B cell functions include activation, expansion, suppression, and modulation of T cell responses; induction of T cell tolerance; regulation of DC development and activation; activation and suppression of macrophage activity; skewing of T helper differentiation; and antibody secretion (Table 3.3). Antibodies in turn serve multiple functions. Tissue-deposited antibodies mediate injury via engagement of Fcγ receptors to activate macrophages, neutrophils, NK cells, DC, or parenchymal cells; through activation of complement cascades; and by directly binding parenchymal cell surfaces. Conversely, regulatory Ig can dampen disease via engagement of target cell inhibitory FcγRIIB receptors, promoting clearance of immune complexes or apoptotic cells by Fc-mediated binding, or by participating in regulatory idiotypic networks.[126] In murine lupus, a predominantly pathogenic role for B cells is suggested by amelioration of disease manifestations by B cell ablation using monoclonal antibody administration or gene deletion.[127] Results of B cell depletion therapy in lupus patients are less uniform, most likely reflecting the multiple and sometimes opposing roles of B cells, although there are multiple reports of efficacy of anti-CD20 therapy in refractory SLE.[128]

Table 3.3 Diverse roles for B cells in immunity and lupus

Produce pathogenic autoantibodies
Produce regulatory antibodies (anti-idiotypic, FcγRIIB-binding, mediator-neutralizing)
Produce immunomodulatory cytokines (IL-10, IL-6, TGFβ, IFNγ, IL-12)
Differentiate into polarized B cell effectors
Process and present antigen to T cells for activation or tolerance induction
Coordinate T cell migration and differentiation
Directly cross-regulate Th1 and Th2 cell differentiation
Inhibit or delete T cell effectors via direct contact or TGFβ
Recruit CD8+ and NKT regulatory T cells
Promote development of follicular dendritic cells
Regulate dendritic cell cytokine production
Maintain secondary lymphoid architecture

Reproduced from Foster, M.H. (2007) T cells and B cells in lupus nephritis. *Semin Nephrol* **27**(1), 47–58, with permission from Elsevier.

B cells promote lupus nephritis through both antibody-dependent and antibody-independent mechanisms. Pathogenic antibodies deposit in glomeruli and tubules, arising either from the circulation, secreted by autoreactive B cells in the spleen or lymph nodes, or from kidney-infiltrating B cells and plasma cells. However, antibody production is not essential for B cell pathogenicity. Whereas complete deficiency of B cells ameliorates disease in MRL/lpr mice, nephritis and early death persist in mice bearing genetically manipulated B cells incapable of secreting antibody.[129,130] Progression of autoimmunity in this setting is attributed in part to a key role for autoreactive B cells in activating CD8 and CD4 effector T cells.

Conversely, regulatory B cells are probably involved in limiting disease in lupus. B cell mediated negative regulation of autoimmunity and inflammation in nonlupus disease models is well described, in some cases revealed by unexpected disease exacerbation after introduction of B cell deficiency (reviewed in[121,122]). Yanaba and colleagues recently identified a rare and phenotypically unique population of CD1d-highCD5+ IL-10-producing regulatory B cells, termed B10 cells, in naïve wild-type mice.[131] B10 cells are responsible for most B cell IL-10 production, and have the ability to inhibit T cell proliferation and T cell mediated inflammatory responses *in vivo*. Abnormalities in B cell IL-10 production are reported in murine lupus.[132] Enhancement of regulatory B cell, or suppressor T cell, numbers or activity offer one of many promising targets for therapeutic intervention in SLE (Table 3.4).

Lupus mice and patients display a variety of B cell abnormalities, in addition to the biochemical anomalies reported above. Unusual circulating B cell populations have been identified in patients, including plasmablasts and cells bearing germinal center markers.[38] Upregulated peripheral B cell CD86 expression correlates with renal involvement.[133] CXCR5+ B cells with an antigen presentation phenotype, plasmablasts, ectopic germinal centers, and organized follicles are reported in lupus kidneys,[134–136] and B cells secreting nephritogenic anti-DNA autoantibodies have been isolated from lupus mouse kidneys.[135] Reports vary on the relative abundance of Ig-producing B cells among renal infiltrating lymphocytes.[134,136] B cell chemoattractant CXCL13 is ectopically expressed in BWF1 mouse kidneys, as well as in other organs, and promotes kidney trafficking of B-1 B cells.[137] Lymphoid chemokine BCA-1 is expressed in nephritic kidneys of SLE patients.[136] Circulating BAFF (or BLyS), a B cell survival and differentiation factor that plays a role in B cell homeostasis and selection, is elevated in a significant proportion of lupus patients (reviewed in[138,139]), and acts in synergy with IL-17 to promote survival and differentiation of human B cells.[114] Mice overexpressing BAFF develop a lupus-like disease with ICGN, even in the complete absence of T cells.[140,141] B cell activating factor rescues autoreactive B cells from peripheral deletion and initiates CD40L-independent IgG isotype class switch.[142]

Nephritogenic autoantibodies and antibody-mediated injury

Glomerular antibody and complement deposition are hallmarks of lupus glomerulonephritis. Immunoglobulin G, IgM, IgA, C3, C4, and C1q are typically present in human lupus kidney biopsies, consistent with activation of the classical pathway. Mechanisms of immune deposition and injury have been reviewed in detail elsewhere[143,144] and are briefly summarized here, with emphasis on recent findings.

Table 3.4 Targeted immunotherapy in lupus nephritis

1. B and T cell signaling and activation thresholds

   Upregulation or stimulation of B cell inhibitory Fcγ RIIB

   B cell tolerance induction (dsDNA oligomers)*

   Inhibition of DNA methylation or histone deacetylation†

2. B and T cell survival, proliferation and differentiation, collaboration and co-stimulation

   Anti-B cell therapy (anti-CD20 and anti-CD19 mAb)

   Blockade of BAFF/BAFF receptor pathway (anti-BAFF mAb; TACI-Ig fusion protein)

   Modulate activating or inhibitory surface receptors (anti-CD22 mAb)

   Anti-T cell subset therapy

   Blockade of B7/CD28 pathway (CTLA4-Ig, single-chain Fv CD28 inhibitor)

   Blockade of CD40/CD40L (anti-CD40L mAb)

   Blockade of ICOS/ICOSL pathway (anti-ICOSL mAb)

   Blockade of CD137 (4-1BB)/4-1BBL pathway

   Stimulation of T cell inhibitory pathways PD-1/PDL-1, CTLA4, BTLA

   Modulation of TLR signaling (inhibitory GpG oligodeoxynucleotides)

   Modified antigen presenting cells (dendritic cell therapy)

3. Regulatory cell function

   In vivo or *ex vivo* induction of regulatory T or B cells

   Administration of tolerizing self-antigen-expressing dendritic or stem cells

4. B and T effector cell function and inflammation

   Blockade of Ig production

   Inhibition of memory or plasma cell differentiation

   Blockade or adsorption of autoantibody reactivity

   Complement inhibition (anti-C5 mAb, soluble Crry or Crry-Fc fusion protein, C5a antagonist)

   Blockade of activatory FcγRI, FcγRIII or FcγRIV

   Stimulation of inhibitory FcγRIIB

   Inhibition of secondary mediators (cytokines, chemokines, NO, ROS, lipid mediators, etc.)

   Antimacrophage or neutrophil therapy

   T helper subset skewing

* Selected examples of interventions currently in preclinical or clinical trials are indicated in parentheses.
† Some interventions modulate multiple checkpoints; for simplicity, only one category is shown.
BLyS, B lymphocyte stimulator (also known as BAFF); TLR, toll-like receptor; Crry, complement receptor-1 related gene/protein Y; PD-1, programmed death-1; CTLA-4, cytotoxic T lymphocyte antigen-4; BTLA, B and T lymphocyte attenuator.
Reproduced from Foster, M.H. (2007) T cells and B cells in lupus nephritis. *Semin Nephrol* **27**(1), 47–58, with permission from Elsevier.

Antibodies isolated from lupus serum, derived as monoclonal antibodies, and eluted from nephritic lupus kidneys encompass multiple IgG subclasses and diverse antigen specificities, binding avidity, and charge.[145] Specificity for DNA or nucleosomes is prominent and important for pathogenesis for a subset of lupus Ig. It has also become clear, however, that anti-DNA activity is neither necessary nor sufficient to induce lupus nephritis, suggesting that other specificities are also engaged in disease pathogenesis.

Nephritogenic antibodies localize to the kidney by several mechanisms. Experimental models suggest that most immune complexes form *in situ*, with only a minority of deposits developing from passive deposition of circulating immune complexes.[146–149] Anti-DNA and antinucleosome antibodies are capable of binding *in situ* to previously deposited nuclear antigens. Basement membrane collagen, laminin, fibronectin, and glomerular cell surfaces have binding sites for DNA, as well as anionic foci that attract cationic immune complexes, histones, and nucleosomes. These planted cationic antigens, in turn, attract anionic DNA through charge–charge interactions. In a similar fashion, previously renal deposited IgG or C1q may be targeted by circulating rheumatoid factors and anti-C1q Ig respectively. Additionally, antigen cross-reactivity is prominent among lupus autoantibodies, as demonstrated for anti-DNA and non-DNA binding Ig eluted from lupus kidneys.[150] Lupus autoantibodies bind to α-actinin, α-enolase, additional unidentified glomerular antigens, and cultured renal parenchymal cells. Renal-bound autoantibodies subsequently activate complement or engage activating Fcγ receptors on macrophages, neutrophils, and renal parenchymal cells to promote leukocyte adhesion and trigger release of inflammatory mediators.[151] Additional pathogenic mechanisms proposed for lupus Ig include direct cellular effects triggered by antibody engagement of renal cell surface ligands; glomerular capillary occlusion by cryoglobulins, a process facilitated by unique self-aggregating properties of murine IgG3; cell uptake of autoantibodies with subsequent disruption of cellular functions by cytoplasmic or nuclear localizing Ig; and thrombus formation by antiphospholipid Ig interference with coagulation.

The diversity of pathogenic mechanisms, cellular effectors, and soluble mediators account in part for the clinical heterogeneity observed in lupus nephritis and for the uncoupling of serum autoantibody titres and renal pathology reported in various experimental models. Disease phenotype depends on both antibody specificity and Ig isotype, and thus Fc, specific effector functions. Each IgG subclass interacts uniquely with complement components and the different Fcγ receptors, expression and activation of which are regulated, in turn, by inflammatory cytokines and a network of regulatory proteins. Furthermore, complement, Fc receptors, autoantibodies, and immune complexes individually play dual and opposing roles in lupus pathogenesis. Complement and Fc receptors are important for immune complex and apoptotic cell clearance, processes that limit inflammation. This key function explains, in part, several perplexing aspects of lupus pathogenesis: the seemingly paradoxical lupus susceptibility imposed by C1q or C4 deficiency;[152,153] the variable capacity of targeted deletion of the common Fc receptor γ-chain gene to attenuate murine lupus nephritis;[154,155] and, the immune deposition observed after deletion of activating Fcγ receptors in nonautoimmune mice.[151] Immunoglobulin and immune complexes also bind to the B cell inhibitory Fcγ RIIB receptor and complement receptor CD21/CD35, respectively, to inhibit B cell signaling; deficiency of either inhibitory receptor interferes with B cell tolerance induction, and, in permissive backgrounds, promotes lupus nephritis.[23,156]

Immune complexes containing antinuclear autoantibodies and antigen (DNA, RNA, or chromatin) are potent amplifiers of autoimmune responses. Dendritic cells and B cells can capture and internalize immune complexes, via either membrane Fcγ receptor/Ig-Fc interactions or via B cell receptor engagement of nucleic acid antigen or binding to Ig Fc regions, for B cells with rheumatoid factor activity. Internalized nucleic acid can activate cytoplasmic TLR9 or TLR7, promoting cell activation, and in B cells, isotype switch.[151,157]

Summary and conclusion

T and B lymphocytes play both pathological effector roles and protective regulatory roles in autoimmune responses, and in the development and progression of lupus nephritis. Their relative contributions, and the relative contributions of their various cell subsets, vary depending on the nature of the particular environmental precipitant, host genetic susceptibility, and stage and time course of disease. T cell–B cell interactions and actions of their soluble products can promote or dampen autoreactivity, and are crucial both to induction of and escape from tolerance and recruitment, activation, and regulation of inflammatory cells. The disease phenotype ultimately depends on the balance of pathogenic and regulatory pathways. Ongoing investigation into the diversity and biology of T cells and B cells in health and in disease promises to reveal numerous new and promising therapeutic targets.

Acknowledgements

This work was supported in part by the Departments of Medicine and the Research Service at the Duke University and Durham Veterans Affairs Medical Centers and by R01DK47424 from the NDDK. The author sincerely apologizes to colleagues for the inability to cite many primary references due to space constraints.

References

1. Wardemann, H., Yurasov, S., Schaefer, A., Young, J.W., Meffre, E., and Nussenzweig, M.C. (2003) Predominant autoantibody production by early human B cell precursors. *Science* **301**(5638), 1374–7.

2. Jacobi, A.M., and Diamond, B. (2005) Balancing diversity and tolerance: lessons from patients with systemic lupus erythematosus. *J Exp Med* **202**(3), 341–4.

3. Goodnow, C., Sprent, J., Fazekas de St Groth, B., and Vinuesa, C. (2005) Cellular and genetic mechanisms of self tolerance and autoimmunity. *Nature* **435**, 590–7.

4. Keir, M., and Sharpe, A. (2005) The B7/CD28 costimulatory family in autoimmunity. *Immunol Rev* **204**, 128–43.

5. Peng, S. (2005) Signaling in B cells via Toll-like receptors. *Curr Opin Immunol* **17**(3), 230–6.

6. Rao, T., and Richardson, B. (1999) Environmentally induced autoimmune diseases: potential mechanisms. *Environ Health Perspect* **107** (Suppl 5), 737–42.

7. Lauwerys, B.R., and Wakeland, E.K. (2005) Genetics of lupus nephritis. *Lupus* **14**(1), 2–12.

8. Lee, B.H., Yegnasubramanian, S., Lin, X., and Nelson, W.G. (2005) Procainamide is a specific inhibitor of DNA methyltransferase 1. *J Biol Chem* **280**(49), 40749–56.

9. Gorelik, G., Fang, J.Y., Wu, A., Sawalha, A.H., and Richardson, B. (2007) Impaired T cell protein kinase C delta activation decreases ERK pathway signaling in idiopathic and hydralazine-induced lupus. *J Immunol* **179**(8), 5553–63.

10. Yung, R., Powers, D., Johnson, K., Amento, E., Carr, D., Laing, T., *et al.* (1996) Mechanisms of drug-induced lupus. II. T cells overexpressing lymphocyte function-associated antigen 1 become autoreactive and cause a lupus-like disease in syngeneic mice. *J Clin Invest* **97**(12), 2866–71.

11. Kretz-Rommel, A., and Rubin, R. (2000) Disruption of positive selection of thymocytes causes autoimmunity. *Nat Med* **6**, 298–305.

12. Lee, P.Y., Kumagai, Y., Li, Y., Takeuchi, O., Yoshida, H., Weinstein, J., *et al.* (2008) TLR7-dependent and FcgammaR-independent production of type I interferon in experimental mouse lupus. *J Exp Med* **205**(13), 2995–3006.

13. Prigent, P., Saoudi, A., Pannetier, C., Graber, P., Bonnefoy, J.Y., Druet, P., *et al.* (1995) Mercuric chloride, a chemical responsible for T helper cell (TH)2-mediated autoimmunity in brown Norway rats, directly triggers T cells to produce interleukin-4. *J Clin Invest* **96**, 1484–9.

14. Kono, D.H., Balomenos, D., Pearson, D.L., Park, M.S., Hildebrandt, B., Hultman, P., *et al.* (1998) The prototypic Th2 autoimmunity induced by mercury is dependent on IFN-gamma and not Th1/Th2 imbalance. *J Immunol* **161**, 234–40.

15. Morel, L. (2007) Genetics of human lupus nephritis. *Semin Nephrol* **27**(1), 2–11.

16. Li, L., and Mohan, C. (2007) Genetic basis of murine lupus nephritis. *Semin Nephrol* **27**(1), 12–21.

17. Rieck, M., Arechiga, A., Onengut-Gumuscu, S., Greenbaum, C., Concannon, P., and Buckner, J.H. (2007) Genetic variation in PTPN22 corresponds to altered function of T and B lymphocytes. *J Immunol* **179**(7), 4704–10.

18. Clark, A.G., Mackin, K.M., and Foster, M.H. (2008) Tracking differential gene expression in MRL/MpJ versus C57BL/6 anergic B cells: Molecular markers of autoimmunity. *Biomarker Insights* **3**, 335–50.

19. Erikson, J., Mandik, L., Bui, A., Eaton, A., Noorchashm, H., Nguyen, K.A., *et al.* (1998) Self-reactive B cells in nonautoimmune and autoimmune mice. *Immunol Res* **17**, 49–61.

20. Michaels, M., Kang, H., Kaliyaperumal, A., Satyaraj, E., Shi, Y., and Datta, S. (2005) A defect in deletion of nucleosome-specific autoimmune T cells in lupus-prone thymus: role of thymic dendritic cells. *J Immunol* **175**(9), 5857–65.

21. Strasser, A., Whittingham, S., Vaux, D.L., Bath, M.L., Adams, J.M., Cory, S., *et al.* (1991) Enforced BCL2 expression in B-lymphoid cells prolongs antibody responses and elicits autoimmune disease. *Proc Natl Acad Sci USA* **88**(19), 8661–5.

22. Hibbs, M.L., Tarlinton, D.M., Armes, J., Grail, D., Hodgson, G., Maglitto, R., *et al.* (1995) Multiple defects in the immune system of lyn-deficient mice, culminating in autoimmune disease. *Cell* **83**, 301–11.

23. Bolland, S., and Ravetch, J. (2000) Spontaneous autoimmune disease in Fc(gamma) RIIB-deficient mice results from strain-specific epistasis. *Immunity* **13**, 277–85.

24. Salvador, J.M., Hollander, M.C., Nguyen, A.T., Kopp, J.B., Barisoni, L., Moore, J.K., *et al.* (2002) Mice lacking the p53-effector gene Gadd45a develop a lupus-like syndrome. *Immunity* **16**(4), 499–508.

25. Bi, Y., Liu, G., and Yang, R. (2009) MicroRNAs: novel regulators during the immune response. *J Cell Physiol* **218**(3), 467–72.

26. Yu, D., Tan, A.H., Hu, X., Athanasopoulos, V., Simpson, N., Silva, D.G., *et al.* (2007) Roquin represses autoimmunity by limiting inducible T-cell co-stimulator messenger RNA. *Nature* **450**(7167), 299–303.

27. Xiao, C., Srinivasan, L., Calado, D.P., Patterson, H.C., Zhang, B., Wang, J., *et al.* (2008) Lymphoproliferative disease and autoimmunity in mice with increased miR-17-92 expression in lymphocytes. *Nat Immunol* **9**(4), 405–14.

28. Nagy, G., Koncz, A., and Perl, A. (2005) T- and B-cell abnormalities in systemic lupus erythematosus. *Crit Rev Immunol* **25**(2), 123–40.

29. Hoffman, R.W. (2004) T cells in the pathogenesis of systemic lupus erythematosus. *Clin Immunol* **113**(1), 4–13.

30. Zielinski, C., Jacob, S., Bouzahzah, F., Ehrlich, B., and Craft, J. (2005) Naive CD4+ T cells from lupus-prone Fas-intact MRL mice display TCR-mediated hyperproliferation due to intrinsic threshold defects in activation. *J Immunol* **174**(8), 5100–9.

31. Crispin, J.C., Kyttaris, V.C., Juang, Y.T., and Tsokos, G.C. (2008) How signaling and gene transcription aberrations dictate the systemic lupus erythematosus T cell phenotype. *Trends Immunol* **29**(3), 110–5.

32. Zhou, Y., and Lu, Q. (2008) DNA methylation in T cells from idiopathic lupus and drug-induced lupus patients. *Autoimmun Rev* **7**(5), 376–83.

33. Fernandez, D., and Perl, A. (2009) Metabolic control of T cell activation and death in SLE. *Autoimmun Rev* **8**(3), 184–9.

34. Xu, L., Zhang, L., Yi, Y., Kang, H.K., and Datta, S.K. (2004) Human lupus T cells resist inactivation and escape death by upregulating COX-2. *Nat Med* **10**(4), 411–5.

35. Sawalha, A.H., Jeffries, M., Webb, R., Lu, Q., Gorelik, G., Ray, D., *et al.* (2008) Defective T-cell ERK signaling induces interferon-regulated gene expression and overexpression of methylation-sensitive genes similar to lupus patients. *Genes Immun* **9**(4), 368–78.

36. Merino, R., Fossati, L., Lacour, M., and Izui, S. (1991) Selective autoantibody production by Yaa+ B cells in autoimmune Yaa+-Yaa- bone marrow chimeric mice. *J Exp Med* **174**, 1023–9.

37. Sobel, E.S., Mohan, C., Morel, L., Schiffenbauer, J., and Wakeland, E.K. (1999) Genetic dissection of SLE pathogenesis: adoptive transfer of Sle1 mediates the loss of tolerance by bone marrow-derived B cells. *J Immunol* **162**, 2415–21.

38. Grammer, A.C., and Lipsky, P.E. (2003) B cell abnormalities in systemic lupus erythematosus. *Arthritis Res Ther* **5** (Suppl 4), S22–7.

39. Renaudineau, Y., Pers, J.O., Bendaoud, B., Jamin, C., and Youinou, P. (2004) Dysfunctional B cells in systemic lupus erythematosus. *Autoimmun Rev* **3**(7-8), 516–23.

40. Tsubata, T. (2005) B cell abnormality and autoimmune disorders. *Autoimmunity* **38**(5), 331–7.

41. Wu, T., Qin, X., Kurepa, Z., Kumar, K.R., Liu, K., Kanta, H., *et al.* (2007) Shared signaling networks active in B cells isolated from genetically distinct mouse models of lupus. *J Clin Invest* **117**(8), 2186–96.

42. Odegard, J.M., DiPlacido, L.D., Greenwald, L., Kashgarian, M., Kono, D.H., Dong, C., *et al.* (2009) ICOS controls effector function but not trafficking receptor expression of kidney-infiltrating effector T cells in murine lupus. *J Immunol* **182**(7), 4076–84.

43. Peng, S.L., Moslehi, J., and Craft, J. (1997) Roles of interferon-gamma and interleukin-4 in murine lupus. *J Clin Invest* **99**, 1936–46.

44. Peng, S.L., Szabo, S.J., and Glimcher, L.H. (2002) T-bet regulates IgG class switching and pathogenic autoantibody production. *Proc Natl Acad Sci U S A* **99**(8), 5545–50.

45. Balomenos, D., Rumold, R., and Theofilopoulos, A. (1998) Interferon-gamma is required for lupus-like disease and lymphoaccumulation in MRL-lpr mice. *J Clin Invest* **101**(2), 364–71.

46. Haas, C., Ryffel, B., and Le Hir, M. (1997) IFN-gamma is essential for the development of autoimmune glomerulonephritis in MRL/lpr mice. *J Immunol* **158**, 5484–91.

47. Haas, C., Ryffel, B., and Le Hir, M. (1998) IFN-gamma receptor deletion prevents autoantibody production and glomerulonephritis in lupus-prone (NZB x NZW)F1 mice. *J Immunol* **160**, 3713–8.

48. Schwarting, A., Wada, T., Kinoshita, K., Tesch, G., and Kelley, V.R. (1998) IFN-gamma receptor signaling is essential for the initiation, acceleration, and destruction of autoimmune kidney disease in MRL-Fas(lpr) mice. *J Immunol* **161**, 494–503.

49. Kelley, V.R. (2007) Leukocyte-renal epithelial cell interactions regulate lupus nephritis. *Semin Nephrol* **27**(1), 59–68.

50. Jevnikar, A.M., Grusby, M.J., and Glimcher, L.H. (1994) Prevention of nephritis in major histocompatibility complex class-II-deficient MRL-lpr mice. *J Exp Med* **179**, 1137–43.

51. Schoop, R., Wahl, P., Le Hir, M., Heemann, U., Wang, M., and Wuthrich, R.P. (2004) Suppressed T-cell activation by IFN-gamma-induced expression of PD-L1 on renal tubular epithelial cells. *Nephrol Dial Transplant* **19**(11), 2713–20.

52. Wahl, P., Schoop, R., Bilic, G., Neuweiler, J., Le Hir, M., Yoshinaga, S.K., *et al.* (2002) Renal tubular epithelial expression of the costimulatory molecule B7RP-1 (inducible costimulator ligand). *J Am Soc Nephrol* **13**(6), 1517–26.

53. Kinoshita, K., Tesch, G., Schwarting, A., Maron, R., Sharpe, A.H., and Kelley, V.R. (2000) Costimulation by B7-1 and B7-2 is required for autoimmune disease in MRL-Faslpr mice. *J Immunol* **164**(11), 6046–56.

54. Kelley, V., Diaz-Gallo, C., Jevnikar, A., and Singer, G. (1993) Renal tubular epithelial and T cell interactions in autoimmune renal disease. *Kidney Int* Suppl 39, S108–15.

55. Yokoyama, H., Zheng, X., Strom, T., and Kelley, V. (1994) B7(+)-transfectant tubular epithelial cells induce T cell anergy, ignorance or proliferation. *Kidney Int* **45**, 1105–12.

56. Lucas, J.A., Menke, J., Rabacal, W.A., Schoen, F.J., Sharpe, A.H., and Kelley, V.R. (2008) Programmed death ligand 1 regulates a critical checkpoint for autoimmune myocarditis and pneumonitis in MRL mice. *J Immunol* **181**(4), 2513–21.

57. Zeller, G., Hirahashi, J., Schwarting, A., Sharpe, A., and Kelley, V. (2006) Inducible co-stimulator null MRL-Faslpr mice: uncoupling of autoantibodies and T cell responses in lupus. *J Am Soc Nephrol* **17**, 122–30.

58. Nguyen, V., Cudrici, C., Zernetkina, V., Niculescu, F., Rus, H., Drachenberg, C., *et al.* (2009) TRAIL, DR4 and DR5 are upregulated in kidneys from patients with lupus nephritis and exert proliferative and proinflammatory effects. *Clin Immunol* **132** (1), 32–42.

59. Kyttaris, V.C., and Tsokos, G.C. (2004) T lymphocytes in systemic lupus erythematosus: an update. *Curr Opin Rheumatol* **16**(5), 548–52.

60. Austin, H.A., 3rd, Boumpas, D.T., Vaughan, E.M., and Balow, J.E. (1994) Predicting renal outcomes in severe lupus nephritis: contributions of clinical and histologic data. *Kidney Int* **45**(2), 544–50.

61. Shivakumar, S., Tsokos, G.C., and Datta, S.K. (1989) T cell receptor alpha/beta expressing double negative (CD4-/CD8-) and CD4+ T helper cells in humans augment the production of pathogenic anti-DNA autoantibodies associated with lupus nephritis. *J Immunol* **143**, 103–12.

62. Rajagopalan, S., Zordan, T., Tsokos, G., and Datta, S. (1990) Pathogenic anti-DNA autoantibody-inducing T helper cell lines from patients with active lupus nephritis: Isolation of CD4-8- T helper cell lines that express the gamma delta T-cell antigen receptor. *Proc Natl Acad Sci USA* **87**, 7020–4.

63. Datta, S.K., Kaliyaperumal, A., and Desai-Mehta, A. (1997) T cells of lupus and molecular targets for immunotherapy. *J Clin Immunol* **17**, 11–20.

64. Theofilopoulos, A.N., and Dixon, F.J. (1985) Murine models of systemic lupus erythematosus. *Adv Immunol* **37**, 269–390.

65. Moore, K., Wada, T., Barbee, S., and Kelley, V. (1998) Gene transfer of RANTES elicits autoimmune renal injury in MRL-Fas(1pr) mice. *Kidney Int* **53**(6), 1631–41.

66. Meyers, C.M., Tomaszewski, J.E., Glass, J.D., and Chen, C.W. (1998) The nephritogenic T cell response in murine chronic graft-versus-host disease. *J Immunol* **161**(10), 5321–30.

67. Harigai, M., Kawamoto, M., Hara, M., Kubota, T., Kamatani, N., and Miyasaka, N. (2008) Excessive production of IFN-gamma in patients with systemic lupus erythematosus and its contribution to induction of B lymphocyte stimulator/B cell-activating factor/TNF ligand superfamily-13B. *J Immunol* **181**(3), 2211–9.

68. Connolly, K., Roubinian, J.R., and Wofsy, D. (1992) Development of murine lupus in CD4-depleted NZB/NZW mice. Sustained inhibition of residual CD4+ T cells is required to suppress autoimmunity. *J Immunol* **149**(9), 3083–8.

69. Peng, S.L., Madaio, M.P., Hughes, D.P.M., Crispe, I.N., Owen, M.J., Wen, L., *et al.* (1996) Murine lupus in the absence of alpha beta T cells. *J Immunol* **156**, 4041–9.

70. Daikh, D.I., Finck, B.K., Linsley, P.S., Hollenbaugh, D., and Wofsy, D. (1997) Long-term inhibition of murine lupus by brief simultaneous blockade of the B7/CD28 and CD40/gp39 costimulation pathways. *J Immunol* **159**, 3104–8.

71. Adachi, Y., Inaba, M., Sugihara, A., Koshiji, M., Sugiura, K., Amoh, Y., *et al.* (1998) Effects of administration of monoclonal antibodies (anti-CD4 or anti-CD8) on the development of autoimmune diseases in (NZW x BXSB)F1 mice. *Immunobiology* **198**(4), 451–64.

72. Iwai, H., Abe, M., Hirose, S., Tsushima, F., Tezuka, K., Akiba, H., *et al.* (2003) Involvement of inducible costimulator-B7 homologous protein costimulatory pathway in murine lupus nephritis. *J Immunol* **171**(6), 2848–54.

73. Stohl, W., Jacob, N., Quinn, W.J., 3rd, Cancro, M.P., Gao, H., Putterman, C., *et al.* (2008) Global T cell dysregulation in non-autoimmune-prone mice promotes rapid development of BAFF-independent, systemic lupus erythematosus-like autoimmunity. *J Immunol* **181**(1), 833–41.

74. Mozes, E., Lovchik, J., Zinger, H., and Singer, D. (2005) MHC class I expression regulates susceptibility to spontaneous autoimmune disease in (NZBxNZW)F1 mice. *Lupus* **14**(4), 308–14.

75. Christianson, G.J., Blankenburg, R.L., Duffy, T.M., Panka, D., Roths, J.B., Marshak-Rothstein, A., *et al.* (1996) Beta2-microglobulin dependence of the lupus-like autoimmune syndrome of MRL-lpr mice. *J Immunol* **156**, 4932–9.

76. Chan, O., Paliwal, V., McNiff, J., Park, S., Bendelac, A., and Shlomchik, M. (2001) Deficiency in beta(2)-microglobulin, but not CD1, accelerates spontaneous lupus skin disease while inhibiting nephritis in MRL-Fas(lpr) mice: an example of disease regulation at the organ level. *J Immunol* **167**(5), 2985–90.

77. Merino, R., Fossati, L., Iwamoto, M., Takahashi, S., Lemoine, R., Ibnou-Zekri, N., *et al.* (1995) Effect of long-term anti-CD4 or anti-CD8 treatment on the development of lpr

CD4- CD8- double negative T cells and of the autoimmune syndrome in MRL-lpr/lpr mice. *J Autoimmun* **8**(1), 33–45.

78. Peng, S.L., Madaio, M.P., Hayday, A.C., and Craft, J. (1996) Propagation and regulation of systemic autoimmunity by gamma delta T cells. *J Immunol* **157**, 5689–98.

79. Godo, M., Sessler, T., and Hamar, P. (2008) Role of invariant natural killer T (iNKT) cells in systemic lupus erythematosus. *Curr Med Chem* **15**(18), 1778–87.

80. Forestier, C., Molano, A., Im, J., Dutronc, Y., Diamond, B., Davidson, A., *et al.* (2005) Expansion and hyperactivity of CD1d-restricted NKT cells during the progression of systemic lupus erythematosus in (New Zealand Black x New Zealand White)F1 mice. *J Immunol* **175**(2), 763–70.

81. Takahashi, T., and Strober, S. (2008) Natural killer T cells and innate immune B cells from lupus-prone NZB/W mice interact to generate IgM and IgG autoantibodies. *Eur J Immunol* **38**(1), 156–65.

82. Tsukamoto, K., Ohtsuji, M., Shiroiwa, W., Lin, Q., Nakamura, K., Tsurui, H., *et al.* (2008) Aberrant genetic control of invariant TCR-bearing NKT cell function in New Zealand mouse strains: possible involvement in systemic lupus erythematosus pathogenesis. *J Immunol* **180**(7), 4530–9.

83. Skaggs, B.J., Singh, R.P., and Hahn, B.H. (2008) Induction of immune tolerance by activation of CD8+ T suppressor/regulatory cells in lupus-prone mice. *Hum Immunol* **69**(11), 790–6.

84. Horwitz, D.A. (2008) Regulatory T cells in systemic lupus erythematosus: past, present and future. *Arthritis Res Ther* **10**(6), 227.

85. Wu, H.Y., and Staines, N.A. (2004) A deficiency of CD4+CD25+ T cells permits the development of spontaneous lupus-like disease in mice, and can be reversed by induction of mucosal tolerance to histone peptide autoantigen. *Lupus* **13**(3), 192–200.

86. Abe, J., Ueha, S., Suzuki, J., Tokano, Y., Matsushima, K., and Ishikawa, S. (2008) Increased Foxp3(+) CD4(+) regulatory T cells with intact suppressive activity but altered cellular localization in murine lupus. *Am J Pathol* **173**(6), 1682–92.

87. Wu, H.Y., Quintana, F.J., and Weiner, H.L. (2008) Nasal anti-CD3 antibody ameliorates lupus by inducing an IL-10-secreting CD4+ CD25- LAP+ regulatory T cell and is associated with down-regulation of IL-17+ CD4+ ICOS+ CXCR5+ follicular helper T cells. *J Immunol* **181**(9), 6038–50.

88. Gerli, R., Nocentini, G., Alunno, A., Bocci, E.B., Bianchini, R., Bistoni, O., *et al.* (2009) Identification of regulatory T cells in systemic lupus erythematosus. *Autoimmun Rev* **8**(5), 426–30.

89. Vargas-Rojas, M.I., Crispin, J.C., Richaud-Patin, Y., and Alcocer-Varela, J. (2008) Quantitative and qualitative normal regulatory T cells are not capable of inducing suppression in SLE patients due to T-cell resistance. *Lupus* **17**(4), 289–94.

90. Parietti, V., Monneaux, F., Decossas, M., and Muller, S. (2008) Function of CD4+,CD25+ Treg cells in MRL/lpr mice is compromised by intrinsic defects in antigen-presenting cells and effector T cells. *Arthritis Rheum* **58**(6), 1751–61.

91. Wang, G., Lai, F.M., Tam, L.S., Li, E.K., Kwan, B.C., Chow, K.M., *et al.* (2009) Urinary FOXP3 mRNA in patients with lupus nephritis–relation with disease activity and treatment response. *Rheumatology (Oxford)* **48**(7), 755–60.

92. La Cava, A., Fang, C., Singh, R., Ebling, F., and Hahn, B. (2005) Manipulation of immune regulation in systemic lupus erythematosus. *Autoimmun Rev* **4**(8), 515–9.

93. Shustov, A., Luzina, I., Nguyen, P., Papadimitriou, J.C., Handwerger, B., Elkon, K.B., *et al.* (2000) Role of perforin in controlling B-cell hyperactivity and humoral autoimmunity. *J Clin Invest* **106**(6), R39–47.

94. Puliaeva, I., Puliaev, R., Shustov, A., Haas, M., and Via, C.S. (2008) Fas expression on antigen-specific T cells has costimulatory, helper, and down-regulatory functions in vivo for cytotoxic T cell responses but not for T cell-dependent B cell responses. *J Immunol* **181**(9), 5912–29.

95. Watanabe-Fukunaga, R., Brannan, C.I., Copeland, N.G., Jenkins, N.A., and Nagata, S. (1992) Lymphoproliferation disorder in mice explained by defects in Fas antigen that mediates apoptosis. *Nature* **356**, 314–7.

96. Peng, S., Moslehi, J., Robert, M., and Craft, J. (1998) Perforin protects against autoimmunity in lupus-prone mice. *J Immunol* **160**(2), 652–60.

97. Jacob, N., Yang, H., Pricop, L., Liu, Y., Gao, X., Zheng, S.G., *et al.* (2009) Accelerated pathological and clinical nephritis in systemic lupus erythematosus-prone New Zealand Mixed 2328 mice doubly deficient in TNF receptor 1 and TNF receptor 2 via a Th17-associated pathway. *J Immunol* **182**(4), 2532–41.

98. Dai, Z., Turtle, C.J., Booth, G.C., Riddell, S.R., Gooley, T.A., Stevens, A.M., *et al.* (2009) Normally occurring NKG2D+CD4+ T cells are immunosuppressive and inversely correlated with disease activity in juvenile-onset lupus. *J Exp Med* **206**(4), 793–805.

99. Yang, D., Wang, H., Ni, B., He, Y., Li, J., Tang, Y., *et al.* (2009) Mutual activation of CD4+ T cells and monocytes mediated by NKG2D-MIC interaction requires IFN-gamma production in systemic lupus erythematosus. *Mol Immunol* **46**(7), 1432–42.

100. Mohan, C., Adams, S., Stanik, V., and Datta, S.K. (1993) Nucleosome: a major immunogen for pathogenic autoantibody-inducing T cells of lupus. *J Exp Med* **177**(5), 1367–81.

101. Kaliyaperumal, A., Mohan, C., Wu, W., and Datta, S.K. (1996) Nucleosomal peptide epitopes for nephritis-inducing T helper cells of murine lupus. *J Exp Med* **183**, 2459–69.

102. Datta, S. (2003) Major peptide autoepitopes for nucleosome-centered T and B cell interaction in human and murine lupus. *Ann N Y Acad Sci* **987**, 79–90.

103. Schwarting, A., Tesch, G., Kinoshita, K., Maron, R., Weiner, H.L., and Kelley, V.R. (1999) IL-12 drives IFN-gamma-dependent autoimmune kidney disease in MRL-Fas(lpr) mice. *J Immunol* **163**, 6884–91.

104. Wada, T., Schwarting, A., Chesnutt, M., Wofsy, D., and Kelley, V. (2001) Nephritogenic cytokines and disease in MRL-Fas(lpr) kidneys are dependent on multiple T-cell subsets. *Kidney Int* **59**(2), 565–78.

105. Kelley, V.R., and Wuthrich, R.P. (1999) Cytokines in the pathogenesis of systemic lupus erythematosus. *Semin Nephrol* **19**(1), 57–66.

106. Bailey, N.C., and Kelly, C.J. (1997) Nephritogenic T cells use granzyme C as a cytotoxic mediator. *Eur J Immunol* **27**(9), 2302–9.

107. Crispin, J.C., Oukka, M., Bayliss, G., Cohen, R.A., Van Beek, C.A., Stillman, I.E., *et al.* (2008) Expanded double negative T cells in patients with systemic lupus erythematosus produce IL-17 and infiltrate the kidneys. *J Immunol* **181**(12), 8761–6.

108. Theofilopoulos, A.N., and Lawson, B.R. (1999) Tumour necrosis factor and other cytokines in murine lupus. *Ann Rheum Dis* **58** (Suppl 1), I49–55.

109. Foster, M.H. (1999) Relevance of Systemic Lupus Erythematosus (SLE) nephritis animal models to human disease. *Semin Nephrol* **19**(1), 12–24.

110. Mishra, N., Reilly, C., Brown, D., Ruiz, P., and Gilkeson, G. (2003) Histone deacetylase inhibitors modulate renal disease in the MRL-lpr/lpr mouse. *J Clin Invest* **111**(4), 539–52.

111. Wang, Y., Ito, S., Chino, Y., Iwanami, K., Yasukochi, T., Goto, D., et al. (2008) Use of laser microdissection in the analysis of renal-infiltrating T cells in MRL/lpr mice. *Mod Rheumatol* **18**(4), 385–93.

112. Zhao, X.F., Pan, H.F., Yuan, H., Zhang, W.H., Li, X.P., Wang, G.H., et al. (2009) Increased serum interleukin 17 in patients with systemic lupus erythematosus. *Mol Biol Rep* **37**(1), 81–5.

113. Yang, J., Chu, Y., Yang, X., Gao, D., Zhu, L., Yang, X., et al. (2009) Th17 and natural Treg cell population dynamics in systemic lupus erythematosus. *Arthritis Rheum* **60**(5), 1472–83.

114. Doreau, A., Belot, A., Bastid, J., Riche, B., Trescol-Biemont, M.C., Ranchin, B., et al. (2009) Interleukin 17 acts in synergy with B cell-activating factor to influence B cell biology and the pathophysiology of systemic lupus erythematosus. *Nat Immunol* **10**(7), 778–85.

115. Vinuesa, C.G., Cook, M.C., Angelucci, C., Athanasopoulos, V., Rui, L., Hill, K.M., et al. (2005) A RING-type ubiquitin ligase family member required to repress follicular helper T cells and autoimmunity. *Nature* **435**(7041), 452–8.

116. Bubier, J.A., Sproule, T.J., Foreman, O., Spolski, R., Shaffer, D.J., Morse, H.C., 3rd, et al. (2009) A critical role for IL-21 receptor signaling in the pathogenesis of systemic lupus erythematosus in BXSB-Yaa mice. *Proc Natl Acad Sci U S A* **106**(5), 1518–23.

117. Shimizu, S., Sugiyama, N., Masutani, K., Sadanaga, A., Miyazaki, Y., Inoue, Y., et al. (2005) Membranous glomerulonephritis development with Th2-type immune deviations in MRL/lpr mice deficient for IL-27 receptor (WSX-1). *J Immunol* **175**(11), 7185–92.

118. Sugiyama, N., Nakashima, H., Yoshimura, T., Sadanaga, A., Shimizu, S., Masutani, K., et al. (2008) Amelioration of human lupus-like phenotypes in MRL/lpr mice by overexpression of interleukin 27 receptor alpha (WSX-1). *Ann Rheum Dis* **67**(10), 1461–7.

119. Madaio, M.P., and Shlomchik, M.J. (1996) Emerging concepts regarding B cells and autoantibodies in murine lupus nephritis. B cells have multiple roles; all autoantibodies are not equal. *J Am Soc Nephrol* **7**(3), 387–96.

120. Shlomchik, M.J., and Madaio, M.P. (2003) The role of antibodies and B cells in the pathogenesis of lupus nephritis. *Springer Semin Immunopathol* **24**(4), 363–75.

121. Mizoguchi, A., and Bhan, A.K. (2006) A case for regulatory B cells. *J Immunol* **176**(2), 705–10.

122. Bouaziz, J.D., Yanaba, K., and Tedder, T.F. (2008) Regulatory B cells as inhibitors of immune responses and inflammation. *Immunol Rev* **224**, 201–14.

123. Clatworthy, M.R., and Smith, K.G. (2007) B cells in glomerulonephritis: focus on lupus nephritis. *Semin Immunopathol* **29**(4), 337–53.

124. Harris, D.P., Haynes, L., Sayles, P.C., Duso, D.K., Eaton, S.M., Lepak, N.M., et al. (2000) Reciprocal regulation of polarized cytokine production by effector B and T cells. *Nat Immunol* **1**(6), 475–82.

125. Pierce, S.K., Morris, J.F., Grusby, M.J., Kaumaya, P., van Buskirk, A., Srinivasan, M., et al. (1988) Antigen-presenting function of B lymphocytes. *Immunol Rev* **106**, 149–80.

126. Sapir, T., and Shoenfeld, Y. (2005) Facing the enigma of immunomodulatory effects of intravenous immunoglobulin. *Clin Rev Allergy Immunol* **29**(3), 185–99.

127. Shlomchik, M.J., Craft, J.E., and Mamula, M.J. (2001) From T to B and back again: positive feedback in systemic autoimmune disease. *Nat Rev Immunol* **1**(2), 147–53.

128. Lu, T.Y., Ng, K.P., Cambridge, G., Leandro, M.J., Edwards, J.C., Ehrenstein, M., *et al.* (2009) A retrospective seven-year analysis of the use of B cell depletion therapy in systemic lupus erythematosus at University College London Hospital: the first fifty patients. *Arthritis Rheum* **61**(4), 482–7.

129. Chan, O., Madaio, M.P., and Shlomchik, M.J. (1997) The roles of B cells in MRL/lpr murine lupus. *Ann N Y Acad Sci* **815**, 75–87.

130. Chan, O.T., Madaio, M.P., and Shlomchik, M.J. (1999) The central and multiple roles of B cells in lupus pathogenesis. *Immunol Rev* **169**, 107–21.

131. Yanaba, K., Bouaziz, J.D., Haas, K.M., Poe, J.C., Fujimoto, M., and Tedder, T.F. (2008) A regulatory B cell subset with a unique CD1dhiCD5+ phenotype controls T cell-dependent inflammatory responses. *Immunity* **28**(5), 639–50.

132. Lenert, P., Brummel, R., Field, E.H., and Ashman, R.F. (2005) TLR-9 activation of marginal zone B cells in lupus mice regulates immunity through increased IL-10 production. *J Clin Immunol* **25**(1), 29–40.

133. Dolff, S., Wilde, B., Patschan, S., Durig, J., Specker, C., Philipp, T., *et al.* (2007) Peripheral circulating activated b-cell populations are associated with nephritis and disease activity in patients with systemic lupus erythematosus. *Scand J Immunol* **66**(5), 584–90.

134. Cassese, G., Lindenau, S., de Boer, B., Arce, S., Hauser, A., Riemekasten, G., *et al.* (2001) Inflamed kidneys of NZB/W mice are a major site for the homeostasis of plasma cells. *Eur J Immunol* **31**(9), 2726–32.

135. Sekine, H., Watanabe, H., and Gilkeson, G.S. (2004) Enrichment of anti-glomerular antigen antibody-producing cells in the kidneys of MRL/MpJ-Fas(lpr) mice. *J Immunol* **172**(6), 3913–21.

136. Steinmetz, O.M., Velden, J., Kneissler, U., Marx, M., Klein, A., Helmchen, U., *et al.* (2008) Analysis and classification of B-cell infiltrates in lupus and ANCA-associated nephritis. *Kidney Int* **74**(4), 448–57.

137. Ito, T., Ishikawa, S., Sato, T., Akadegawa, K., Yurino, H., Kitabatake, M., *et al.* (2004) Defective B1 cell homing to the peritoneal cavity and preferential recruitment of B1 cells in the target organs in a murine model for systemic lupus erythematosus. *J Immunol* **172**(6), 3628–34.

138. Binard, A., Le Pottier, L., Saraux, A., Devauchelle-Pensec, V., Pers, J.O., and Youinou, P. (2008) Does the BAFF dysregulation play a major role in the pathogenesis of systemic lupus erythematosus? *J Autoimmun* **30**(1-2), 63–7.

139. Stadanlick, J.E., and Cancro, M.P. (2008) BAFF and the plasticity of peripheral B cell tolerance. *Curr Opin Immunol* **20**(2), 158–61.

140. Mackay, F., Woodcock, S.A., Lawton, P., Ambrose, C., Baetscher, M., Schneider, P., *et al.* (1999) Mice transgenic for BAFF develop lymphocytic disorders along with autoimmune manifestations. *J Exp Med* **190**(11), 1697–710.

141. Groom, J.R., Fletcher, C.A., Walters, S.N., Grey, S.T., Watt, S.V., Sweet, M.J., *et al.* (2007) BAFF and MyD88 signals promote a lupuslike disease independent of T cells. *J Exp Med* **204**(8), 1959–71.

142. Thien, M., Phan, T., Gardam, S., Amesbury, M., Basten, A., Mackay, F., *et al.* (2004) Excess BAFF rescues self-reactive B cells from peripheral deletion and allows them to enter forbidden follicular and marginal zone niches. *Immunity* **20**(6), 785–98.

143. Su, W., and Madaio, M. (2003) Recent advances in the pathogenesis of lupus nephritis: autoantibodies and B cells. *Semin Nephrol* **23**, 564–8.

144. Foster M.H. (1999) Nephritogenic properties of lupus autoantibodies. In: *Lupus Nephritis* (eds EJ Lewis, MM Schwartz, SM Korbet), pp. 22–78. Oxford University Press, New York.

145. Madaio, M.P. (2003) Lupus autoantibodies 101: one size does not fit all; however, specificity influences pathogenicity. *Clin Exp Immunol* **131**(3), 396–7.

146. Vlahakos, D.V., Foster, M.H., Adams, S., Katz, M., Ucci, A.A., Barrett, K.J., *et al.* (1992) Anti-DNA antibodies form immune deposits at distinct glomerular and vascular sites. *Kidney Int* **41**, 1690–700.

147. Raz, E., Brezis, M., Rosenmann, E., and Eilat, D. (1989) Anti-DNA antibodies bind directly to renal antigens and induce kidney dysfunction in the isolated perfused rat kidney. *J Immunol* **142**, 3076–82.

148. Bernstein, K.A., Divalerio, R., and Lefkowith, J.B. (1995) Glomerular binding activity in MRL lpr serum consists of antibodies that bind to a DNA histone type IV collagen complex. *J Immunol* **154**, 2424–33.

149. Berden, J.H., Licht, R., van Bruggen, M.C., and Tax, W.J. (1999) Role of nucleosomes for induction and glomerular binding of autoantibodies in lupus nephritis. *Curr Opin Nephrol Hypertens* **8**, 299–306.

150. Pankewycz, O.G., Migliorini, P., and Madaio, M.P. (1987) Polyreactive autoantibodies are nephritogenic in murine lupus nephritis. *J Immunol* **139**, 3287–94.

151. Nimmerjahn, F., and Ravetch, J. (2006) Fcgamma receptors: old friends and new family members. *Immunity* **24**, 19–28.

152. Slingsby, J.H., Norsworthy, P., Pearce, G., Vaishnaw, A.K., Issler, H., Morley, B.J., *et al.* (1996) Homozygous hereditary C1q deficiency and systemic lupus erythematosus. A new family and the molecular basis of C1q deficiency in three families. *Arthritis Rheum* **39**(4), 663–70.

153. Chen, Z., Koralov, S.B., and Kelsoe, G. (2000) Complement C4 inhibits systemic autoimmunity through a mechanism independent of complement receptors CR1 and CR2. *J Exp Med* **192**, 1339–52.

154. Clynes, R., Dumitru, C., and Ravetch, J.V. (1998) Uncoupling of immune complex formation and kidney damage in autoimmune glomerulonephritis. *Science* **279**, 1052–4.

155. Matsumoto, K., Watanabe, N., Akikusa, B., Kurasawa, K., Matsumura, R., Saito, Y., *et al.* (2003) Fc receptor-independent development of autoimmune glomerulonephritis in lupus-prone MRL/lpr mice. *Arthritis Rheum* **48**(2), 486–94.

156. Prodeus, A.P., Goerg, S., Shen, L.M., Pozdnyakova, O.O., Chu, L., Alicot, E.M., *et al.* (1998) A critical role for complement in maintenance of self-tolerance. *Immunity* **9**(5), 721–31.

157. Leadbetter, E.A., Rifkin, I.R., Hohlbaum, A.M., Beaudette, B.C., Shlomchik, M.J., and Marshak-Rothstein, A. (2002) Chromatin-IgG complexes activate B cells by dual engagement of IgM and Toll-like receptors. *Nature* **416**(6881), 603–7.

Chapter 4

The many effects of complement in lupus nephritis

Lihua Bao[*] and Richard J. Quigg[*]

The complement system consists of three pathways and over 30 proteins, including those with biological activity that directly or indirectly mediate the effects of this system, along with a set of regulatory proteins necessary to prevent injudicious complement activation on host tissue. The role for complement in the pathogenesis of systemic lupus erythematosus (SLE) is paradoxical. On one hand, the complement system appears to have protective features, as hereditary homozygous deficiencies of classical pathway components are associated with an increased risk for SLE. On the other hand, immune complex-mediated activation of complement in affected tissues is clearly evident in both experimental and human SLE, along with pathological features that are logical consequences of complement activation. By using accurate mouse models of SLE, we have gained remarkable insights into pathogenic features likely relevant to the human disease, as well as the ability to test potential therapies, some of which have made it to standard clinical use. Studies in genetically altered mice and using recombinant protein inhibitors of complement have confirmed what was believed but unproven—early complement proteins C1q and C4 are protective whereas complement activation later in the pathways is proinflammatory and deleterious. Complement-targeted drugs, including soluble complement receptor 1 (TP10), C1 esterase inhibitor (C1-INH), and a monoclonal anti-C5 antibody (eculizumab) have been shown to inhibit complement safely are now being investigated in a variety of clinical conditions. Although these and others earlier in their clinical development hold promise to be used therapeutically in lupus nephritis, this optimism must be tempered by the fact that the clinical trials to prove this remain fraught with obstacles.

The complement system is an important part of innate immunity that defends the host against infectious microorganisms, clears immune complexes (ICs) and dead cells, and connects innate to adaptive immunity.[1-3] Complement can be activated through classical, alternative, and mannose-binding lectin (MBL) pathways, each with different initiators (shown schematically in Figure 4.1).

The classical pathway is activated when C1q of C1 binds with high affinity to the Fc portion of immunoglobulin (Ig) M (CH3 domain) or IgG (CH2 domain) in ICs.

[*] Supported by a grant from the National Institutes of Health (R01DK055357).

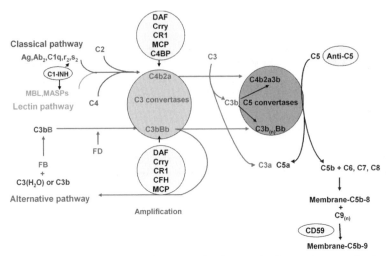

Fig. 4.1 The complement system. Shown are the three activation pathways—classical, MBL and alternative pathways and the common intermediates of activation, C3 and C5 convertases. The main effectors of complement's actions, C1q, C3a, C3b, C5a and C5b-9 are in bold type. Regulatory proteins are in the unshaded circles, as is anti-C5 antibody.

Besides Igs, C1q also binds to a wide range of targets to activate the classical pathway. Of particular recent interest is the ability of C1q to bind and facilitate the removal of apoptotic cells, which provides it with an important role in immune tolerance. C1q binds to apoptotic cells through C1q ligands such as DNA,[4] phosphatidylserine,[5] IgM,[6] and altered self structures like β-amyloid fibrils.[7] One of the C1q binding molecules that has been extensively studied is C-reactive protein (CRP), which itself binds to microbes,[8] host cells,[9] and chromatin.[10] C1q also has important biological effects. The cell surface protein CD93 was once considered to be a specific cellular C1q receptor (C1qR),[11] which more recently was disproved;[12] the roles for other C1qRs, including globular C1qR (gC1qR) and calreticulin (cC1qR) are still under investigation.[13]

C1q itself has no enzymatic function; instead, binding of C1q to its target triggers its conformational change and self-activation of C1r, followed by the activation of C1s.[14] Activated C1 (as the multi-protein C1qr$_2$s$_2$ complex) cleaves both C4 and C2 to generate C4a/C4b and C2a/C2b. C4b2a acts as a C3 convertase, which cleaves and activates C3.

The alternative pathway is spontaneously activated, which is called "tickover". This "tickover" process of C3 conformation occurs slowly but continuously to generate hydrolyzed C3 (C3(H$_2$O)). C3(H$_2$O) then binds factor B (CFB) in the fluid phase. Upon cleavage by factor D (CFD, adipsin), an initial C3 convertase C3(H$_2$O)Bb is formed, which can be stabilized by properdin and amplify itself to form C3bBb, the alternative pathway C3 convertase.[2]

The MBL pathway is another antibody-independent complement activation pathway. Mannose-binding lectin is a plasma lectin that consists of multimers of an identical 32 kDa polypeptide chain. The binding of MBL to terminal carbohydrate groups on certain microbes leads to the activation of the MBL-associated serine proteases (MASP). Activated MASP cleaves C4 to C4a and C4b. Immobilized C4b induces the binding of C2, which is also cleaved by MASP and generates the C4b2a C3 convertase.[15]

Irrespective of the pathway of activation, cleavage of C3 and C5 ultimately occurs, with the generation of the C3a and C5a anaphylatoxins, C3b opsonins, and C5b to start the nonenzymatic assembly of the C5b-9 membrane attack complex. The main effectors of the complement system act through specific cellular receptors—the G protein-coupled C3a and C5a receptors (C3aR and C5aR) and complement receptors 1–4 (CR1–4) for C3b, iC3b, and C3dg. The latter two are specific products of factor I (CFI), which requires a cofactor from CR1 (CD35), factor H (CFH), and membrane cofactor protein (MCP, CD46). Although these various receptors are traditionally on effectors of the immune system, such as neutrophils and monocyte/macrophages, there is growing appreciation for effects on other immune cells, such as B and T lymphocytes, and follicular dendritic cells, as well as what can be considered a local organ-specific immune system. For example, in the kidney, epithelial cells of the glomerulus and proximal tubule bear C3aR and CR1.[16–18] In contrast to the specificity of cellular receptors for C3a, C3b, and C5a, C5b-9 is promiscuous in its cellular binding, requiring simply a receptive lipid bilayer for insertion.[19] C5b-9 can result in cellular death by its insertion, which occurs in *Neisseria* sp. bacteria[20] and erythrocytes (E) in paroxysmal nocturnal hemoglobinuria (PNH),[21] as well as recruiting and activating specific signaling cascades in nucleated cells to result in a number of cellular events.[22–24]

Given the potency of the complement system, natural fluid-phase and cell membrane-bound regulatory proteins acting throughout the three cascades are essential to prevent activation and injury to host tissues (Figure 4.1).[1,2] The regulators of complement activation (RCA) gene family on human chromosome 1q3.2 (and a comparable location in mouse chromosome 1) include MCP, CR1, decay accelerating factor (DAF, CD55), C4b-binding protein (C4bp), and CFH.[25,26] These proteins inhibit complement activation through interactions of their conserved short consensus repeats (SCRs) with fragments of C3 and/or C4.[27]

Membrane cofactor protein is a cell surface glycoprotein that serves as a cofactor for factor I-mediated cleavage of C3b and C4b, thereby inhibiting the formation of C3/C5 convertases. Membrane cofactor protein has been identified in all cell types in humans except erythrocytes,[28] whereas in rodents, MCP appears restricted predominantly to testicular germ cells.[29–31] Decay accelerating factor is a glycosylphosphatidylinositol (GPI)-anchored membrane protein, which binds C3b and C4b and accelerates the decay of C3 (C4b2a in classical pathway and C3bBb in alternative pathway) and C5 (C4b2a3b in classical pathway and C3bBb3b in alternative pathway) convertases.[32]

Complement receptor 1 is a single chain transmembrane glycoprotein, which has the combined functions of DAF and MCP: it accelerates the decay of C3 and C5 convertases like DAF and it also serves as a cofactor for factor I-mediated inactivation of C3b and C4b into iC3b and iC4b like MCP.[33]

The plasma proteins, C4bp and CFH have cofactor activity for factor I-mediated inactivation of C4b and C3b into iC4b and iC3b, respectively. C4bp also accelerates the decay of the C3 convertase C4b2a of the classical pathway. Factor H inhibits the formation of the alternative pathway C3 convertase by binding to C3b or promoting the dissociation of this C3 convertase. Specific to rodents is the 65-kDa rodent complement regulatory protein, p65,[34] more commonly referred to as CR1-related gene/protein y (Crry) because of its protein and nucleotide similarity to human CR1.[35] At the "ends" of the complement cascades are C1-inhibitor (C1-INH) and CD59, which inhibit C1 activation and C5b-9 formation respectively.[36,37]

In humans, CR1 and CR2 are products of separate genes, whereas in mice CR1 and CR2 are encoded in the same single gene *Cr2* and produced by alternative splicing.[38] Complement receptor 1 is expressed in all peripheral blood cell types except platelets in humans, whereas in the mouse it is predominantly expressed on B cells and follicular dendritic cells.[39] Although CR2 (CD21) is a RCA member, it has highest affinity for C3dg and does not inhibit C3 convertases. Similarly, the β_2 integrins CR3 (*Itgam*, CD11b/CD18, Mac-1) and CR4 (*Itgax*, CD11c/CD18) have binding affinity for iC3b and are also not complement inhibitors.[40]

The involvement of the complement system in the pathogenesis of a number of autoimmune diseases is well accepted, yet its exact roles are still unclear. On one hand, hereditary deficiencies of early classical pathway complement components predispose patients to SLE. On the other hand, activation of complement by ICs is certainly a prominent feature in SLE. Therefore, an imbalance of the complement system in either way can be relevant to the development of this disease. In this chapter, we will discuss the dual roles of complement in SLE, and in particular in lupus nephritis. The relevance of what we now know of this system to potential treatment of human SLE will be emphasized.

Why complement in human SLE?

Initially, complement caught people's attention based on the observations of hypocomplementemia in patients with active SLE. Low total complement hemolytic activity (CH_{50}) and decreased C3 and C4 levels have been found in about 75% of SLE patients with focal nephritis and 90% of patients with diffuse nephritis.[41] The co-localization of Ig isotypes IgG, IgA, and IgM with C1q, C4, and C3 (and C5b-9) is called a "full house," which is almost exclusively present in glomeruli of patients with lupus nephritis.[42] Complement split products such as C3d and C5b-9 can also be detected in the urine of SLE patients, and provide further circumstantial evidence that complement is involved in lupus nephritis.[43]

Impairment of IC handling is also believed to be pathogenic and relevant to the complement system in SLE patients.[44,45] Immune complexes can form in glomeruli through the passive trapping of preformed circulating ICs and/or the binding of plasma antibodies directly with intrinsic or extrinsic antigens in glomeruli.[46] As the complement system is required at all steps of normal IC metabolism, any number of alterations can lead to pathological glomerular IC accumulation, particularly in conditions of IC excess, as in SLE.[44,47] The first step is classical pathway activation on ICs, leading to incorporation of C4b and C3b, which can profoundly affect the physicochemical characteristics of both circulating and tissue-bound (glomerular) ICs.[45,48,49]

The next key complement protein is CR1 present on Es (or CFH on the rodent platelet[50]) where it has binding affinity for C3b, and serves as a CFI-cofactor for the cleavage of C3b to iC3b. Immune complexes bound to human E CR1 (or mouse platelet CFH) are transported and transferred to cells of the mononuclear phagocyte system, such as liver or spleen. The ICs are removed and the Es return to the circulation. Studies have shown the association of low levels of E-CR1 with SLE,[51,52] suggesting that a defective E/IC-clearing system may be related to SLE pathogenesis. Acquired low levels of E-CR1 in SLE patients[53] can be improved by stimulating erythropoiesis.[54,55] In neutrophils from SLE patients, IC downregulates and interferon (IFN) γ upregulates the levels of CR1 transcripts, and ICs inhibit IFNγ-induced CR1 expression.[56] Abnormally high levels of erythrocyte C4d (E-C4d) can also be found in SLE patients.[57] The value of E-C4d and E-CR1 to diagnose or indicate SLE disease activity has been questioned by findings that high levels of E-C4d and low levels of CR1 are also seen in rheumatic diseases other than SLE, and they do not correlate with SLE disease activity.[58] Glomerular podocytes also bear CR1, which may play a role in IC processing locally and is similarly decreased in lupus nephritis.[16]

In contrast to CR1, the role of CR2 in SLE development is less well known. A strong association of CR2 polymorphism to lupus susceptibility genes has been found in both humans and mice.[59,60] Functionally, IFNα, an important lupus-prone cytokine,[61,62] was found to be a ligand of CR2. Interferon α binds to CR2 with the same high affinity and at the same sites as the other ligands of CR2, yet the biological consequences of this binding still need to be clarified.[63]

As a paradox to the widespread belief that generation of complement activation products in kidney and other disease sites is proinflammatory, patients with homozygous deficiencies of the C1 proteins (C1q or C1r/s) or C4 have a high prevalence (>80%) of autoantibodies and SLE-like disease.[64,65] Despite the strongest association of C1q deficiency with SLE, as >90% of such patients can develop disease features, neither heterozygous deficiency of C1q nor single nucleotide polymorphism in *C1qA* leading to reduced C1q levels associate with an increased risk for lupus nephritis.[66] It is also noteworthy that autoantibodies to C1q and coexistent hypocomplementemia are associated with, though not specific to, lupus nephritis. In SLE patients, anti-C1q antibodies are associated with proliferative lupus nephritis and their levels may indicate renal disease activity.[67]

Interestingly, homozygous deficiency of C3, the most critical protein that affects all three pathways of complement activation, is not associated with SLE.[68] The finding that homozygous deficiency of early components of the classical pathway other than C3 predispose to SLE suggests that the physiological function of these molecules are protective in SLE. Although the exact mechanism is still unknown, one very plausible explanation is the clearance hypothesis proposed by Walport and colleagues. In their well-designed studies, they found that mice with generated C1q and C4 deficiencies had impaired ability to clear apoptotic debris,[69] leading to the accumulation of potentially immunogenic autoantigens and initiation of an autoimmune reaction in the right genetic setting. In further support of this, C1q-deficient mice had increased mortality and higher titers of autoantibodies, with 25% of the mice developing glomerulonephritis, characterized by glomerular IC deposits and apoptotic debris.[70] The mechanisms indicate that C1q and DNase1 are important in the degradation of chromatin derived from necrotic cells.[71] More recently, it was reported that in the presence of sera from individuals deficient in C1q, C4, C2, or C3, phagocytosis of apoptotic cells was decreased compared with studies using normal sera, indicating important roles of all these complement classical pathway components in clearance of apoptotic and necrotic cells.[72]

Complement also plays important roles in thrombotic complications associated with SLE. The risk of thrombosis is particularly high in SLE patients with antiphospholipid autoantibodies (APL). One explanation is that APL-containing ICs bind to platelets, which can subsequently activate the classical complement pathway. Vascular injury in SLE patients may predispose this process. This mechanism is supported by the finding that sera from SLE patients with APL had a higher capacity to activate the classical pathway on heterologous platelets.[73] In SLE patients, glomerular deposition of C4d was found to be strongly correlated to the presence of thrombotic microangiopathy, though not correlated with APL status, supporting the idea that the classical pathway of complement is critical in the development of thrombosis in lupus nephritis and that glomerular C4d deposition in renal biopsy tissues could have predictive value for the risk of developing thrombotic microangiopathy.[74]

Mouse models of human SLE

There are several murine models that spontaneously develop lupus-like syndromes. Two of the best studied models are the F_1 cross between New Zealand Black and New Zealand White mice (NZB/W) and the MRL/MpJ-$Tnfrsf6^{lpr/lpr}$/J (MRL/lpr) strain.[75] Similar to the female predominance in humans, only female NZB/W mice develop SLE. MRL/lpr mice are on the autoimmune MRL/Mp background with a retrotransposon in the $Tnfrsf6$ (Fas) gene leading to nearly complete absence of the proapoptotic Fas protein.[76] Both models have B cell hyperactivity, autoantibodies, hypocomplementemia, circulating and glomerular-bound ICs, and severe nephritis. As in humans, there is plenty of circumstantial evidence that complement activation is actively involved in the pathogenesis of glomerular disease in these mice. In the early stages (4 and 5 months in MRL/lpr and NZB/W mice respectively), granular deposition of mouse IgG, IgA, IgM, and C3 are present largely in the mesangium, coincident with histopathology showing mesangial proliferation. As the disease progresses, there are glomerular capillary wall IC deposits, proliferation of intrinsic endothelial and mesangial cells, and infiltration with inflammatory cells. Eventually, crescent formation (more often in MRL/lpr mice) and glomerulosclerosis (more often in NZB/W mice) occurs, and mice die of renal failure.[75]

Other spontaneous mouse models (e.g. BXSB and congenic strains derived from New Zealand mice[77]), and those induced by antibodies[78] or with deficiency of certain genes such as TGF-β1,[79] have been generated and studied. Lupus-prone NZM2410 mice on the C57BL/6 background show different characteristics of lupus when carrying different lupus susceptibility genes (sle1-sle3). Congenic mice with coexpression of sle1, sle2, and sle3 developed severe systemic autoimmunity and fatal glomerulonephritis.[80] These models will not be discussed in this chapter as they are less frequently used in complement research. MRL/Mp mice with normal Fas protein (MRL/Mp+/+) or animals of the nonautoimmune C57BL/6 background with the *lpr* gene (C57BL/6$^{lpr/lpr}$) can be considered autoimmune-prone, and are useful to test whether a given alteration accelerates autoimmunity. For instance, deficiency of C1q in MRL/Mp+/+ mice hastens the development of SLE disease features.[81]

Functional studies of complement in experimental lupus models

The manipulation of individual complement proteins through genetic techniques in lupus mouse strains has provided considerable insight into how complement is involved in this disease. In addition, functional inhibition through the use of specific antibodies or antagonists using recombinant or transgenic techniques can be extremely illuminating. Given that C3 is the common point connecting all three pathways in complement activation, there are more naturally occurring proteins regulating its activation than anywhere else. As such, many of the studies in lupus mice performed to date have concentrated on activators and regulators of C3.

Decay accelerating factor is a ubiquitously expressed GPI-anchored membrane protein that inhibits C3 activation through all pathways by inhibiting formation and accelerating decay of the C3/C5 convertase.[32] Histochemically, DAF is mainly present in the juxtaglomerular apparatus.[82] It is notable that human, rat, and mouse podocytes do appear to have functional DAF, as shown through a variety of *in vivo* and *in vitro* experiments.[83–85] The relevance of DAF to kidney diseases is suggested by enhanced expression in mesangial cells, tubular cells, vascular endothelium, and infiltrating inflammatory cells in disease states.[82,86,87] The Song group showed that DAF-deficient MRL/*lpr* mice had exacerbated lymphoproliferation, antichromatin autoantibody production, and dermatitis, particularly evident in females, whereas lupus nephritis appeared to be unaffected.[88] Furthermore, DAF-deficient MRL/*lpr* mice also deficient in C3 developed comparable lymphadenopathy, splenomegaly, and antichromatin autoantibodies as seen in the complement-sufficient mice, suggesting the protective effect of DAF in MRL/*lpr* autoimmunity is complement-independent. Decay accelerating factor-sufficient MRL/*lpr* chimeras with DAF-deficient MRL/*lpr* bone marrow developed significantly attenuated dermatitis compared with that in DAF-deficient MRL/*lpr* chimeras with DAF-sufficient MRL/*lpr* bone marrow, indicating that the protective effect of DAF on dermatitis is attributable to local expression.[89] Overall, it seems likely that DAF is not the most important glomerular complement regulator in lupus nephritis, given the coexistent strong expression of Crry in mouse glomeruli, which could compensate for those instances in which DAF was deficient. The exacerbated dermatitis can be explained by the fact that DAF is strongly expressed in the skin, whereas Crry is not.

The finding of enhanced autoimmunity in DAF-deficient MRL/*lpr* mice, together with the fact that DAF is also a ligand for the activation-associated lymphocyte antigen CD97,[90] also suggests that DAF may function as a negative regulator of adaptive immunity. This intriguing hypothesis was supported by the same group by showing deficiency of DAF significantly enhanced T lymphocyte responses to active immunization, and exacerbated the T lymphocyte-dependent experimental autoimmune encephalomyelitis model.[91] Functionally, the regulatory impact of DAF on adaptive immunity can significantly affect renal disease development. Recently, our group developed a novel sheep antimouse podocyte antibody-induced murine focal and segmental glomerulosclerosis (FSGS) model, which was dependent on an abnormal immune response of T cells lacking DAF.[92]

Like human CR1, Crry is an intrinsic membrane complement inhibitor that inhibits C3 convertases of all pathways through decay-accelerating and factor I cofactor activities for C3b and C4b, combining activities of human DAF and MCP.[93] CR1-related gene/protein y is widely expressed in most mouse tissues, particularly at potential sites of IC deposition and damage, such as the mesangium and arterial endothelium.[94] The role for Crry in limiting complement activation in these sites is supported by a series of insightful studies from the Matsuo and Okada labs.[95–98] Given that the Crry-deficient mice generated by Molina *et al.* have complete embyronic lethality from unrestricted maternal complement activation,[99] the exact role for Crry in murine SLE and lupus nephritis awaits the generation of Crry-deficient lupus mice. This will require fairly elaborate experimental strategies to surmount the problem of embryonic lethality. That Crry will be relevant in lupus nephritis seems almost inescapable based upon what we know already. Additional support for this comes from our recent studies of chronic serum sickness in $Crry^{-/-}C3^{+/-}$ mice and transplantation of $Crry^{-/-}C3^{-/-}$ kidneys into wild-type hosts.[100,101] In the former, the glomerular disease phenotype was worsened compared to controls, whereas in the latter there was marked inflammation in the tubulointerstitium, which led to complete failure of the transplanted kidney within weeks (whereas the appropriate controls, including wild-type kidneys transplanted into wild-type or $Crry^{-/-}C3^{-/-}$ mice remained normal).

Soluble CR1 is a recombinant form of human CR1 lacking its transmembrane region and short cytoplasmic tail. Like native CR1, soluble CR1 inhibits complement activation by accelerating the decay of both alternative and classical pathway C3/C5 convertases and by acting as a factor I cofactor for the cleavage and inactivation of C3b. That inhibiting complement activation at the C3/C5 convertase step would be worthwhile in lupus nephritis was suggested by studies performed by Couser *et al.* in three rat models of glomerular diseases, which collectively had manifestations comparable to lupus nephritis.[102] Transgenic mice developed by our group, which over-expressed a soluble form of Crry had inhibited complement activation systemically and locally in the kidney.[103] When crossed into the MRL/*lpr* strain, Crry-complement inhibited MRL/*lpr* mice had less severe lupus nephritis as determined by blood urea nitrogen (BUN) and albuminuria measurements. As the spontaneous mortality in lupus mice is largely due to kidney disease, this translated into prolonged survival, whereas the underlying abnormal autoimmunity was not affected.[104] To make this complement inhibition more applicable to human SLE treatment, a recombinant soluble form of Crry fused to the hinge CH2 and CH3 domains of mouse IgG1 (Crry-Ig)[105] was also used in MRL/*lpr* mice. In chronic usage from early in the autoimmune disease until the end stage, inhibited complement activation by Crry-Ig ameliorated lupus nephritis.[106] Interestingly, transcript profiling experiments showed that excessive matrix components such as collagens I, III, IV, and VI were overexpressed in control MRL/*lpr* mice compared with MRL/Mp+/+ strain controls, which could be suppressed by complement inhibition with Crry-Ig. Potential explanations for these phenomena were that Crry-Ig mediated reductions in connective tissue growth factor and transforming growth factor (TGF)β1 expression, suggesting that these profibrotic agents may contribute to the progressive glomerulosclerosis in MRL/*lpr* mice in a complement-dependent manner.[107]

As CR1 and CR2 are the alternatively spliced product of a single *Cr2* gene,[108] knockout of the mouse *Cr2* gene leads to CR1 and CR2 protein deficiencies. In both human and experimental SLE, CR1/CR2 expression decreases, suggesting a relevance for, or at least involvement with, disease.[109,110] In C57BL/6*lpr/lpr* mice, deficiencies of C4 or CR1/CR2 result in autoimmune disease,[111,112] suggesting that classical pathway activation on antigenic material (such as that derived from apoptotic debris in lupus) can maintain tolerance via B lymphocyte CR1/CR2 signaling.[113,114] Yet, MRL/*lpr* mice deficient in CR1/CR2 had significantly lower levels of total IgG3 and specific IgG3 rheumatoid factor, supporting the role of CR1/CR2 in production of IgG3 in response to autoantigens. Nonetheless, this decrease of IgG3 autoantibodies did not lead to a reduction in features of lupus nephritis.[41]

C4bp is a major soluble complement inhibitor of the classical pathway. C4bp is mainly expressed in the liver in both humans and mice.[115] It was reported that C4bp serum levels are elevated in SLE patients, which supports its involvement.[116] More detailed studies came from the Braun group in their MRL/lpr mouse model with deficiency of C4bp. Although serum C4 levels were lower in MRL/lpr mice compared with normal C57BL/6 mice, starting as early as 3 weeks of age (i.e. prior to autoimmune disease), surprisingly, deficiency of C4bp affected neither serum C4 levels nor the classical pathway hemolytic activity. With an unaffected complement classical pathway, C4bp deficiency did not lead to a significantly different outcome in these mice, including glomerular C3 and IgG deposition, glomerulonephritis, tubulointerstitial inflammation, proteinuria, and renal function. Moreover, the systemic immune response was not affected by the absence of C4bp in these mice.[117] One explanation for the negligible role of C4bp in lupus development in MRL/lpr mice is that the extensively activated classical pathway in this model overwhelmed the absence of C4bp. In this situation, "a gain of function" of C4bp may reveal more information. For instance, in two murine models of arthritis, purified human C4bp successfully inhibited the classical complement pathway, which led to delayed or reduced disease development in these models.[118]

In physiological situations, there is spontaneous continuous low-level alternative pathway activation that is restrained by effective complement regulation. Observational studies in humans, and more recently in animals with spontaneous or targeted CFH deficiencies, have clearly illustrated the primary role of CFH as the alternative pathway regulator[119–121]; yet, even fully functional CFH can be overwhelmed by the tempo of complement activation. Although the traditional thinking is that SLE is induced through IC-directed classical pathway activation without involvement of the alternative pathway, Gilkeson *et al.* demonstrated that CFB- or CFD-deficient MRL/*lpr* mice had reduced glomerular C3 deposition associated with less severe glomerular histopathology.[122,123] These results imply that IC-directed classical pathway activation can recruit the potent alternative pathway to further amplify generation of C3 and C5 activation products.

C5b-9 was localized in diseased lupus kidneys more than two decades ago.[124] Yet, compared with extensive studies focusing on C3 activation and its regulation, fewer studies have been done to investigate the downstream events following C3 activation in the pathogenesis of SLE. One exception was the important study of Wang *et al.* using a specific monoclonal antibody to inhibit C5 function in NZB/W mice.[125] Six months of continuous therapy led to significantly delayed onset of proteinuria, improved renal pathological changes, and prolonged survival, implicating products of the terminal complement pathway, namely C5a and C5b-9, in lupus nephritis.

The C3a and C5a anaphylatoxins are generated through complement activation when C3 and C5 are activated and cleaved. By signaling through C3aR and C5aR, they play a role in leukocyte accumulation occurring in various inflammatory diseases, including glomerulonephritis.[43] Greater expression of C3aR expression was found in glomeruli in human lupus nephritis.[126] C3aR and C5aR expression was significantly upregulated at both the mRNA and protein levels and accompanied by a wider cellular distribution in MRL/*lpr* mouse kidneys.[17,127] This upregulated expression started before the onset of kidney disease, suggesting C3aR and C5aR may be involved in the development of disease, rather than simply a consequence.

Chronic administration of a specific C3aR antagonist (SB290157) led to significantly reduced kidney disease and prolonged survival in MRL/*lpr* mice.[17] Similarly, when C5a signaling was blocked in our studies with a specific antagonist[127] or in those by Michael Braun's group through gene targeting,[128] MRL/*lpr* mice animals displayed attenuated renal disease and prolonged viability. The effects of blocking C3aR and C5aR in lupus mice had certain features in common, including a reduction in renal neutrophil and macrophage infiltration, apoptosis, and interleukin (IL)1β expression.[17,127] Effects on chemokine expression were distinct, with C3aR- and C5aR-inhibited MRL/*lpr* mice having reduced CCL5 (RANTES) and CXCL2 (MIP-2) expression respectively. C3aR-inhibited mice also had increased phosphorylation of protein kinase B (Akt), which we considered suggestive that C3aR signals promote renal cell apoptosis through an Akt pathway.[17] In C5aR-deficient MRL/*lpr* mice, there was a reduction in CD4+ T cell renal infiltration, lower titers of anti-double stranded DNA antibodies, and inhibition of IL-12 p20 and IFN-γ production, suggesting that Th1 responses are important to link C5a signaling in lupus nephritis.[128] In contrast, C3aR-deficient MRL/*lpr* mice had elevated autoantibody titers, more glomerular crescents, and more severe intrarenal vasculitis, although it did not affect long-term renal injury or survival.[129] The mechanisms of different outcomes from short-term (by using antagonist) and long-term (by using gene-targeting) blockade of C3aR signaling in this lupus model still need to be clarified. The reported agonist effect of the particular C3aR antagonist (SB290157) may play a role in its beneficial effect in this lupus model.[130]

As discussed above, C3 is the converging point for all three complement pathways. Alterations in C3 activation through manipulating its regulators, such as Crry or DAF, or blockade of the effects of C3 activation with inhibitors of C3aR, C5aR, and C5 have shown C3 activation is an important factor in the development of SLE. Surprisingly, C3 deficiency did not affect the development of nephritis in MRL/*lpr* mice, whereas glomerular IgG deposition was significantly increased.[131] This study is consistent with the important role of complement, and in particular C3, in the clearance of ICs.[49,132] The most likely explanation why there was still inflammatory glomerular disease is that excessive IC deposition resulted in a greater degree of cellular accumulation via FcγRs. The relative roles of complement activation products and their receptors and FcγRs remains an unsettled area in lupus nephritis.[133,134]

As discussed before, the complement system is an important part of innate immunity, which provides a number of benefits, such as imparting resistance towards infectious agents, processing of naturally generated ICs and apoptotic material,[44,47] and the development of an optimal and directed humoral immune response.[135,136] In theory, each of these may be affected with chronic systemic complement inhibition, which is supported by some experimental evidence.[106,137] The alternative approach of selectively targeting the desired complement regulator to the site of tissue injury has been advanced largely through the work of the Tomlinson group, first in proof-of-principle experiments[138,139] and more recently in disease states.[137,140,141] Given that sites of complement activation in the glomerulus and elsewhere are "marked" by the presence of C3d,[142] this represents an ideal target for therapy, as can be accomplished with CR2, given its natural affinity for C3d. Thus, low doses of chimeric CR2–DAF and CR2–CD59 efficiently protected target cells from complement attack.[141] CR2–DAF was targeted to the glomerulus in lupus nephritis, whereas soluble DAF failed.[141] Long-term (8 weeks) treatment of diseased MRL/*lpr* mice with low doses of CR2–Crry provided significant complement inhibition locally in the lupus glomerulus, which conferred significant reduction of glomerulonephritis and renal vasculitis, as well as prolonged survival in these mice.[143] Relevant to proteinuric renal diseases, in general, is that Crry and CD59 targeted to the rat proximal tubule using a monoclonal antibody approach protected rats from tubular injury in puromycin-induced proteinuria.[140]

What we've learned from animals can be used in the treatment of humans

Strategies to manipulate the complement system in different human diseases have followed from successful animal studies, including those using recombinant intrinsic complement regulators and blocking antibodies. In addition to the treatment approaches indicated in studies using experimental models discussed above, we will focus on several promising therapeutic approaches that have been used in the treatment of human diseases, and may potentially extend to the treatment of human SLE and lupus nephritis.

Soluble CR1 was first developed in 1990, and has both decay accelerator and cofactor activity in classical and alternative complement pathways. It showed a protective effect in a rat model of reperfusion injury of ischemic myocardium.[144] A current therapeutic form of soluble CR1 designated as TP10 (Avant Immunotherapeutic, Nedham, MA, USA) has been used in clinical trials in several human diseases. In a Phase I clinical trial in patients with acute respiratory distress syndrome, the half-life of TP10 was 33.4–94.5 hours with a dose-dependent reduction in CH50 values.[145] More recently, two separate randomized, multi-centre, placebo-controlled, double-blind Phase II clinical trials showed protective effects of TP10 in ischemia–reperfusion injury in patients undergoing lung transplantation or cardiac surgery. The first involved 33 medical centers in the USA. A total of 564 high-risk patients undergoing cardiac surgery received an intravenous bolus of sCR1 (at 1, 3, 5, or 10 mg/kg) or placebo immediately before cardiopulmonary bypass. TP10 reduced the incidence of death or myocardial infarction in males by 36%, although the beneficial effect did not extend to female patients.[146] This gender specificity in the treatment effect was confirmed by a subsequent Phase II clinical trial that included only 297 female patients.[147] The other clinical trial was conducted at four North American lung transplant centers in which a total of 59 patients were given a single 10 mg/kg TP10 dose intravenously. Of the variables examined, TP10 significantly reduced the number of patients who were ventilator-dependent at 24 hours (50% versus 81%), indicating that TP10 decreases the severity of ischemia–reperfusion injury in patients after lung transplantation.[148]

C1 esterase inhibitor (C1-INH) is the only complement-associated protease inhibitor that has been used in clinical trials for hereditary angio-edema (HAE) and ischemia–reperfusion injury. In a randomized controlled trial, plasma derived C1-INH provided relief twice as fast as placebo to HAE patients having acute attacks.[149] Plasma-derived C1-INH was also shown to be an effective prophylactic in patients with severe and frequent attacks of HAE who discontinued long-term treatment with danazol, commonly used for prophylaxis from HAE, because of lack of efficacy, intolerance, and/or severe side effects.[150] Recombinant human C1-INH also proved to be effective in the treatment of HAE patients during acute attacks.[151] Beneficial effects of C1-INH were also shown in two separate clinical trials of 57 and 80 patients with ST-elevation myocardial infarction who underwent emergent reperfusion with coronary artery bypass grafting.[152,153]

The most extensively used antibody targeting the complement system is a monoclonal antibody that directly binds human C5 and prevents its cleavage to C5a and C5b, either as a humanized monoclonal antibody (eculizumab, Alexion Pharmaceuticals, Inc., Cheshire, CT, USA) or its single chain (ScFv) form (pexelizumab, Alexion Pharmaceuticals, Inc.). The latter has had some efficacy in attenuating post-operative myocardial injury for patients undergoing cardiopulmonary bypass and coronary artery bypass grafting.[154,155] Paroxysmal nocturnal hemoglobinuria is an acquired disorder of GPI-linked proteins, including DAF and CD59, characterized by spontaneous complement activation and C5b-9-mediated hemolysis.[21] In March 2007, eculizumab (Soliris) became the first US Food and Drug Administration (FDA) approved complement-specific drug and the only FDA-approved drug for the treatment of PNH, a life-threatening disorder. Based on the known pathophysiology of

PNH, it is gratifying that eculizumab has been shown to be effective therapy for this condition,[156] and should be effective for long-term use.[157]

Moving to the kidney, idiopathic membranous nephropathy is also a disease in which C5b-9-mediated effects (in this case on the podocyte) are predicted, from a large amount of animal data, to be pathogenic.[158] A multi-centre Phase II trial in the USA in which 122 patients with idiopathic membranous nephropathy were enrolled in a randomized placebo-controlled study of eculizumab has been completed. Unfortunately, there was no difference, comparing treatment with placebo, in the primary outcome variable of urinary protein excretion. Because of the short-term treatment strategy in a long-term disease, the study design may have been insufficient to uncover a true therapeutic effect. This is supported by the finding of an apparent benefit in patients enrolled in an open-label extension. As noted earlier, long-term treatment with anti-C5 had impressive effects on lupus nephritis in NZB/W lupus mice.[125] Given this, as well as favourable Phase I safety data in patients with SLE, we designed a multi-centre Phase II trial using eculizumab in proliferative lupus nephritis supported by the United States National Institutes of Health. Unfortunately, after enrollment of our first patient, this study encountered logistical delays and ultimately came to a complete halt. Although this reflects the difficulties in clinical trials for a disorder such as lupus nephritis, based on what is known about the pathophysiology we remain interested in the potential efficacy of this drug in the treatment of lupus nephritis.

References

1. Walport, M.J. (2001) Advances in Immunology: Complement (First of Two Parts). *N Engl J Med* **344**, 1058–66.
2. Liszewski, M.K., and Atkinson, J.P. (1993) The complement system. In: *Fundamental Immunology*, 3rd ed. (Paul, W.E., ed.), pp. 917–39. Raven Press, New York.
3. Holers, V.M. (2001) Complement deficiencies. In: *Clinical Immunology: Principles and Practices* (Rich, R., ed.), p 36.1–36.10. Mosby, St. Louis.
4. Elward, K., Griffiths, M., Mizuno, M., Harris, C.L., Neal, J.W., Morgan, B.P. *et al.* (2005) CD46 plays a key role in tailoring innate immune recognition of apoptotic and necrotic cells. *J Biol Chem* **280**, 36342–54.
5. Paidassi, H., Tacnet-Delorme, P., Garlatti, V., Darnault, C., Ghebrehiwet, B., Gaboriaud, C. *et al.* (2008) C1q binds phosphatidylserine and likely acts as a multiligand-bridging molecule in apoptotic cell recognition. *J Immunol* **180**, 2329–38.
6. Ogden, C.A., Kowalewski, R., Peng, Y., Montenegro, V., and Elkon, K.B. (2005) IGM is required for efficient complement mediated phagocytosis of apoptotic cells in vivo. *Autoimmunity* **38**, 259–64.
7. Tacnet-Delorme, P., Chevallier, S., and Arlaud, G.J. (2001) Beta-amyloid fibrils activate the C1 complex of complement under physiological conditions: evidence for a binding site for A beta on the C1q globular regions. *J Immunol* **167**, 6374–81.
8. Suresh, M.V., Singh, S.K., Ferguson, D.A., Jr., and Agrawal, A. (2006) Role of the property of C-reactive protein to activate the classical pathway of complement in protecting mice from pneumococcal infection. *J Immunol* **176**, 4369–74.
9. Kim, S.J., Gershov, D., Ma, X., Brot, N., and Elkon, K.B. (2003) Opsonization of apoptotic cells and its effect on macrophage and T cell immune responses. *Ann N Y Acad Sci* **987**, 68–78.

10. Robey, F.A., Jones, K.D., Tanaka, T., and Liu, T.Y. (1984) Binding of C-reactive protein to chromatin and nucleosome core particles. A possible physiological role of C-reactive protein. *J Biol Chem* **259**, 7311–6.

11. Nepomuceno, R.R., Henschen-Edman, A.H., Burgess, W.H., and Tenner, A.J. (1997) cDNA cloning and primary structure analysis of C1qR(P), the human C1q/MBL/SPA receptor that mediates enhanced phagocytosis in vitro. *Immunity* **6**, 119–29.

12. McGreal, E.P., Ikewaki, N., Akatsu, H., Morgan, B.P., and Gasque, P. (2002) Human C1qRp is identical with CD93 and the mNI-11 antigen but does not bind C1q. *J Immunol* **168**, 5222–32.

13. Vegh, Z., Kew, R.R., Gruber, B.L., and Ghebrehiwet, B. (2006) Chemotaxis of human monocyte-derived dendritic cells to complement component C1q is mediated by the receptors gC1qR and cC1qR. *Mol Immunol* **43**, 1402–7.

14. Gaboriaud, C., Thielens, N.M., Gregory, L.A., Rossi, V., Fontecilla-Camps, J.C., and Arlaud, G.J. (2004) Structure and activation of the C1 complex of complement: unraveling the puzzle. *Trends Immunol* **25**, 368–73.

15. Wallis, R., Dodds, A.W., Mitchell, D.A., Sim, R.B., Reid, K.B., and Schwaeble, W.J. (2007) Molecular interactions between MASP-2, C4, and C2 and their activation fragments leading to complement activation via the lectin pathway. *J Biol Chem* **282**, 7844–51.

16. Kazatchkine, M.D., Fearon, D.T., Appay, M.D., Mandet, C., and Bariety, J. (1982) Immunohistochemical study of the human glomerular C3b receptor in normal kidney and in seventy-five cases of renal diseases. *J Clin Invest* **69**, 900–12.

17. Bao, L., Osawe, I., Haas, M., and Quigg, R.J. (2005) Signaling through up-regulated C3a receptor is key to the development of experimental lupus nephritis. *J Immunol* **175**, 1947–55.

18. Braun, M.C., Reins, R.Y., Li, T.B., Hollmann, T.J., Dutta, R., Rick, W.A., *et al.* (2004) Renal expression of the C3a receptor and functional responses of primary human proximal tubular epithelial cells. *J Immunol* **173**, 4190–6.

19. Müller-Eberhard, H.J. (1986) The membrane attack complex of complement. *Ann Rev Immunol* **4**, 503–28.

20. Densen, P., Brown, E.J., O'Neill, G.J., Tedesco, F., Clark, R.A., Frank, M.M., *et al.* (1983) Inherited deficiency of C8 in a patient with recurrent meningococcal infections: Further evidence for a dysfunctional C8 molecule and nonlinkage to the HLA system. *J Clin Immunol* **3**, 90–9.

21. Johnson, R.J., and Hillmen, P. (2002) Paroxysmal nocturnal haemoglobinuria: Nature's gene therapy? *Mol Pathol* **55**, 145–52.

22. Morgan, B.P. (1992) Effects of the membrane attack complex of complement on nucleated cells. *Curr Top Microbiol Immunol* **178**, 115–40.

23. Fosbrink, M., Niculescu, F., and Rus, H. (2005) The role of C5b-9 terminal complement complex in activation of the cell cycle and transcription. *Immunol Res* **31**, 37–46.

24. Bohana-Kashtan, O., Ziporen, L., Donin, N., Kraus, S., and Fishelson, Z. (2004) Cell signals transduced by complement. *Mol Immunol* **41**, 583–97.

25. Carroll, M.C., Alicot, E.M., Katzman, P.J., Klickstein, L.B., Smith, J.A., and Fearon, D.T. (1988) Organization of the genes encoding complement receptors type 1 and 2, decay-accelerating factor, and C4-binding protein in the RCA locus on human chromosome 1. *J Exp Med* **167**, 1271–80.

26. Bora, N.S., Lublin, D.M., Kumar, B.V., Hockett, R.D., Holers, V.M., and Atkinson, J.P. (1989) Structural gene for human membrane cofactor protein (MCP) of complement maps to within 100 kb of the 3' end of the C3b/C4b receptor gene. *J Exp Med* **169**, 597–602.

27. Hourcade, D., Holers, V.M., and Atkinson, J.P. (1989) The regulators of complement activation (RCA) gene cluster. *Adv Immunol* **45**, 381–416.

28. Liszewski, M.K., Post, T.W., and Atkinson, J.P. (1991) Membrane cofactor protein (MCP or CD46): newest member of the regulators of complement activation gene cluster. *Annu Rev Immunol* **9**, 31–55.

29. Mead, R., Hinchliffe, S.J., and Morgan, B.P. (1999) Molecular cloning, expression and characterization of the rat analogue of human membrane cofactor protein (MCP/CD46). *Immunology* **98**, 137–43.

30. Tsujimura, A., Shida, K., Kitamura, M., Nomura, M., Takeda, J., Tanaka, H., *et al.* (1998) Molecular cloning of a murine homologue of membrane cofactor protein (CD46): preferential expression in testicular germ cells. *Biochem J* **330** (Pt 1), 163–8.

31. Miwa, T., Nonaka, M., Okada, N., Wakana, S., Shiroishi, T., and Okada, H. (1998) Molecular cloning of rat and mouse membrane cofactor protein (MCP, CD46): preferential expression in testis and close linkage between the mouse Mcp and Cr2 genes on distal chromosome 1. *Immunogenetics* **48**, 363–71.

32. Lublin, D.M., and Atkinson, J.P. (1989) Decay-accelerating factor: biochemistry, molecular biology, and function. *Annu Rev Immunol* **7**, 35–58.

33. Ahearn, J.M., and Fearon, D.T. (1989) Structure and function of the complement receptors, CR1 (CD35) and CR2 (CD21). *Adv Immunol* **46**, 183–219.

34. Wong, W., and Fearon, D.T. (1985) p65: A C3b-binding protein on murine cells that shares antigenic determinants with the human C3b receptor (CR1) and is distinct from murine C3b receptor. *J Immunol* **134**, 4048–56.

35. Paul, M.S., Aegerter, M., O'Brien, S.E., Kurtz, C.B., and Weis, J.H. (1989) The murine complement receptor gene family. I. Analysis of mCRY gene products and their homology to human CR1. *J Immunol* **142**, 582–9.

36. Morgan, B.P., and Harris, C.L. (1999) Regulation in the activation pathways. In: *Complement Regulatory Proteins*, pp. 41–136. Academic Press, San Diego.

37. Morgan, B.P., and Harris, C.L. (1999) Regulation in the terminal pathway. In: *Complement Regulatory Proteins*, pp. 137–70. Academic Press, San Diego.

38. Kurtz, C.B., O'Toole, E., Christensen, S.M., and Weis, J.H. (1990) The murine complement receptor gene family. IV. Alternative splicing of Cr2 gene transcripts predicts two distinct gene products that share homologous domains with both human CR2 and CR1. *J Immunol* **144**, 3581–91.

39. Jacobson, A.C., and Weis, J.H. (2008) Comparative functional evolution of human and mouse CR1 and CR2. *J Immunol* **181**, 2953–9.

40. Xia, Y., Vetvicka, V., Yan, J., Hanikyrov, M., Mayadas, T., Ross, *et al.* (1999) The beta-glucan-binding lectin site of mouse CR3 (CD11b/CD18) and its function in generating a primed state of the receptor that mediates cytotoxic activation in response to iC3b-opsonized target cells. *J Immunol* **162**, 2281–90.

41. Valentijn, R.M., van, O.H., Hazevoet, H.M., Hermans, J., Cats, A., Daha, M.R., *et al.* (1985) The value of complement and immune complex determinations in monitoring disease activity in patients with systemic lupus erythematosus. *Arthritis Rheum* **28**, 904–13.

42. Dalmasso A.P. (1986) Complement in the pathophysiology and diagnosis of human diseases. *Crit Rev Clin Lab Sci* **24**, 123–83.

43. Manzi, S., Rairie, J.E., Carpenter, A.B., Kelly, R.H., Jagarlapudi, S.P., Sereika, S.M., *et al.* (1996) Sensitivity and specificity of plasma and urine complement split products as indicators of lupus disease activity. *Arthritis Rheum* **39**, 1178–88.

44. Schifferli, J.A., and Taylor, R.P. (1989) Physiological and pathological aspects of circulating immune complexes. *Kidney Int* **35**, 993–1003.

45. Davies, K.A., Schifferli, J.A., and Walport, M.J. (1994) Complement deficiency and immune complex disease. *Springer Sem Immunopathol* **15**, 397–416.

46. Nangaku, M., and Couser, W.G. (2005) Mechanisms of immune-deposit formation and the mediation of immune renal injury. *Clin Exp Nephrol* **9**, 183–91.

47. Hebert, L.A. (1991) The clearance of immune complexes from the circulation of man and other primates. *Am J Kidney Dis* **27**, 352–61.

48. Schifferli, J.A., Ng, Y.C., and Peters, D.K. (1986) The role of complement and its receptor in the elimination of immune complexes. *N Engl J Med* **315**, 488–95.

49. Quigg, R.J., Lim, A., Haas, M., Alexander, J.J., He, C., and Carroll, M.C. (1998) Immune complex glomerulonephritis in C4- and C3-deficient mice. *Kidney Int* **53**, 320–30.

50. Alexander, J.J., Hack, B.K., Cunningham, P.N., and Quigg, R.J. (2001) A protein with characteristics of factor H is present on rodent platelets and functions as the immune adherence receptor. *J Biol Chem* **276**, 32129–35.

51. Ross, G.D., Yount, W.J., Walport, M.J., Winfield, J.B., Parker, C.J., Fuller, C.R. *et al.* (1985) Disease-associated loss of erythrocyte complement receptors (CR1, C3b receptors) in patients with systemic lupus erythematosus and other diseases involving autoantibodies and/or complement activation. *J Immunol* **135**, 2005–14.

52. Fyfe, A., Holme, E.R., Zoma, A., and Whaley, K. (1987) C3b receptor (CR1) expression on the polymorphonuclear leukocytes from patients with systemic lupus erythematosus. *Clin Exp Immunol* **67**, 300–8.

53. Kiss, E., Csipo, I., Cohen, J.H., Reveil, B., Kavai, M., and Szegedi, G. (1996) CR1 density polymorphism and expression on erythrocytes of patients with systemic lupus erythematosus. *Autoimmunity* **25**, 53–8.

54. Hebert, L.A., Birmingham, D.J., Shen, X.P., and Cosio, F.G. (1992) Stimulating erythropoiesis increases complement receptor expression on primate erythrocytes. *Clin Immunol Immunopathol* **62**, 301–6.

55. Kiss, E., Kavai, M., Csipo, I., and Szegedi, G. (1998) Recombinant human erythropoietin modulates erythrocyte complement receptor 1 functional activity in patients with lupus nephritis. *Clin Nephrol* **49**, 364–9.

56. Arora, V., Mondal, A.M., Grover, R., Kumar, A., Chattopadhyay, P., and Das, N. (2007) Modulation of CR1 transcript in systemic lupus erythematosus (SLE) by IFN-gamma and immune complex. *Mol Immunol* **44**, 1722–8.

57. Manzi, S., Navratil, J.S., Ruffing, M.J., Liu, C.C., Danchenko, N., Nilson, S.E., *et al.* (2004) Measurement of erythrocyte C4d and complement receptor 1 in systemic lupus erythematosus. *Arthritis Rheum* **50**, 3596–604.

58. Singh, V., Mahoney, J.A., and Petri, M. (2008) Erythrocyte C4d and complement receptor 1 in systemic lupus erythematosus. *J Rheumatol* **35**, 1989–93.

59. Wu, H., Boackle, S.A., Hanvivadhanakul, P., Ulgiati, D., Grossman, J.M., Lee, Y. *et al.* (2007) Association of a common complement receptor 2 haplotype with increased risk of systemic lupus erythematosus. *Proc Natl Acad Sci U S A* **104**, 3961–6.

60. Boackle, S.A., Holers, V.M., Chen, X., Szakonyi, G., Karp, D.R., Wakeland, E.K., *et al.* (2001) Cr2, a candidate gene in the murine Sle1c lupus susceptibility locus, encodes a dysfunctional protein. *Immunity* **15**, 775–85.

61. Baechler, E.C., Batliwalla, F.M., Karypis, G., Gaffney, P.M., Ortmann, W.A., Espe, K.J., *et al.* (2003) Interferon-inducible gene expression signature in peripheral blood cells of patients with severe lupus. *Proc Natl Acad Sci U S A* **100**, 2610–5.

62. Santiago-Raber, M.L., Baccala, R., Haraldsson, K.M., Choubey, D., Stewart, T.A., Kono, D.H. *et al.* (2003) Type-I interferon receptor deficiency reduces lupus-like disease in NZB mice. *J Exp Med* **197**, 777–88.

63. Asokan, R., Hua, J., Young, K.A., Gould, H.J., Hannan, J.P., Kraus, D.M., *et al.* (2006) Characterization of human complement receptor type 2 (CR2/CD21) as a receptor for IFN-alpha: a potential role in systemic lupus erythematosus. *J Immunol* **177**, 383–94.

64. Navratil, J.S., Korb, L.C., and Ahearn, J.M. (1999) Systemic lupus erythematosus and complement deficiency: clues to a novel role for the classical complement pathway in the maintenance of immune tolerance. *Immunopharmacology* **42**, 47–52.

65. Manderson, A.P., Botto, M., and Walport, M.J. (2004) The role of complement in the development of systemic lupus erythematosus. *Annu Rev Immunol* **22**, 431–56.

66. Racila, D.M., Sontheimer, C.J., Sheffield, A., Wisnieski, J.J., Racila, E., and Sontheimer, R.D. (2003) Homozygous single nucleotide polymorphism of the complement C1QA gene is associated with decreased levels of C1q in patients with subacute cutaneous lupus erythematosus. *Lupus* **12**, 124–32.

67. Kallenberg, C.G. (2008) Anti-C1q autoantibodies. *Autoimmun Rev* **7**, 612–5.

68. Pickering, M.C., Botto, M., Taylor, P.R., Lachmann, P.J., and Walport, M.J. (2000) Systemic lupus erythematosus, complement deficiency, and apoptosis. *Adv Immunol* **76**, 227–324.

69. Taylor, P.R., Carugati, A., Fadok, V.A., Cook, H.T., Andrews, M., Carroll, M.C., *et al.* (2000) A hierarchical role for classical pathway complement proteins in the clearance of apoptotic cells in vivo. *J Exp Med* **192**, 359–66.

70. Botto, M., Dell'Agnola, C., Bygrave, A.E., Thompson, E.M., Cook, H.T., Petry, F., *et al.* (1998) Homozygous C1q deficiency causes glomerulonephritis associated with multiple apoptotic bodies. *Nat Genet* **19**, 56–9.

71. Gaipl, U.S., Beyer, T.D., Heyder, P., Kuenkele, S., Bottcher, A., Voll, R.E. *et al.* (2004) Cooperation between C1q and DNase I in the clearance of necrotic cell-derived chromatin. *Arthritis Rheum* **50**, 640–9.

72. Gullstrand, B., Martensson, U., Sturfelt, G., Bengtsson, A.A., and Truedsson, L. (2009) Complement classical pathway components are all important in clearance of apoptotic and secondary necrotic cells. *Clin Exp Immunol* **156**, 303–11.

73. Peerschke, E., Yin, W., Alpert, D., Roubey, R., Salmon, J., and Ghebrehiwet, B. (2009) Serum complement activation on heterologous platelets is associated with arterial thrombosis in patients with systemic lupus erythematosus and antiphospholipid antibodies. *Lupus* **18**, 530–8.

74. Cohen, D., Koopmans, M., Kremer, H.I., Berger, S.P., Roos van, G.M., Steup-Beekman, G.M. *et al.* (2008) Potential for glomerular C4d as an indicator of thrombotic microangiopathy in lupus nephritis. *Arthritis Rheum* **58**, 2460–9.

75. Hahn, B.H. (2001) Animal models of systemic lupus erythematosus. In: *Dubois' Lupus Erythematosus*, 6 edn (Wallace, D.J., and Hahn, B.H., eds), pp. 339–388. Williams and Wilkins, Baltimore, MD, USA.

76. Watanabe-Fukunaga, R., Brannan, C.I., Copeland, N.G., Jenkins, N.A., and Nagata, S. (1992) Lymphoproliferation disorder in mice explained by defects in Fas antigen that mediates apoptosis. *Nature* **356**, 314–7.

77. Drake, C.G., Rozzo, S.J., Vyse, T.J., Palmer, E., and Kotzin, B.L. (1995) Genetic contributions to lupus-like disease in (NZB x NZW)F1 mice. *Immunol Rev* **144**, 51–74.

78. Blank, M., Mendlovic, S., Mozes, E., Coates, A.R., and Shoenfeld, Y. (1991) Induction of systemic lupus erythematosus in naive mice with T-cell lines specific for human anti-DNA

antibody SA-1 (16/6 Id+) and for mouse tuberculosis antibody TB/68 (16/6 Id+). *Clin Immunol Immunopathol* **60**, 471–83.

79. Dang, H., Geiser, A.G., Letterio, J.J., Nakabayashi, T., Kong, L., Fernandes, G., *et al.* (1995) SLE-like autoantibodies and Sjogren's syndrome-like lymphoproliferation in TGF-beta knockout mice. *J Immunol* **155**, 3205–12.

80. Morel, L., Croker, B.P., Blenman, K.R., Mohan, C., Huang, G., Gilkeson, G., *et al.* (2000) Genetic reconstitution of systemic lupus erythematosus immunopathology with polycongenic murine strains. *Proc Natl Acad Sci USA* **97**, 6670–5.

81. Mitchell, D.A., Pickering, M.C., Warren, J., Fossati-Jimack, L., Cortes-Hernandez, J., Cook, H.T., *et al.* (2002) C1q deficiency and autoimmunity: the effects of genetic background on disease expression. *J Immunol* **168**, 2538–43.

82. Cosio, F.G., Sedmak, D.D., Mahan, J.D., and Nahman, N.S., Jr. (1989) Localization of decay accelerating factor in normal and diseased kidneys. *Kidney Int* **36**, 100–7.

83. Bao, L., Spiller, O.B., St, J.P., Haas, M., Hack, B.K., Ren, G., *et al.* (2002) Decay-accelerating factor expression in the rat kidney is restricted to the apical surface of podocytes. *Kidney Int* **62**, 2010–21.

84. Quigg, R.J., Nicholson-Weller, A., Cybulsky, A.V., Badalamenti, J., and Salant, D.J. (1989) Decay accelerating factor regulates complement activation on glomerular epithelial cells. *J Immunol* **142**, 877–82.

85. Sogabe, H., Nangaku, M., Ishibashi, Y., Wada, T., Fujita, T., Sun, X., *et al.* (2001) Increased susceptibility of decay-accelerating factor deficient mice to anti-glomerular basement membrane glomerulonephritis. *J Immunol* **167**, 2791–7.

86. Abe, K., Miyazaki, M., Koji, T., Furusu, A., Ozono, Y., Harada, T., *et al.* (1998) Expression of decay accelerating factor mRNA and complement C3 mRNA in human diseased kidney. *Kidney Int* **54**, 120–30.

87. Arora, M., Arora, R., Tiwari, S.C., Das, N., and Srivastava, L.M. (2000) Expression of complement regulatory proteins in diffuse proliferative glomerulonephritis. *Lupus* **9**, 127–31.

88. Miwa, T., Maldonado, M.A., Zhou, L., Sun, X., Luo, H.Y., Cai, D., *et al.* (2002) Deletion of decay-accelerating factor (CD55) exacerbates autoimmune disease development in MRL/lpr mice. *Am J Pathol* **161**, 1077–86.

89. Miwa, T., Maldonado, M.A., Zhou, L., Yamada, K., Gilkeson, G.S., Eisenberg, R.A., *et al.* (2007) Decay-accelerating factor ameliorates systemic autoimmune disease in MRL/lpr mice via both complement-dependent and -independent mechanisms. *Am J Pathol* **170**, 1258–66.

90. Qian, Y.M., Haino, M., Kelly, K., and Song, W.C. (1999) Structural characterization of mouse CD97 and study of its specific interaction with the murine decay-accelerating factor (DAF, CD55). *Immunology* **98**, 303–11.

91. Liu, J., Miwa, T., Hilliard, B., Chen, Y., Lambris, J.D., Wells, A.D., *et al.* (2005) The complement inhibitory protein DAF (CD55) suppresses T cell immunity in vivo. *J Exp Med* **201**, 567–77.

92. Bao, L., Haas, M., Pippin, J., Wang, Y., Miwa, T., Chang, A. *et al.* (2009) Focal and segmental glomerulosclerosis induced in mice lacking decay-accelerating factor in T cells. *J Clin Invest* **119**, 1264–74.

93. Kim, Y.-U., Kinoshita, T., Molina, H., Hourcade, D., Seya, T., Wagner, L.M., *et al.* (1995) Mouse complement regulatory protein Crry/p65 uses the specific mechanisms of both human decay-accelerating factor and membrane cofactor protein. *J Exp Med* **181**, 151–9.

94. Li, B., Sallee, C., Dehoff, M., Foley, S., Molina, H., and Holers, V.M. (1993) Mouse Crry/p65: Characterization of monoclonal antibodies and the tissue distribution of a functional homologue of human MCP and DAF. *J Immunol* **151**, 4295–305.

95. Nishikage, H., Baranyi, L., Okada, H., Okada, N., Isobe, K., Nomura, A., *et al.* (1995) Role of a complement regulatory protein in rat mesangial glomerulonephritis. *J Am Soc Nephrol* **6**, 234–42.

96. Matsuo, S., Ichida, S., Takizawa, H., Okada, N., Baranyi, L., Iguchi, A., *et al.* (1994) In vivo effects of monoclonal antibodies that functionally inhibit complement regulatory proteins in rats. *J Exp Med* **180**, 1619–27.

97. Hatanaka, Y., Yuzawa, Y., Nishikawa, K., Fukatsu, A., Okada, N., Okada, H., *et al.* (1995) Role of a rat membrane inhibitor of complement in anti-basement membrane antibody-induced renal injury. *Kidney Int* **48**, 1728–37.

98. Mizuno, M., Nishikawa, K., Goodfellow, R.M., Piddlesden, S.J., Morgan, B.P., and Matsuo, S. (1997) The effects of functional suppression of a membrane-bound complement regulatory protein, CD59, in the synovial tissue in rats. *Arthritis Rheum* **40**, 527–33.

99. Xu, C., Mao, D., Holers, V.M., Palanca, B., Cheng, A.M., and Molina, H. (2000) A critical role for murine complement regulator Crry in fetomaternal tolerance. *Science* **287**, 498–501.

100. Bao, L., Wang, Y., Chang, A., Minto, A.W., Zhou, J., Kang, H., *et al.* (2007) Unrestricted C3 activation occurs in Crry-deficient kidneys and rapidly leads to chronic renal failure. *J Am Soc Nephrol* **18**, 811–22.

101. Bao, L., Wang, Y., Chen, P., Sarav, M., Haas, M., Minto, A.W., *et al.* (2009) Mesangial cell Crry limits complement-dependent neutrophil accumulation in immune complex glomerulonephritis. *Immunology* **128**, e895–904.

102. Couser, W.G., Johnson, R.J., Young, B.A., Yeh, C.G., Toth, C.A., and Rudolph, A.R. (1995) The effects of soluble recombinant complement receptor 1 on complement-mediated experimental glomerulonephritis. *J Am Soc Nephrol* **5**, 1888–94.

103. Quigg, R.J., He, C., Lim, A., Berthiaume, D., Alexander, J.J., Kraus, D., *et al.* (1998) Transgenic mice overexpressing the complement inhibitor Crry as a soluble protein are protected from antibody-induced glomerular injury. *J Exp Med* **188**, 1321–31.

104. Bao, L., Haas, M., Boackle, S.A., Kraus, D.M., Cunningham, P.N., Park, P., *et al.* (2002) Transgenic expression of a soluble complement inhibitor protects against renal disease and promotes survival in MRL/lpr mice. *J Immunol* **168**, 3601–7.

105. Quigg, R.J., Kozono, Y., Berthiaume, D., Lim, A., Salant, D.J., Weinfeld, A., *et al.* (1998) Blockade of antibody-induced glomerulonephritis with Crry-Ig, a soluble murine complement inhibitor. *J Immunol* **160**, 4553–60.

106. Bao, L., Haas, M., Kraus, D.M., Hack, B.K., Rakstang, J.K., Holers, V.M., *et al.* (2003) Administration of a soluble recombinant complement C3 inhibitor protects against renal disease in MRL/lpr mice. *J Am Soc Nephrol* **14**, 670–9.

107. Bao, L., Zhou, J., Holers, V.M., and Quigg, R.J. (2003) Excessive matrix accumulation in the kidneys of MRL/lpr lupus mice Is dependent on complement activation. *J Am Soc Nephrol* **14**, 2516–25.

108. Molina, H., Kinoshita, T., Inoue, K., Carel, J.C., and Holers, V.M. (1990) A molecular and immunochemical characterization of mouse CR2. Evidence for a single gene model of mouse complement receptors 1 and 2. *J Immunol* **145**, 2974–83.

109. Wilson, J.G., Ratnoff, W.D., Schur, P.H., and Fearon, D.T. (1986) Decreased expression of the C3b/C4b receptor (CR1) and the C3d receptor (CR2) on B lymphocytes and of CR1 on neutrophils of patients with systemic lupus erythematosus. *Arthritis Rheum* **29**, 739–47.

110. Takahashi, K., Kozono, Y., Waldschmidt, T.J., Berthiaume, D., Quigg, R.J., Baron, A., *et al.* (1997) Mouse complement receptors type 1 (CR1, CD35) and 2 (CR2, CD21). Expression on normal B cell subpopulations and decreased levels during the development of autoimmunity in MRL/lpr mice. *J Immunol* **159**, 1557–69.

111. Einav, S., Pozdnyakova, O.O., Ma, M., and Carroll, M.C. (2002) Complement C4 is protective for lupus disease independent of C3. *J Immunol* **168**, 1036–41.

112. Prodeus, A.P., Goerg, S., Shen, L.M., Pozdnyakova, O.O., Chu, L., Alicot, E.M., et al. (1998) A critical role for complement in maintenance of self-tolerance. *Immunity* **9**, 721–31.

113. Carroll, M.C. (2000) A protective role for innate immunity in autoimmune disease. *Clin Immunol* **95**, S30–S38.

114. Pickering, M.C., and Walport, M.J. (2000) Links between complement abnormalities and systemic lupus erythematosus. *Rheumatology (Oxford)* **39**, 133–41.

115. Blom, A.M., Villoutreix, B.O., and Dahlback, B. (2004) Complement inhibitor C4b-binding protein-friend or foe in the innate immune system? *Mol Immunol* **40**, 1333–46.

116. Barnum, S.R., and Dahlback, B. (1990) C4b-binding protein, a regulatory component of the classical pathway of complement, is an acute-phase protein and is elevated in systemic lupus erythematosus. *Complement Inflamm* **7**, 71–7.

117. Wenderfer, S.E., Soimo, K., Wetsel, R.A., and Braun, M.C. (2007) Analysis of C4 and the C4 binding protein in the MRL/lpr mouse. *Arthritis Res Ther* **9**, R114.

118. Blom, A.M., Nandakumar, K.S., and Holmdahl, R. (2009) C4b-binding protein (C4BP) inhibits development of experimental arthritis in mice. *Ann Rheum Dis* **68**, 136–42.

119. Pickering, M.C., Cook, H.T., Warren, J., Bygrave, A.E., Moss, J., Walport, M.J., et al. (2002) Uncontrolled C3 activation causes membranoproliferative glomerulonephritis in mice deficient in complement factor H. *Nat Genet* **31**, 424–8.

120. Hogasen, K., Jansen, J.H., Mollnes, T.E., Hovdenes, J., and Harboe, M. (1995) Hereditary porcine membranoproliferative glomerulonephritis type II is caused by factor H deficiency. *J Clin Invest* **95**, 1054–61.

121. Zipfel, P.F. (2001) Complement factor H: physiology and pathophysiology. *Semin Thromb Hemost* **27**, 191–9.

122. Watanabe, H., Garnier, G., Circolo, A., Wetsel, R.A., Ruiz, P., Holers, V.M., et al. (2000) Modulation of renal disease in MRL/lpr mice genetically deficient in the alternative complement pathway factor B. *J Immunol* **164**, 786–94.

123. Elliott, M.K., Jarmi, T., Ruiz, P., Xu, Y., Holers, V.M., and Gilkeson, G.S. (2004) Effects of complement factor D deficiency on the renal disease of MRL/lpr mice. *Kidney Int* **65**, 129–38.

124. Biesecker, G., Katz, S., and Koffler, D. (1981) Renal localization of the membrane attack complex in systemic lupus erythematosus nephritis. *J Exp Med* **154**, 1779–94.

125. Wang, Y., Hu, Q., Madri, J.A., Rollins, S.A., Chodera, A., and Matis, L.A. (1996) Amelioration of lupus-like autoimmune disease in NZB/W F1 mice after treatment with a blocking monoclonal antibody specific for complement component C5. *Proc Natl Acad Sci USA* **93**, 8563–8.

126. Mizuno, M., Blanchin, S., Gasque, P., Nishikawa, K., and Matsuo, S. (2007) High levels of complement C3a receptor in the glomeruli in lupus nephritis. *Am J Kidney Dis* **49**, 598–606.

127. Bao, L., Osawe, I., Puri, T., Lambris, J.D., Haas, M., and Quigg, R.J. (2005) C5a promotes development of experimental lupus nephritis which can be blocked with a specific receptor antagonist. *Eur J Immunol* **35**, 3012–20.

128. Wenderfer, S.E., Ke, B., Hollmann, T.J., Wetsel, R.A., Lan, H.Y., and Braun, M.C. (2005) C5a receptor deficiency attenuates T cell function and renal disease in MRLlpr mice. *J Am Soc Nephrol* **16**, 3572–82.

129. Wenderfer, S.E., Wang, H., Ke, B., Wetsel, R.A., and Braun, M.C. (2009) C3a receptor deficiency accelerates the onset of renal injury in the MRL/lpr mouse. *Mol Immunol* **46**, 1397–404.

130. Mathieu, M.C., Sawyer, N., Greig, G.M., Hamel, M., Kargman, S., Ducharme, Y., *et al.* (2005) The C3a receptor antagonist SB 290157 has agonist activity. *Immunol Lett* **100**, 139–45.

131. Sekine, H., Reilly, C.M., Molano, I.D., Garnier, G., Circolo, A., Ruiz, P., *et al.* (2001) Complement component C3 is not required for full expression of immune complex glomerulonephritis in MRL/lpr mice. *J Immunol* **166**, 6444–51.

132. Sheerin, N.S., Springall, T., Carroll, M., and Sacks, S.H. (1999) Altered distribution of intraglomerular immune complexes in C3-deficient mice. *Immunology* **97**, 393–9.

133. Clynes, R., Dumitru, C., and Ravetch, J.V. (1998) Uncoupling of immune complex formation and kidney damage in autoimmune glomerulonephritis. *Science* **279**, 1052–4.

134. Matsumoto, K., Watanabe, N., Akikusa, B., Kurasawa, K., Matsumura, R., Saito, Y., *et al.* (2003) Fc receptor-independent development of autoimmune glomerulonephritis in lupus-prone MRL/lpr mice. *Arthritis Rheum* **48**, 486–94.

135. Pepys, M.B. (1974) Role of complement in induction of antibody production in vivo. Effect of cobra factor and other C3-reactive agents on thymus- dependent and thymus-independent antibody responses. *J Exp Med* **140**, 126–45.

136. Carroll, M.C. (1998) The role of complement and complement receptors in induction and regulation of immunity. *Ann Rev Immunol* **16**, 545–68.

137. Atkinson, C., Song, H., Lu, B., Qiao, F., Burns, T.A., Holers, V.M., *et al.* (2005) Targeted complement inhibition by C3d recognition ameliorates tissue injury without apparent increase in susceptibility to infection. *J Clin Invest* **115**, 2444–53.

138. Zhang, H., Lu, S., Morrison, S.L., and Tomlinson, S. (2001) Targeting of functional antibody-decay-accelerating factor fusion proteins to a cell surface. *J Biol Chem* **276**, 27290–5.

139. Zhang, H., Yu, J., Bajwa, E., Morrison, S.L., and Tomlinson, S. (1999) Targeting of functional antibody-CD59 fusion proteins to a cell surface. *J Clin Invest* **103**, 55–61.

140. He, C., Imai, M., Song, H., Quigg, R.J., and Tomlinson, S. (2005) Complement inhibitors targeted to the proximal tubule prevent injury in experimental nephrotic syndrome and demonstrate a key role for C5b-9. *J Immunol* **174**, 5750–7.

141. Song, H., He, C., Knaak, C., Guthridge, J.M., Holers, V.M., and Tomlinson, S. (2003) Complement receptor 2-mediated targeting of complement inhibitors to sites of complement activation. *J Clin Invest* **111**, 1875–85.

142. Schulze, M., Pruchno, C.J., Burns, M., Baker, P.J., Johnson, R.J., and Couser, W.G. (1993) Glomerular C3c localization indicates ongoing immune deposit formation and complement activation in experimental glomerulonephritis. *Am J Pathol* **142**, 179–87.

143. Atkinson, C., Qiao, F., Song, H., Gilkeson, G.S., and Tomlinson, S. (2008) Low-dose targeted complement inhibition protects against renal disease and other manifestations of autoimmune disease in MRL/lpr mice. *J Immunol* **180**, 1231–8.

144. Weisman, H.F., Bartow, T., Leppo, M.K., Marsh, H.C., Jr., Carson, G.R., Concino, M.F., *et al.* (1990) Soluble human complement receptor type 1: In vivo inhibitor of complement suppressing post-ischemic myocardial inflammation and necrosis. *Science* **249**, 146–51.

145. Zimmerman, J.L., Dellinger, R.P., Straube, R.C., and Levin, J.L. (2000) Phase I trial of the recombinant soluble complement receptor 1 in acute lung injury and acute respiratory distress syndrome. *Crit Care Med* **28**, 3149–54.

146. Lazar, H.L., Bokesch, P.M., van, L.F., Fitzgerald, C., Emmett, C., Marsh, H.C., Jr. *et al.* (2004) Soluble human complement receptor 1 limits ischemic damage in cardiac surgery patients at high risk requiring cardiopulmonary bypass. *Circulation* **110**, II274–II279.

147. Lazar, H.L., Keilani, T., Fitzgerald, C.A., Shapira, O.M., Hunter, C.T., Shemin, R.J., *et al.* (2007) Beneficial effects of complement inhibition with soluble complement receptor 1 (TP10) during cardiac surgery: is there a gender difference? *Circulation* **116**, I83–I88.

148. Keshavjee, S., Davis, R.D., Zamora, M.R., de, P.M., and Patterson, G.A. (2005) A randomized, placebo-controlled trial of complement inhibition in ischemia-reperfusion injury after lung transplantation in human beings. *J Thorac Cardiovasc Surg* **129**, 423–8.

149. Kunschak, M., Engl, W., Maritsch, F., Rosen, F.S., Eder, G., Zerlauth, G., *et al.* (1998) A randomized, controlled trial to study the efficacy and safety of C1 inhibitor concentrate in treating hereditary angioedema. *Transfusion* **38**, 540–9.

150. Kreuz, W., Martinez-Saguer, I., ygoren-Pursun, E., Rusicke, E., Heller, C., and Klingebiel, T. (2009) C1-inhibitor concentrate for individual replacement therapy in patients with severe hereditary angioedema refractory to danazol prophylaxis. *Transfusion* **49**, 1987–95.

151. Choi, G., Soeters, M.R., Farkas, H., Varga, L., Obtulowicz, K., Bilo, B., *et al.* (2007) Recombinant human C1-inhibitor in the treatment of acute angioedema attacks. *Transfusion* **47**, 1028–32.

152. Fattouch, K., Bianco, G., Speziale, G., Sampognaro, R., Lavalle, C., Guccione, F., *et al.* (2007) Beneficial effects of C1 esterase inhibitor in ST-elevation myocardial infarction in patients who underwent surgical reperfusion: a randomised double-blind study. *Eur J Cardiothorac Surg* **32**, 326–32.

153. Thielmann, M., Marggraf, G., Neuhauser, M., Forkel, J., Herold, U., Kamler, M., *et al.* (2006) Administration of C1-esterase inhibitor during emergency coronary artery bypass surgery in acute ST-elevation myocardial infarction. *Eur J Cardiothorac Surg* **30**, 285–93.

154. Shernan, S.K., Fitch, J.C., Nussmeier, N.A., Chen, J.C., Rollins, S.A., Mojcik, C.F., *et al.* (2004) Impact of pexelizumab, an anti-C5 complement antibody, on total mortality and adverse cardiovascular outcomes in cardiac surgical patients undergoing cardiopulmonary bypass. *Ann Thorac Surg* **77**, 942–9.

155. Fitch, J.C., Rollins, S., Matis, L., Alford, B., Aranki, S., Collard, C.D., *et al.* (1999) Pharmacology and biological efficacy of a recombinant, humanized, single-chain antibody C5 complement inhibitor in patients undergoing coronary artery bypass graft surgery with cardiopulmonary bypass. *Circulation* **100**, 2499–506.

156. Hillmen, P., Hall, C., Marsh, J.C., Elebute, M., Bombara, M.P., Petro, B.E., *et al.* (2004) Effect of eculizumab on hemolysis and transfusion requirements in patients with paroxysmal nocturnal hemoglobinuria. *N Engl J Med* **350**, 552–9.

157. Hill, A., Hillmen, P., Richards, S.J., Elebute, D., Marsh, J.C., Chan, J., *et al.* (2005) Sustained response and long-term safety of eculizumab in paroxysmal nocturnal hemoglobinuria. *Blood* **106**, 2259–65.

158. Cybulsky, A.V., Quigg, R.J., and Salant, D.J. (2005) Experimental membranous nephropathy redux. *Am J Physiol Renal, Fluid Electrolyte Physiol* **289**, F660–F671.

Chapter 5

Pathways of cellular adaptive immunity in autoimmune crescentic glomerulonephritis and lupus nephritis

Stephen R. Holdsworth and Peter G. Tipping

Human crescentic glomerulonephritis (GN) is frequently associated with systemic or organ-specific autoimmunity, which results from disturbance of the delicate balance between immune effector responses and immune tolerance. T cell subsets and antigen presenting cells (APCs) have central roles in initiating and regulating adaptive nephritogenic immune responses that result in crescentic renal injury. There is strong functional evidence from experimental models and circumstantial evidence from human studies to implicate Th1 immune responses and cellular effector pathways leading to crescent formation. The contribution of the more recently described Th17 pathway has been explored in human and experimental studies, but the functional importance of Th17 responses is not yet clear. Recent studies of the involvement of natural killer T (NKT) cells in crescentic GN provide conflicting data suggesting either injurious or protective roles. Knowledge of the complexity of immune tolerance mechanisms is rapidly increasing and some evidence for the disturbances of T regulatory cell function in crescentic GN is emerging. Dendritic cells play a central role in initiation of immune responses and modulating the direction of subsequent immune effector pathway activation. Their involvement in GN is just beginning to be explored, but their involvement at the interface between innate and adaptive immune responses raises the prospect of new therapeutic strategies directed at molecules such as type I interferons and toll-like receptors, that control their function.

Introduction

The presence of T cells and/or immunoglobulin in glomeruli in the majority of cases of human GN implicates the involvement of adaptive immunity in initiation of glomerular inflammation. The disease processes associated with crescentic GN in humans often involve autoimmunity, either organ-specific to glomerular antigens (e.g. in anti-glomerular basement membrane (GBM) GN) or systemic to nonglomerular antigens (e.g. in lupus nephritis and ANCA-associated crescentic GN), implicating loss of immune tolerance in disease initiation. The consistent local participation of

T cells and macrophages, frequently unaccompanied by antibody deposition, provides strong evidence for a central role for cellular adaptive immunity in the effector pathway leading to glomerular injury.

Adaptive immune responses result from the complex interactions between APCs and various effector T cell subsets and T regulatory cells. The contributions of T helper (Th)1 and Th2 cells have received considerable attention over many years in a variety of diseases, including crescentic GN. More recently, the important effector role of Th17 cells, the identity and function of regulatory T cells, the contribution of "natural killer" (NK) T cells and the immunomodulatory role of dendritic cells in adaptive immunity is becoming better understood. Evidence from experimental models and human glomerular pathology suggests a prominent role for CD4+ T cell-driven Th1-type responses in crescentic GN with delayed type hypersensitivity (DTH), like cellular effectors (T cells and macrophages) and Th1 immunoglobulin isotypes in glomeruli. Recent studies are beginning to explore the role of other T cell subsets and the involvement of dendritic cells in immune renal injury.

The concept of T helper cell subsets now extends beyond Th1 and Th2 cells. The balance of environmental signals (e.g. cytokines, co-stimulatory molecules, type I interferons and toll-like receptor (TLR) ligands, etc.) at the time of antigen presentation can direct T cells towards three additional pathways of differentiation: Th17, T regulatory cells (Treg) and ThFH (follicular helper) cells. Transforming growth factor β (TGFβ) is a major determinant of T cell differentiation towards Th17 and Treg pathways, through effects directly on T cells and indirectly via dendritic cells. Transforming growth factor β signals through signal transducer and activator of transcription 4 (STAT4) to induce expression of Foxp3 and promote Treg cell development. However, TGFβ stimulation combined with interleukin-6 (IL-6) induces the transcription factor RORγt that drives production of IL-17 and T cell differentiation down the Th17 effector pathway. In the absence of IL-6, IL-21 can promote Th17 development.[1] Interleukin-23 serves as a cofactor, enhancing the survival and subsequent proliferation of Th17 cells.[2] T helper 17 cells play an important role in host defense against extracellular bacteria, and IL-17 mobilizes neutrophils from the bone marrow and induces the production of chemokines by IL-17 receptor-bearing cells that direct neutrophil recruitment to inflammatory sites.

T follicular helper cells are a recently discovered subset of CD4+ effector T cells that play a primary role in providing B cell help and stimulating humoral immunity during immune responses. They are defined by their expression of CXCR5, which directs migration to the germinal centers by interaction with the B cell follicle chemokine, CXCL13.[3] This differentiation pathway is directed by IL-6 and IL-21, which upregulate the transcription factor STAT3.[4] T follicular helper cells may be an important source of IL-21,[5] but their contribution to GN is unknown.

T helper pathways in experimental crescentic GN

Th1 and Th2 pathways

The prominent glomerular accumulation of CD4+ T cells and macrophages in human crescentic GN suggests a potential "helper" T cell role in directing crescentic injury.[6,7]

The role of CD4+ T cells has been extensively explored in planted antigen models of crescentic GN,[8–10] as well as in models involving organ-specific[11,12] and systemic autoimmunity.[13,14] These demonstrate that the Th1 or Th2 bias of the CD4+ T cell response exerts a major influence on immune effector mechanisms and resultant patterns of glomerular injury. T helper 1 cells develop from naïve CD4+ (Th0) cells under the influence of IL-12 and IL-18, and play a key role in directing DTH and augmenting production of opsonizing and complement fixing subclasses of IgG. T helper 2 cells develop under the influence of IL-4 and IL-13 and promote allergic responses, mast cell/IgE-mediated hypersensitivity responses and production of IgE and IgG with lower complement fixing capacity (Figure 5.1).

The propensity of Th1-biased responses to direct crescentic patterns of injury has been demonstrated in autoimmune crescentic GN induced in rodents by immunization with α3 chains of type IV collagen.[12,15] In anti-GBM antibody induced GN (anti-GBM GN) T helper 1 cytokine deficiencies, for example IL-12[16] and interferon (IFN)γ,[17] attenuate crescentic injury, as does blocking Th1 cytokines using antibodies. Conversely, administration of IL-12, the key Th1 cytokine, exacerbates disease.[18] Interleukin-18 enhances crescentic GN even in the absence of IL-12.[19] Mice with deficiencies of Th2 cytokines (IL-4 and IL-10) show greater susceptibility to crescentic GN[20,21] and administration of these Th2 cytokines, either during the initiation of disease[22] or after glomerular injury is established,[23] provides protection from development of crescents. Interleukin-4 administration also attenuates crescent formation in anti-GBM GN in rats.[24] The role of T helper subsets in models involving systemic

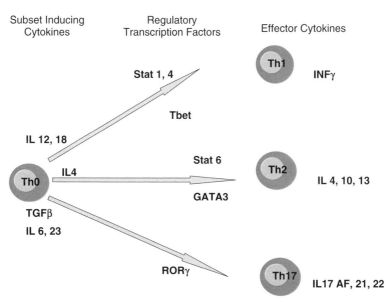

Fig. 5.1 A simplified depiction of the major elements in T helper subset differentiation and effector cytokines. Th1 directed effector mechanisms play a dominant role in development of crescentic GN.

autoimmunity appears more complex. Interferon γ receptor-deficient MRL/*lpr* lupus prone mice show protection from development of crescentic GN,[25] whereas blocking IL-4 but not IL-12 provides protection from GN.[26] In human lupus nephritis, there is conflicting evidence for the involvement of Th1/Th2 subsets. Taken together, these data suggest that Th1 polarized systemic immune responses directing cell-mediated immune glomerular injury play a major role in the development of crescentic GN.

In addition to their critical role in initiation of immune responses in crescentic GN, CD4+ T cells also have key effector roles, in particular via their capacity to recruit macrophages. In experimental anti-GBM GN induced by heterologous antibody, CD4+ T cell depletion in the effector phase of the disease (after the nephritogenic immune response is established) is effective in preventing glomerular macrophage recruitment and crescentic injury.[27] Potential contributions of proinflammatory cytokines such as (IFNγ,[28] IL-12,[29] IL-1β,[30] and tumor necrosis factor (TNF))[30] from T cells, macrophages, and intrinsic renal cells during the effector phase crescentic GN have been demonstrated in murine models. Intrinsic cells produce chemokines and IL-23 that attract and activate leukocytes. T cell expression of CD40 and intrinsic cell-produced IFNγ activate macrophages to produce IL-1 which, in turn, drives intrinsic cells to produce injurious TNF (Figure 5.2).

Experimental studies have demonstrated that autoimmune responses leading to murine lupus are T cell dependent.[14,31] Deficiency of α/β T cells inhibits development of lupus nephritis in some experimental models,[31,32] but α/β T cell-independent mechanisms may also be involved.[33,34] Failure of deletion of B cells following polyclonal activation by superantigens has been suggested as an alternative mechanism for development of autoantibodies.[35] Reduced apoptosis of B cells is a feature of some murine models of lupus but has not been detected in human lupus.[36] The involvement of Treg imbalance in human disease induction is suggested by decreased Treg cells in the blood of patients with systemic lupus erythematosus (SLE),[37] although this is not a consistent finding. Deficiency of CD25+ Treg cells does not appear to be involved in murine lupus.[38]

The role of T cells as effectors of injury in lupus nephritis is less clear. The presence of T cells in crescentic glomeruli and the interstitium in lupus-prone mice is consistent with a local effector role.[38] In MRL/*lpr* mice, B cells are necessary for development of GN.[39] However, this role may be independent of their involvement in autoantibody production,[39] as lupus-prone mice with B cells that fail to make immunoglobulin still develop GN. This may be explained by the ability of B cells to allow persistence of autoimmune responses via their capacity to present antigen to T cells. Depletion of kidney-autoreactive T cells by intrathymic injection of syngeneic renal cells (but not splenocytes) into neonatal MRL/*lpr* mice attenuated development of GN without altering the levels of autoantibodies.[40] In lupus-prone NZ mixed 2410 (NZM2410) mice, deficiency of the T cell intracellular signaling molecule STAT6 or treatment with anti-IL-4 antibody decreased Th2 responses and GN despite enhanced levels of anti-DNA antibodies.[41] STAT 4 deficiency decreased Th1 cytokines and accelerated development of GN in the absence of high levels of anti-DNA antibodies.[41] The dissociation of GN from autoantibody production in these models of lupus nephritis is consistent with an effector role for T cells in directing glomerular inflammation.

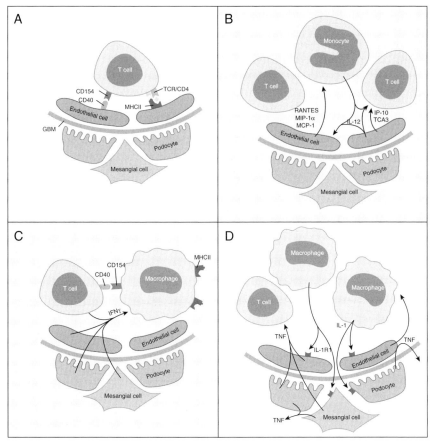

Fig. 5.2 Mechanisms of effector T cell-directed injury in crescentic nephrotoxic nephritis (NTN) have been demonstrated using chimeric mice with selective leukocyte or intrinsic renal cell deletions of major histocompatibility complex (MHC)II,[176] CD40,[177] interleukin (IL)12,[29] interferon (IFN)γ,[44] tumor necrosis factor (TNF),[178] IL1β and IL1 receptor I.[179] Effector T cells require MHCII and CD40 expression by intrinsic renal cells to recognize nephritogenic antigens and initiate injury (A). Intrinsic renal cell production of monocyte and T cell chemoattractant chemokines and IL12 directs further leukocyte influx (B). T cell expression of CD40 and IFNγ from T cells and intrinsic renal cells activates monocytes to macrophages (C). Macrophages produce IL1, which acts via IL1 receptor I on intrinsic renal cells to induce TNF production and crescentic injury (D) (see Plate 1).

Th17 pathways in GN

Evidence is now emerging through experimental models and human studies for the participation of IL-17 in GN. Studies in IL-17 and IL-23 p19-deficient mice demonstrate that the IL-23/Th17 pathway contributes to glomerular injury and crescent formation in murine nephrotoxic nephritis.[42] In IL-23 p35-deficient mice developing autoimmune anti-GBM nephritis, renal injury is attenuated in association with reduced autoantibody and IL-17A levels, without changes in Treg cell numbers.[43]

In lupus-prone MRL/*lpr* mice, cytokine profiles of T cells from renal lesions show enhanced IL-17 mRNA expression, indicating the involvement of Th17 cells, although the presence of IFNγ and IL-13 is consistent with Th1 and Th2 participation.[44] Further indirect evidence for a proinflammatory role of IL-17 in murine lupus comes from studies of TNF receptor-deficient New Zealand mixed 2328 mice. Deletion of both TNF receptors (TNFR1 and TNFR2) on this strain background increased circulating anti-dsDNA antibody levels and accelerated development of nephritis, and was associated with increased numbers of CD44 (high),CD62L(low),CD4+ T cells that expressed a gene profile (increased RORγt, IL-23, IL-17A and F) consistent with Th17 cells.[45]

Inbred BXD2 mice show high levels of IL-17 production, which results in spontaneous germinal center formation and development of pathogenic autoantibodies,[46] whereas mice lacking the IL-17 receptor have reduced humoral immunity.[46] Deletion of the IL-21 receptor in lupus-prone BXSB-Yaa mice prevents development of autoantibodies and nephritis, although the IL-21 production in this model was not from Th17 cells and was not limited to CXCR5+ TFH cells.[47] These data raise the possibility that the Th17 lineage may induce lupus nephritis by humoral means rather than through Th17-driven cellular effector pathways of injury. Although intriguing, this hypothesis remains to be formally tested.[48] Interestingly, IL-21 receptor-deficient mice were not protected from injury in models previously thought to involve the Th17 pathway.[49] Further studies are necessary to clarify these results.[50]

T helper cells in autoimmune human GN

Recognition of the important role of autoimmunity in most forms of human crescentic GN has led to renewed interest in identification of the antigenic epitopes and the mechanisms of initiation and regulation of autoimmune (nephritogenic) responses. Recent work has characterized some of the autoantigens in human crescentic GN at molecular level. Target antigens may be endogenous glomerular antigens (e.g. the noncollagenous domain (NC1) of the α3 chain of type IV collagen [α3(IV)NC1] in anti-GBM disease) or endogenous systemic antigens (myeloperoxidase (MPO), proteinase 3 (PR3), and lysosome-associated membrane protein-2 (LAMP2) in vasculitis, and nuclear epitopes in lupus nephritis). These nonrenal antigens may be targeted to glomeruli as immune complexes, antineutrophil cytoplasmic antibody (ANCA), or passively deposited antigens in the glomerular filter where they subsequently bind antibody and thereby act as *in situ* immune complexes.

T cells in autoimmune anti-GBM GN

Characterization of the nephritogenic peptides of α3(IV)NC1 has highlighted the role of T cells in this uncommon form of autoimmune crescentic GN. Studies in Wky rats have demonstrated the capacity of recombinant α3(IV)NC1 to elicit nephritogenic responses[51] and the ability of transferred Th1 cell lines to induce crescentic disease in the absence of glomerular antibody deposition,[52] confirming the primary role of autoreactive T cells in this model of autoimmune crescentic GN. Peptide mapping has defined a potent T cell epitope pCol(28-40), which induced severe glomerulonephritis in rats.[53]

Experimental studies in mice have demonstrated the role of major histocompatibility complex (MHC) Class II in susceptibility to autoimmunity and the ability of splenocytes and Th1 antibody isotypes to transfer disease.[12] Human studies show association between HLA DRB1*15 and DRB1*04 and susceptibility to anti-GBM disease, whereas expression of DRB1*07 confers protection.[54] T cells from patients with acute disease react to a limited number of peptides of α3(IV)NC1 (α3 71–90 and α3 131–150), suggesting that these are the likely natural immunodominant peptides.[55,56] However, these are not the peptides inducing the strongest responses in T cells from patients with anti-GBM GN when presented by DR15 on Epstein–Barr virus-transformed human B cells, suggesting that factors other than T cell receptor affinity determine selection of immunodominant autoreactive epitopes.[56] The cytokine profile of autoreactive α3(IV)NC1 T cells from patients in the acute phase of the disease is Th1 predominant (producing IFNγ); during resolution of disease IL-10 production is predominant.[57] Studies of anti-GBM antibody from patients with anti-GBM GN[58] suggest that the B cell epitope is quite different to that seen by T cells.

The maintenance of tolerance involves peripheral mechanisms including antigen ignorance, Th2 deviation, and T regulatory cells. The mechanisms for maintaining tolerance to autoantigens like α3(IV)NC1 are both central (clonal deletion) and peripheral. α3(IV)NC1 is expressed in the thymus,[59] so clonal deletion would be expected. However, deletion is incomplete and patients with anti-GBM GN (as well as normal individuals) have nondeleted T cells reactive with α3(IV)NC1.[60] The unexpected reduced MHC II presentation of immunodominant α3(IV)NC1 epitopes by human antigen presenting cells suggests peripheral tolerance through ignorance. The absence of CD25+Foxp3+Tregs during acute disease and appearance during the recovery phase of human anti-GBM GN suggests that changes in the regulatory T cell balance may be involved in the development of Goodpasture's disease.[61] The predominance of IL-10-secreting T cells during the resolution of anti-GBM GN is also consistent with the appearance of Tregs.[57] Mucosal presentation of autoantigens has been shown to be effective in induction of tolerance and, in experimental autoimmune anti-GBM GN in rats, oral feeding of α3(IV)NC1 collagen provides protection.[62] These human and experimental observations suggest the possibility of immune modulation therapy for this rare but severe form of autoimmune crescentic GN.

T cells in ANCA-associated crescentic GN

A number of observations suggest a role for CD4+ T cell-directed autoimmunity in crescentic GN, associated with small vessel vasculitis and ANCA. Perhaps the most obvious is the presence of circulating antibodies to neutrophil MPO and PR3 in this group of diseases and the presence of CD4+ T cells and DTH effectors and relative paucity of antibody in affected glomeruli.[63–65] The capacity for MPO autoimmunity to induce crescentic GN has been established in experimental models. Rats immunized with MPO develop crescentic GN following infusion of a crude preparation of this antigen into their kidneys.[66] Splenocytes or antibody from MPO-deficient mice immunized with murine MPO induce a necrotizing and crescentic GN following passive transfer to immunodeficient mice.[67]

The prominent isotype switching observed with ANCA[68] and the predominance of Th1 isotypes of ANCA in Wegener's granulomatosis[65] are consistent with Th1-directed responses in the genesis of the autoimmunity. The cytokine profile of mononuclear cells (high IFNγ, IL-12, and TNFα, which is suppressed by IL-10) in the blood and affected tissues of patients with ANCA-associated GN is consistent with a Th1 response.[69] The phenotype of T cells from blood, bronchial lavage, and nasal biopsy specimens of patients with Wegener's granulomatosis is also consistent with Th1-driven cell-mediated immunity.[69,70] Immunohistochemistry of affected tissues also demonstrates the presence of IFNγ[70] and IL-8.[70,71] However, these observations are not uniform, and predominance of CD3+ cells, eosinophils, and Th2 cytokines has been reported in a study of nasal biopsies from patients with Wegner's granulomatosis.[72]

The presence of T cells responding to the likely target antigens, MPO and PR3, in patients with ANCA-associated GN provides evidence for the involvement of T cell-directed autoimmunity.[73–77] The immunodominant T cell epitopes have not been precisely defined but, for PR3, predominant T cell-reactive residues in three peptide regions involving the C terminus of the propeptide and the signal sequence have been identified.[78] The efficacy of therapies targeted to T cells, including anti-CD4 monoclonal antibodies[79] and T cell leukapheresis[80] also suggest involvement of cell-mediated immunity.

T cells in human lupus nephritis

T cells are present in glomeruli in crescentic human lupus nephritis,[81,82] and there is a positive correlation between interstitial T cell accumulation, the histological severity of injury, and renal function.[83] The presence of a restricted Vβ usage by T cells in renal biopsies of patients with lupus nephritis suggests that these T cells are not nonspecifically recruited but are oligoclonal and potentially antigen-specific.[81,84] Human studies provide conflicting evidence for the role of Th1- and Th2-biased responses in human lupus nephritis. Higher serum and glomerular IL-18 levels in patients with lupus nephritis compared to non-nephritic patients, and high IFNγ and low IL-4 levels in peripheral blood lymphocytes, suggest that a Th1-biased response is associated with development of nephritis.[85] Glomerular expression of CD40 and a high ratio of Th1/Th2 cytokine-expressing cells in crescentic/proliferative lupus nephritis compared to non-crescentic nephritis[86] is consistent with involvement of Th1 responses in crescentic injury. However, in children with lupus nephritis, both Th1 and Th2 antibody isotypes were observed in glomeruli.[87] Expression of IL-4 and IL-10 mRNA in the absence of IFNγ[84] in patients with crescentic nephritis is consistent with a Th2 phenotype, as is expression of the CCR4 chemokine receptor on intrarenal CD4+ cells.[88] However, another study of Class IV lupus nephritis has reported high expression of the Th1-associated chemokine receptor CCR5 in extracapillary lesions and decreased expression following glucocorticoid therapy.[89]

Evidence is now emerging for the participation of Th17 cells in human lupus nephritis. Increased serum levels of IL-17 have been found in patients with SLE,[90] although these levels did not correlate with disease activity of SLE (SLEDAI) or the presence of lupus nephritis.[91] Elispot analysis has confirmed that increased numbers of IL-17-producing CD4+ cells were present in the circulation of lupus patients.[92] These authors were able to show increased levels of IL-23 and IL-17 in the serum of patients, correlating with activity (SLEDAI) and renal impairment. Furthermore, *in vitro*, these IL-17 producing blood mononuclear cells responded to IL-23 with increased IL-17 secretion, consistent with a Th17 response. However, these responses were not antigen-specific and the patients also had elevated IL-12 levels. Lupus patients have been shown to have circulating double-negative T cells that respond to CD3 stimulation with enhanced IL-17 production, and double-negative cells and IL-17 positive cells in their kidneys, supporting a role for Th17 cells in lupus nephritis.[93] Analysis of gene polymorphisms has been used to provide evidence for dysregulated or enhanced expression of genes involved in CD4+ T cell differentiation. Such analysis has been applied to the IL-23 receptor genes in lupus patients; however, this failed to show differences between these patients and normal populations.[94]

T regulatory cells in crescentic GN

T regulatory cells (Tregs) are a subset of T cells involved in the induction and maintenance of peripheral tolerance. T cells with immunosuppressive capacities were described in the 1970s[95] as ill-defined heterogeneous populations. The field progressed slowly until specific phenotypic markers were discovered. Candidate markers now number over 30.[95] Several subtypes of Tregs have been described, including CD4+,CD25+ T cells, T regulatory cells (Tr1) and Th3 cells. The best known are naturally occurring Tregs. These can be thymically derived or generated in the periphery. Thymically derived "naturally" occurring Tregs are CD4+ CD25+ and express Foxp3. They suppress both CD4+ and CD8+ effector cells in an antigen- and cytokine-independent, but cell–cell contact-dependent, manner.[96] Adaptive or induced Tregs are generated from CD4+ CD25- cells in the periphery in the presence of TGFβ, which induces Foxp3 expression. They have the same phenotype and function as thymically derived Tregs, but use TGFβ and IL-10 in their suppressive effects.[97]

Th3 cells have been reported in the context of murine autoimmunity and the generation of oral tolerance in experimental autoimmune encephalomyelitis (EAE), where they can adoptively transfer suppression by antigen-independent, cell–cell contact- and TGFβ-dependent mechanisms. Tr1 cells are induced from CD4+ cells by repeated antigenic stimulation in the presence of IL-10 or antigen presentation by immature APCs. They function by IL-10 generation and induce suppression by cell–cell-independent mechanisms.[98]

Although regulatory cells are traditionally regarded as T cells, it is now apparent that other cells, including B cells, CD8 cells, NK cells, and APCs, can also serve immunoregulatory roles.[99] Impairment of Treg function has the potential to contribute to the development of autoimmune forms of GN and augmentation of Treg function has been suggested as a potential therapeutic strategy. Regulatory T cell activity has been demonstrated in the peripheral blood of patients following remission of Goodpasture's syndrome, but not during the acute illness.[61] These cells were capable of suppressing autoreactive T cells, and their activity was associated with a CD4+,CD25+ phenotype. The potential for CD4+,CD25+ Tregs to attenuate experimental anti-GBM GN has been demonstrated in mice developing nephrotoxic nephritis.[100] Transfer of CD4+,CD25+ cells from naïve mice decreases glomerular T cells and macrophage accumulation and suppresses development of GN, but CD4+,CD25+ cells from nephritic mice aggravated disease.[100] Transferred cells traffick predominantly to secondary lymphoid organs.

The role of Tregs in lupus has been examined through clinical observations and studies in lupus-prone mouse strains. As yet, there is no clear evidence for a single common abnormality of Tregs that could make a major contribution to the immunopathogenesis of the disease. Murine studies allow proof-of-concept experiments, through deletion or transfer of Treg populations. Neonatal thymectomy at day 3 results in systemic Treg depletion. In lupus-prone SNF1 mice, neonatal thymectomy resulted in initial acceleration of autoantibody production, but organ-specific autoimmune injury was reduced.[101] Genetically autoimmune prone mice developed organ-specific autoimmunity and lupus with expanded autoreactive T cell populations and enhanced autoantibody production. Transfer of CD4+,CD25+ T cells (enriched for Tregs) from syngeneic mice suppressed these effects.[102] Transfer of other Treg subpopulations, including *ex vivo* TGFβ-generated Tregs[103] and *ex vivo* expanded Tregs, have similarly shown beneficial effects.[104]

Clinical studies of patients with active lupus have reported reduced percentages of circulating Tregs,[105] but this is not confirmed in other studies.[106] At least some of these discrepancies relate to difficulties in defining and enumerating Tregs in the circulation. Other differences in these studies relate to the patterns of disease and disease activity, as well as the therapeutic agents used in the patients. The availability and specificity of Foxp3 and other phenotypic markers are now allowing more precise and standardized functional analysis. Research studies employing these strategies have, in general, failed to demonstrate abnormal reduction in Tregs in lupus.[107] Some studies even show an increase in Tregs in active disease.[108]

Although studies show few abnormalities of Treg numbers and function in lupus patients, abnormal suppression of T and B effectors is clearly present. This may be due to a failure of suppressibility of effector cells themselves, rather than changes in Tregs. Several factors may contribute to these abnormalities. Vigorous production of inflammatory cytokines can antagonize the capacity of regulatory T cells to attenuate chronic inflammation.[109] These cytokines may overactivate intracellular signaling pathways, inducing hyporesponsiveness to Treg suppression.[110] There is also evidence that APCs from patients with lupus can suppress Treg function through excessive IFNα production.[108]

NK cells and NKT cells in crescentic GN and lupus

Natural killer cells comprise 5–15% of circulating leukocytes, and also reside in bone marrow, lymph nodes, spleen, and liver.[111,112] They were originally identified as important effector cells in viral infections and tumor cytotoxicity. Recently, subpopulations of NK cells with distinct phenotypic and functional properties have been identified in humans and mice.[113] The major subgroup in the blood and spleen are strongly cytotoxic NK cells that express high levels of CD16, dim CD56, and produce IFNγ.[113] They recognize cells expressing reduced levels of MHC I (the "missing self" hypothesis[114]) and/or "stress ligands," and their activation is regulated by a balance of activating and inhibitory receptors.[115] Unlike T cells and B cells, they do not require priming and thus have the capacity to be early responders. A second subgroup of CD56(high),

CD16- NK cells are present in lymph nodes and have important immunomodulatory functions. They show poor cytotoxic activity, but have high cytokine production. They have the capacity to regulate dendritic cell function and modulate T cell priming and effector responses by direct cellular interactions and via cytokine production.[116] Despite the significant numerical contribution of NK cells to leukocyte subsets and increasing knowledge of their immunoregulatory functions, there is very little known about their role in GN. Circulating NK cell numbers and cytotoxicity activity have been reported to be reduced in patients with lupus[117] and in first-degree relatives of patients with lupus,[118,119] and, conversely, increased numbers of immunoregulatory, CD56(bright),CD16- NK cells have been demonstrated in the blood of patients with lupus.[120] There are no studies of the functional contribution of NK cells to GN.

In contrast to our knowledge of the role of NK cells, there is increasing interest in the role of NKT cells in GN. A number of studies of their functional contribution have recently been published, although a clear consensus on their contribution to injury has not yet emerged. Natural killer T cells are a subset of T cells with a restricted T cell receptor (TCR) repertoire, which recognize lipid and glycolipid antigens presented on an MHC I-like molecule, CD1d. In C57BL/6 mice, NKT cells express the cell surface marker NK1.1.[121] Two subsets of NKT cells have been identified, invariant NKT cells (iNKT cells), which have a highly restricted T cell receptor containing Vα14-Jα18 in mice and Vα24-Jα18 in humans, and type II or non-iNKT cells, which express a more diverse TCR repertoire. Invariant natural killer T cells respond to the marine sponge-derived glycolipid α-galactosylceramide (α-GalCer), closely related to microbial glycolipids and the self-antigen iGb3.[121] Following TCR ligation, they rapidly produce a variety of Th1 and Th2 cytokines, which can result in activation of dendritic cells, NK cells, B cells, and conventional T cells.[122] The antigen specificity of the more diverse TCR repertoire of type II NKT cells is unknown.

The roles of NKT cells and the iNKT cell subset have been investigated in murine models of GN. Whereas genetic CD1d deficiency, which results in failure of development of all NKT cells, exacerbates the development of pristine-induced lupus-like nephritis,[123] NZB-NZW lupus nephritis,[124] and nephrotoxic nephritis[125] in mice, administration of blocking anti-CD1d antibodies has been shown to augment Th2 responses, delay onset of proteinuria, and prolong survival in NZB/W mice.[126] Prolonged inhibition of NKT cells by administration of anti-NK1.1 antibodies in NZB/W mice also ameliorated lupus.[127]

Circulating iNKT cell numbers have been shown to correlate with disease activity in patients with lupus, with a reduction in active disease and return towards normal with disease remission.[128] However, in NZB/W mice, expansion and hyperactivity of iNKT cells has been reported during the development and progression of lupus.[129] Invariant natural killer T cell activation by administration of α-GalCer enhanced Th1 responses and aggravated lupus in NZB/W mice.[126] In experimental models involving Jα18-deficient mice, iNKT cells have also been shown to be associated with protection from GN. Jα281 (now known as Jα18)-deficient mice spontaneously developed anti-DNA and anticardiolipin antibodies, and glomerular damage on aging,[130] and Jα18-deficient mice developed more severe anti-GBM GN, which was attributed to loss of the reno-protective effect mediated via TGFβ production.[131]

Dendritic cells, TLRs, and type I interferons

Dendritic cells play a pivotal role in initiation of immune responses through their ability to present antigen to naïve T cells in secondary lymphoid organs and to influence the effector pathways adopted by T cells following activation. They share many functional and phenotypic properties with macrophages,[132] and it has been suggested that these two cell types may be considered as different ends of a common lineage spectrum.[133] A number of subsets of dendritic cells, with different phenotypic and functional attributes have been recognized. Human and murine dendritic cell subsets share many similarities but are not entirely analogous. Conventional (myeloid) dendritic cells are widely distributed throughout the body. They express high levels of CD11c and are classical APCs. In mice, they have been further divided into CD11b+,CD8-,CD24- cells that migrate from peripheral tissues and present antigen to CD4+ T cells in lymph nodes and CD11b-,CD8+,CD24+ dendritic cells, which reside in lymphatic tissues and are involved antigen cross-presentation, activation, or tolerization of T cells.[134] Other dendritic cell subsets include plasmacytoid dendritic cells and Langerhans cells. Plasmacytoid dendritic cells express low levels of CD11c, as well as the B cell marker, B220 and Gr-1, a myeloid lineage marker, and produce type I interferons on stimulation by bacterial CpG or viral infections. Langerhans cells reside in the skin, express langerin, and migrate to regional lymph nodes upon activation. The antigen presentation capacity of Langerhans cells is greatly enhanced following maturation by exposure to granulocyte macrophage colony-stimulating factor.[135]

Recent advances in techniques to identify and isolate dendritic cells in renal tissues have facilitated investigation of their role in crescentic GN. CD11c-positive cells have been isolated from normal mouse kidneys and functionally characterized as dendritic cells.[136] Many of these cells express low or intermediate levels of F4/80 and CD11b, and have been previously assumed to be resident tissue macrophages.[137] Morphological examination of kidneys from CX3CR1[GFP/+] "knock-in" mice, which express green fluorescent protein (GFP) in CX3CR1+ (fractalkine receptor) cells, revealed an intricate contiguous network of dendritic cells in the renal interstitium.[138] CX3CR1 is expressed on a common dendritic cell/macrophage precursor cell.[139] As flow cytometry of isolated renal leukocytes revealed significant mismatch between GFP and CD11c expression,[138] the identity of GFP+ cells in glomeruli that lacked stellate morphology is uncertain. In human crescentic GN, glomerular CX3CR1+ cells appear to correspond with infiltrating macrophages and T cells.[140]

Kidney dendritic cells have been shown to traffic to the renal lymph node following lipopolysaccharide challenge and to stimulate CD4+ T cell proliferation.[141] Interstitial CD11c+ dendritic cell numbers increase during the development of nephrotoxic nephritis in periglomerular and perivascular locations.[136] Renal dendritic cells from nephritic mice express inducible co-stimulator ligand (ICOSL, an inducer of IL-10) and stimulate antigen-specific proliferation and IL-10 secretion by CD4+ T cells ex vivo.[142] Depletion of dendritic cells in CD11c-DTR/GFP mice developing nephrotoxic nephritis showed no effect on macrophage recruitment after a single dose of diphtheria toxin 4 days after disease initiation, but aggravation of histological and functional injury following a second dose later in the disease (day 11–14), suggesting that renal dendritic cells may ameliorate CD4+T cell-dependent renal injury by stimulating IL-10 production. Functional evidence for a proinflammatory role for renal dendritic cells has been provided in a model of renal inflammation induced by co-administration of ovalbumin-specific CD4+ and CD8+ T cell lines to mice, which express ovalbumin in their podocytes.[143] In this model, dendritic cells in the renal lymph node were shown to be involved in antigen cross-presentation. Dendritic cells in the renal interstitium were shown to contribute to development of perivascular leukocyte infiltration. In murine lupus nephritis, reduction of circulating, splenic, and renal dendritic cells by inhibition of p38 mitogen activated protein kinase (MAPK) has been associated with reduced renal injury.[144]

In normal human kidneys, different subtypes of dendritic cells have been identified in interstitial areas and often around, but rarely within, glomeruli.[145] The staining pattern of the myeloid dendritic cell marker DC-SIGN extensively overlapped with CD68, suggesting that most interstitial macrophages are, in fact, dendritic cells. A more recent study suggests that the population of DC-SIGN+ renal interstitial cells is smaller than the CD68+ cell population,[146] meaning that not all interstitial CD68+ cells are dendritic cells. Plasmacytoid (BDCA-2+) dendritic cells were also identified in the renal interstitium. Their frequency was approximately one-quarter that of myeloid (BDCA-1+) dendritic cells.[145] In human proliferative GN, including lupus nephritis and necrotizing GN, CD68+ cells were abundant in glomeruli and the tubulointerstitium.[146] In the interstitium, the majority of CD68+ cells were also DC-SIGN+, but DC-SIGN+ cells were not detected in glomerular tufts despite prominent presence of CD68+ macrophages. In non-proliferative forms of GN (focal and segmental glomerulosclerosis (FSGS) and minimal change disease), although CD68+ macrophage numbers were not increased, interstitial CD-SIGN+ cells appeared mildly increased.

Signals such as those provided via TLRs and type I interferons play an important role in modulating dendritic cell function and provide a link between innate and adaptive immunity.[147] Toll-like receptors comprise a family of 11 receptors that have the capacity to recognize highly conserved exogenous ligands associated with pathogenic microorganisms ("pattern associated molecular patterns" or PAMPS) and to augment innate immune mechanisms, such as opsonization and phagocytosis of bacteria and viruses, activation of the complement and coagulation cascades, and production of type 1 interferons. They can also recognize a number of endogenous ligands, including components of necrotic and apoptotic cells[148] and Tamm–Horsfall protein in urine[149] and have the capacity to modulate adaptive immune responses, via effects on dendritic cells, T helper subset differentiation, and immune tolerance.[147]

Studies, particularly in murine lupus nephritis, indicate relevance of these effects to crescentic GN, although the precise nature of their role is controversial. Toll-like receptor 9 is of particular interest because of evidence that some currently effective therapies for human lupus (e.g. chloroquine) inhibit TLR9[150] and because of the use of synthetic TLR9 agonist in humans,[151] but reports of its role are inconsistent. Toll-like receptor 9 agonist ligands augment autoimmune responses and GN in lupus-prone MRL[lpr/lpr] mice,[152] and inhibitory ligands block disease.[153] Toll-like receptor 9 deficiency in lupus-prone mice has been reported to increase autoimmunity and

GN,[154] and to reduce anti-DNA antibodies without protecting from renal disease.[155] Currently, TLR9 is regarded as a potential therapeutic target in SLE.[156] There is also conflicting evidence for the involvement of TLR3 in lupus nephritis. Toll-like receptor 3 agonists aggravated nephritis in MRL[lpr/lpr] mice without altering anti-DNA antibodies[157] (suggesting the possibility of direct effects on mesangial cells), whereas anti-DNA antibodies and renal injury were unaffected in TLR3-deficient lupus-prone mice.[155] The ability of a TLR7 ligand to aggravate nephritis in MRL[lpr/lpr] mice has also been reported.[158,159] In B6.Sle1Yaa mice development of lupus is associated with over-expression of TLR7, whereas disease is prevented by genetic deletion of TLR7.[160]

There is accumulating evidence for an important role of type I interferons in autoimmunity and lupus. Elevated serum levels of IFNα in patients with active lupus suggest it may have a functional role in modulation of disease activity.[161,162] Serum of patients with lupus has been shown to induce production of IFNα by plasmacytoid dendritic cells[163] and to induce monocyte differentiation to dendritic cells via IFNα.[164] Microarray analysis of peripheral blood mononuclear cells shows induction of IFNα-responsive genes in patients with SLE, establishing the signature of IFNα involvement consistent with the resulting pattern of inflammation.[165–167] Furthermore, type I interferon treatment of patients with hepatitis C and carcinoid tumors can result in development of lupus-associated autoantibodies, autoimmune manifestations, and, in some cases, clinical SLE.[168,169] At the experimental level, immune complexes containing DNA and RNA have been shown to be potent inducers of IFNα.[170] Blocking studies suggest that these events require the FcγR2 receptor.[171] In murine models of lupus, deficiency of type I interferon receptors reduced autoantibody production and clinical manifestations of lupus, including GN.[172]

These data suggest that in lupus, autoantibodies can combine with DNA antigens to engage Fc receptors on dendritic cells. Internalization of these antigens allows their presentation to intracytoplasmic TLRs, including TLR7, 8 and 9, resulting in IFNα production, which upregulates proinflammatory response genes in immune cells, and enhances immune complex formation and inflammatory injury in target organs. These observations have led to the view that type I interferons are a potential therapeutic target in lupus. This hypothesis is currently being tested by clinical trials in lupus using neutralizing monoclonal antibodies to IFNα. A cautionary note is provided by observations that in some circumstances IFNα can inhibit immune activation, for example in Th1-mediated inflammation.[173–175]

Thus, in the normal kidney, dendritic cells provide an intricate interstitial network of processes anatomically suited to sampling filtered antigens. Their presence is enhanced in proliferative GN and their activation is modulated by TLR-activating ligands and type I interferons. They have the capacity to traffic to the renal lymph node, to stimulate T cell proliferation, and to modulate inflammatory responses involved in the development of renal injury in lupus and other forms of GN.

Conclusion

T cell-directed adaptive immunity underpins many forms of GN and particularly crescentic GN. T cell-driven autoimmunity and Th1 cell-driven effector mechanisms play an important role in crescentic human GN. The involvement of Th17 cells and regulatory T cells is currently poorly understood. There is an increasing awareness of the important role of dendritic cells, TLRs, and type I interferons in autoimmunity and lupus, which is revealing potential new therapeutic targets that may result in new therapies for autoimmune crescentic GN.

References

1. Korn, T., Bettelli, E., Gao, W., Awasthi, A., *et al.* (2007) IL-21 initiates an alternative pathway to induce proinflammatory T(H)17 cells. *Nature* **448**, 484–7.

2. Bettelli, E., Korn, T., and Kuchroo, V.K. (2007) Th17: the third member of the effector T cell trilogy. *Curr Opin Immunol* **19**, 652–7.

3. King, C., Tangye, S.G., and Mackay, C.R. (2008) T follicular helper (TFH) cells in normal and dysregulated immune responses. *Annu Rev Immunol* **26**, 741–66.

4. Eddahri, F., Denanglaire, S., Bureau, F., Spolski, R., *et al.* (2009) Interleukin-6/STAT3 signaling regulates the ability of naive T cells to acquire B-cell help capacities. *Blood* **113**, 2426–33.

5. Vogelzang, A., McGuire, H.M., Yu, D., Sprent, J., *et al.* (2008) A fundamental role for interleukin-21 in the generation of T follicular helper cells. *Immunity* **29**, 127–37.

6. Stachura, I., Si, L., and Whiteside, T.L. (1984) Mononuclear-cell subsets in human idiopathic crescentic glomerulonephritis (ICGN): analysis in tissue sections with monoclonal antibodies. *J Clin Immunol* **4**, 202–8.

7. Neale, T.J., Tipping, P.G., Carson, S.D., and Holdsworth, S.R. (1988) Participation of cell-mediated immunity in deposition of fibrin in glomerulonephritis. *Lancet* **2**, 421–4.

8. Huang, X.R., Holdsworth, S.R., and Tipping, P.G. (1994) Evidence for delayed-type hypersensitivity mechanisms in glomerular crescent formation. *Kidney Int* **46**, 69–78.

9. Tipping, P.G., Huang, X.R., Qi, M., Van, G.Y., *et al.* (1998) Crescentic glomerulonephritis in CD4- and CD8-deficient mice. Requirement for CD4 but not CD8 cells. *Am J Pathol* **152**, 1541–8.

10. Li, S., Holdsworth, S.R., and Tipping, P.G. (1997) Antibody independent crescentic glomerulonephritis in mu chain deficient mice. *Kidney Int* **51**, 672–8.

11. Reynolds, J., and Pusey, C.D. (1994) In vivo treatment with a monoclonal antibody to T helper cells in experimental autoimmune glomerulonephritis in the BN rat. *Clin Exp Immunol* **95**, 122–7.

12. Kalluri, R., Danoff, T.M., Okada, H., and Neilson, E.G. (1997) Susceptibility to anti-glomerular basement membrane disease and Goodpasture syndrome is linked to MHC class II genes and the emergence of T cell-mediated immunity in mice. *J Clin Invest* **100**, 2263–75.

13. Jabs, D.A., Burek, C.L., Hu, Q., Kuppers, R.C., *et al.* (1992) Anti-CD4 monoclonal antibody therapy suppresses autoimmune disease in MRL/Mp-lpr/lpr mice. *Cell Immunol* **141**, 496–507.

14. Connolly, K., Roubinian, J.R., and Wofsy, D. (1992) Development of murine lupus in CD4-depleted NZB/NZW mice. Sustained inhibition of residual CD4+ T cells is required to suppress autoimmunity. *J Immunol* **149**, 3083–8.

15. Hopfer, H., Maron, R., Butzmann, U., Helmchen, U., *et al.* (2003) The importance of cell-mediated immunity in the course and severity of autoimmune anti-glomerular basement membrane disease in mice. *Faseb J* **17**, 860–8.

16. Kitching, A.R., Turner, A.L., Wilson, G.R., Semple, T., *et al.* (2005) IL-12p40 and IL-18 in crescentic glomerulonephritis: IL-12p40 is the key Th1-defining cytokine chain, whereas IL-18 promotes local inflammation and leukocyte recruitment. *J Am Soc Nephrol* **16**, 2023–33.

17. Kitching, A.R., Holdsworth, S.R., and Tipping, P.G. (1999) IFN-gamma mediates crescent formation and cell-mediated immune injury in murine glomerulonephritis. *J Am Soc Nephrol* **10**, 752–9.

18. Kitching, A.R., Tipping, P.G., and Holdsworth, S.R. (1999) IL-12 directs severe renal injury, crescent formation and Th1 responses in murine glomerulonephritis. *Eur J Immunol* **29**, 1–10.

19. Kitching, A.R., Tipping, P.G., Kurimoto, M., and Holdsworth, S.R. (2000) IL-18 has IL-12-independent effects in delayed-type hypersensitivity: studies in cell-mediated crescentic glomerulonephritis. *J Immunol* **165**, 4649–57.

20. Kitching, A.R., Tipping, P.G., Mutch, D.A., Huang, X.R., *et al.* (1998) Interleukin-4 deficiency enhances Th1 responses and crescentic glomerulonephritis in mice. *Kidney Int* **53**, 112–18.

21. Kitching, A.R., Tipping, P.G., Timoshanko, J.R., and Holdsworth, S.R. (2000) Endogenous interleukin-10 regulates Th1 responses that induce crescentic glomerulonephritis. *Kidney Int* **57**, 518–25.

22. Tipping, P.G., Kitching, A.R., Huang, X.R., Mutch, D.A., *et al.* (1997) Immune modulation with interleukin-4 and interleukin-10 prevents crescent formation and glomerular injury in experimental glomerulonephritis. *Eur J Immunol* **27**, 530–7.

23. Kitching, A.R., Tipping, P.G., Huang, X.R., Mutch, D.A., *et al.* (1997) Interleukin-4 and interleukin-10 attenuate established crescentic glomerulonephritis in mice. *Kidney Int* **52**, 52–9.

24. Cook, H.T., Singh, S.J., Wembridge, D.E., Smith, J., *et al.* (1999) Interleukin-4 ameliorates crescentic glomerulonephritis in Wistar Kyoto rats. *Kidney Int* **55**, 1319–26.

25. Haas, C., Ryffel, B., and Le Hir, M. (1997) IFN-gamma is essential for the development of autoimmune glomerulonephritis in MRL/Ipr mice. *J Immunol* **158**, 5484–91.

26. Santiago, M.L., Fossati, L., Jacquet, C., Muller, W., *et al.* (1997) Interleukin-4 protects against a genetically linked lupus-like autoimmune syndrome. *J Exp Med* **185**, 65–70.

27. Huang, X.R., Tipping, P.G., Apostolopoulos, J., Oettinger, C., *et al.* (1997) Mechanisms of T cell-induced glomerular injury in anti-glomerular basement membrane (GBM) glomerulonephritis in rats. *Clin Exp Immunol* **109**, 134–42.

28. Timoshanko, J.R., Holdsworth, S.R., Kitching, A.R., and Tipping, P.G. (2002) IFN-gamma production by intrinsic renal cells and bone marrow-derived cells is required for full expression of crescentic glomerulonephritis in mice. *J Immunol* **168**, 4135–41.

29. Timoshanko, J.R., Kitching, A.R., Holdsworth, S.R., and Tipping, P.G. (2001) Interleukin-12 from intrinsic cells is an effector of renal injury in crescentic glomerulonephritis. *J Am Soc Nephrol* **12**, 464–71.

30. Timoshanko, J.R., Kitching, A.R., Iwakura, Y., Holdsworth, S.R., *et al.* (2004) Contributions of IL-1beta and IL-1alpha to crescentic glomerulonephritis in mice. *J Am Soc Nephrol* **15**, 910–18.

31. Lawson, B.R., Koundouris, S.I., Barnhouse, M., Dummer, W., *et al.* (2001) The role of alpha beta+ T cells and homeostatic T cell proliferation in Y-chromosome-associated murine lupus. *J Immunol* **167**, 2354–60.

32. Seery, J.P., Wang, E.C., Cattell, V., Carroll, J.M., *et al.* (1999) A central role for alpha beta T cells in the pathogenesis of murine lupus. *J Immunol* **162**, 7241–8.

33. Peng, S.L., Madaio, M.P., Hughes, D.P., Crispe, I.N., *et al.* (1996) Murine lupus in the absence of alpha beta T cells. *J Immunol* **156**, 4041–9.

34. Peng, S.L., McNiff, J.M., Madaio, M.P., Ma, J., *et al.* (1997) alpha beta T cell regulation and CD40 ligand dependence in murine systemic autoimmunity. *J Immunol* **158**, 2464–70.

35. Drake, C.G., and Kotzin, B.L. (1992) Superantigens: biology, immunology, and potential role in disease. *J Clin Immunol* **12**, 149–62.

36. Mysler, E., Bini, P., Drappa, J., Ramos, P., *et al.* (1994) The apoptosis-1/Fas protein in human systemic lupus erythematosus. *J Clin Invest* **93**, 1029–34.

37. Liu, M.-F., Wang, C.-R., Fung, L.-L., and Wu, C.-R. (2004) Decreased CD4+CD25+ T Cells in Peripheral Blood of Patients with Systemic Lupus Erythematosus. *Scand J Immunol* **59**, 198–202.

38. Bagavant, H., Deshmukh, U.S., Gaskin, F., and Fu, S.M. (2004) Lupus glomerulonephritis revisited 2004: autoimmunity and end-organ damage. *Scand J Immunol* **60**, 52–63.

39. Chan, O.T., Hannum, L.G., Haberman, A.M., Madaio, M.P., *et al.* (1999) A novel mouse with B cells but lacking serum antibody reveals an antibody-independent role for B cells in murine lupus. *J Exp Med* **189**, 1639–48.

40. Bloom, R.D., O'Connor, T., Cizman, B., Kalluri, R., *et al.* (2002) Intrathymic kidney cells delay the onset of lupus nephritis in MRL-lpr/lpr mice. *Int Immunol* **14**, 867–71.

41. Singh, R.R., Saxena, V., Zang, S., Li, L., *et al.* (2003) Differential contribution of IL-4 and STAT6 vs STAT4 to the development of lupus nephritis. *J Immunol* **170**, 4818–25.

42. Paust, H.J., Turner, J.E., Steinmetz, O.M., Peters, A., *et al.* (2009) The IL-23/Th17 axis contributes to renal injury in experimental glomerulonephritis. *J Am Soc Nephrol* **20**, 969–79.

43. Ooi, J.D., Phoon, R.K., Holdsworth, S.R., and Kitching, A.R. (2009) IL-23, not IL-12, directs autoimmunity to the Goodpasture antigen. *J Am Soc Nephrol* **20**, 980–9.

44. Wang, Y., Ito, S., Chino, Y., Iwanami, K., *et al.* (2008) Use of laser microdissection in the analysis of renal-infiltrating T cells in MRL/lpr mice. *Mod Rheumatol* **18**, 385–93.

45. Jacob, N., Yang, H., Pricop, L., Liu, Y., *et al.* (2009) Accelerated pathological and clinical nephritis in systemic lupus erythematosus-prone New Zealand Mixed 2328 mice doubly deficient in TNF receptor 1 and TNF receptor 2 via a Th17-associated pathway. *J Immunol* **182**, 2532–41.

46. Hsu, H.C., Yang, P., Wang, J., Wu, Q., *et al.* (2008) Interleukin 17-producing T helper cells and interleukin 17 orchestrate autoreactive germinal center development in autoimmune BXD2 mice. *Nat Immunol* **9**, 166–75.

47. Bubier, J.A., Sproule, T.J., Foreman, O., Spolski, R., *et al.* (2009) A critical role for IL-21 receptor signaling in the pathogenesis of systemic lupus erythematosus in BXSB-Yaa mice. *Proc Natl Acad Sci U S A* **106**, 1518–23.

48. Tarlinton, D. (2008) IL-17 drives germinal center B cells? *Nat Immunol* **9**, 124–6.

49. Sonderegger, I., Kisielow, J., Meier, R., King, C., *et al.* (2008) IL-21 and IL-21R are not required for development of Th17 cells and autoimmunity in vivo. *Eur J Immunol* **38**, 1833–8.

50. Holmdahl, R. (2008) IL-21 and autoimmune disease–hypothesis and reality? *Eur J Immunol* **38**, 1800–2.

51. Wu, J., Hicks, J., Ou, C., Singleton, D., *et al.* (2001) Glomerulonephritis induced by recombinant collagen IV alpha 3 chain noncollagen domain 1 is not associated with glomerular basement membrane antibody: a potential T cell-mediated mechanism. *J Immunol* **167**, 2388–95.

52. Wu, J., Hicks, J., Borillo, J., Glass, W.F., 2nd, *et al.* (2002) CD4(+) T cells specific to a glomerular basement membrane antigen mediate glomerulonephritis. *J Clin Invest* **109**, 517–24.

53. Wu, J., Borillo, J., Glass, W.F., Hicks, J., *et al.* (2003) T-cell epitope of alpha3 chain of type IV collagen induces severe glomerulonephritis. *Kidney Int* **64**, 1292–301.

54. Fisher, M., Pusey, C.D., Vaughan, R.W., and Rees, A.J. (1997) Susceptibility to anti-glomerular basement membrane disease is strongly associated with HLA-DRB1 genes. *Kidney Int* **51**, 222–9.

55. Derry, C.J., Ross, C.N., Lombardi, G., Mason, P.D., *et al.* (1995) Analysis of T cell responses to the autoantigen in Goodpasture's disease. *Clin Exp Immunol* **100**, 262–8.

56. Phelps, R.G., Jones, V.L., Coughlan, M., Turner, A.N., *et al.* (1998) Presentation of the Goodpasture autoantigen to CD4 T cells is influenced more by processing constraints than by HLA class II peptide binding preferences. *J Biol Chem* **273**, 11440–7.

57. Cairns, L.S., Phelps, R.G., Bowie, L., Hall, A.M., *et al.* (2003) The fine specificity and cytokine profile of T-helper cells responsive to the alpha3 chain of type IV collagen in Goodpasture's disease. *J Am Soc Nephrol* **14**, 2801–12.

58. Netzer, K.O., Leinonen, A., Boutaud, A., Borza, D.B., *et al.* (1999) The goodpasture autoantigen. Mapping the major conformational epitope(s) of alpha3(IV) collagen to residues 17-31 and 127-141 of the NC1 domain. *J Biol Chem* **274**, 11267–74.

59. Wong, D., Phelps, R.G., and Turner, A.N. (2001) The Goodpasture antigen is expressed in the human thymus. *Kidney Int* **60**, 1777–83.

60. Salama, A.D., Chaudhry, A.N., Ryan, J.J., Eren, E., *et al.* (2001) In Goodpasture's disease, CD4(+) T cells escape thymic deletion and are reactive with the autoantigen alpha3(IV) NC1. *J Am Soc Nephrol* **12**, 1908–15.

61. Salama, A.D., Chaudhry, A.N., Holthaus, K.A., Mosley, K., *et al.* (2003) Regulation by CD25+ lymphocytes of autoantigen-specific T-cell responses in Goodpasture's (anti-GBM) disease. *Kidney Int* **64**, 1685–94.

62. Reynolds, J., and Pusey, C.D. (2001) Oral administration of glomerular basement membrane prevents the development of experimental autoimmune glomerulonephritis in the WKY rat. *J Am Soc Nephrol* **12**, 61–70.

63. Cunningham, M.A., Huang, X.R., Dowling, J.P., Tipping, P.G., *et al.* (1999) Prominence of cell-mediated immunity effectors in 'pauci-immune' glomerulonephritis. *J Am Soc Nephrol* **10**, 499–506.

64. Weidner, S., Geuss, S., Hafezi-Rachti, S., Wonka, A., *et al.* (2004) ANCA-associated vasculitis with renal involvement: an outcome analysis. *Nephrol Dial Transplant* **19**, 1403–11.

65. Brouwer, E., Tervaert, J.W., Horst, G., Huitema, M.G., *et al.* (1991) Predominance of IgG1 and IgG4 subclasses of anti-neutrophil cytoplasmic autoantibodies (ANCA) in patients with Wegener's granulomatosis and clinically related disorders. *Clin Exp Immunol* **83**, 379–86.

66. Brouwer, E., Huitema, M.G., Klok, P.A., de Weerd, H., *et al.* (1993) Antimyeloperoxidase-associated proliferative glomerulonephritis: an animal model. *J Exp Med* **177**, 905–14.

67. Xiao, H., Heeringa, P., Hu, P., Liu, Z., *et al.* (2002) Antineutrophil cytoplasmic autoantibodies specific for myeloperoxidase cause glomerulonephritis and vasculitis in mice. *J Clin Invest* **110**, 955–63.

68. Mellbye, O.J., Mollnes, T.E., and Steen, L.S. (1994) IgG subclass distribution and complement activation ability of autoantibodies to neutrophil cytoplasmic antigens (ANCA). *Clin Immunol Immunopathol* **70**, 32–9.

69. Csernok, E., Trabandt, A., Muller, A., Wang, G.C., *et al.* (1999) Cytokine profiles in Wegener's granulomatosis: predominance of type 1 (Th1) in the granulomatous inflammation. *Arthritis Rheum* **42**, 742–50.

70. Muller, A., Trabandt, A., Gloeckner-Hofmann, K., Seitzer, U., *et al.* (2000) Localized Wegener's granulomatosis: predominance of CD26 and IFN-gamma expression. *J Pathol* **192**, 113–20.

71. Cockwell, P., Brooks, C.J., Adu, D., and Savage, C.O. (1999) Interleukin-8: A pathogenetic role in antineutrophil cytoplasmic autoantibody-associated glomerulonephritis. *Kidney Int* **55**, 852–63.

72. Balding, C.E., Howie, A.J., Drake-Lee, A.B., and Savage, C.O. (2001) Th2 dominance in nasal mucosa in patients with Wegener's granulomatosis. *Clin Exp Immunol* **125**, 332–9.

73. Rasmussen, N., and Petersen, J. (1993) Cellular immune responses and pathogenesis in c-ANCA positive vasculitides. *J Autoimmun* **6**, 227–36.

74. Griffith, M.E., Coulthart, A., and Pusey, C.D. (1996) T cell responses to myeloperoxidase (MPO) and proteinase 3 (PR3) in patients with systemic vasculitis. *Clin Exp Immunol* **103**, 253–8.

75. Popa, E.R., Franssen, C.F., Limburg, P.C., Huitema, M.G., *et al.* (2002) In vitro cytokine production and proliferation of T cells from patients with anti-proteinase 3- and antimyeloperoxidase-associated vasculitis, in response to proteinase 3 and myeloperoxidase. *Arthritis Rheum* **46**, 1894–904.

76. Mathieson, P.W., Lockwood, C.M., and Oliveira, D.B. (1992) T and B cell responses to neutrophil cytoplasmic antigens in systemic vasculitis. *Clin Immunol Immunopathol* **63**, 135–41.

77. Brouwer, E., Stegeman, C.A., Huitema, M.G., Limburg, P.C., *et al.* (1994) T cell reactivity to proteinase 3 and myeloperoxidase in patients with Wegener's granulomatosis (WG). *Clin Exp Immunol* **98**, 448–53.

78. van der Geld, Y.M., Huitema, M.G., Franssen, C.F., van der Zee, R., *et al.* (2000) In vitro T lymphocyte responses to proteinase 3 (PR3) and linear peptides of PR3 in patients with Wegener's granulomatosis (WG). *Clin Exp Immunol* **122**, 504–13.

79. Mathieson, P.W., Cobbold, S.P., Hale, G., Clark, M.R., *et al.* (1990) Monoclonal-antibody therapy in systemic vasculitis. *N Engl J Med* **323**, 250–4.

80. Yokoyama, H., Wada, T., and Furuichi, K. (2003) Immunomodulation effects and clinical evidence of apheresis in renal diseases. *Ther Apher Dial* **7**, 513–19.

81. Massengill, S.F., Goodenow, M.M., and Sleasman, J.W. (1998) SLE nephritis is associated with an oligoclonal expansion of intrarenal T cells. *Am J Kidney Dis* **31**, 418–26.

82. Masutani, K., Akahoshi, M., Tsuruya, K., Tokumoto, M., *et al.* (2001) Predominance of Th1 immune response in diffuse proliferative lupus nephritis. *Arthritis Rheum* **44**, 2097–106.

83. Alexopoulos, E., Seron, D., Hartley, R.B., and Cameron, J.S. (1990) Lupus nephritis: correlation of interstitial cells with glomerular function. *Kidney Int* **37**, 100–9.

84. Murata, H., Matsumura, R., Koyama, A., Sugiyama, T., *et al.* (2002) T cell receptor repertoire of T cells in the kidneys of patients with lupus nephritis. *Arthritis Rheum* **46**, 2141–7.

85. Calvani, N., Richards, H.B., Tucci, M., Pannarale, G., *et al.* (2004) Up-regulation of IL-18 and predominance of a Th1 immune response is a hallmark of lupus nephritis. *Clin Exp Immunol* **138**, 171–8.

86. Uhm, W.S., Na, K., Song, G.W., Jung, S.S., *et al.* (2003) Cytokine balance in kidney tissue from lupus nephritis patients. *Rheumatology (Oxford)* **42**, 935–8.

87. Kawasaki, Y., Suzuki, J., Sakai, N., Isome, M., *et al.* (2004) Evaluation of T helper-1/-2 balance on the basis of IgG subclasses and serum cytokines in children with glomerulonephritis. *Am J Kidney Dis* **44**, 42–9.

88. Yamada, M., Yagita, H., Inoue, H., Takanashi, T., *et al.* (2002) Selective accumulation of CCR4+ T lymphocytes into renal tissue of patients with lupus nephritis. *Arthritis Rheum* **46**, 735–40.

89. Furuichi, K., Wada, T., Sakai, N., Iwata, Y., *et al.* (2000) Distinct expression of CCR1 and CCR5 in glomerular and interstitial lesions of human glomerular diseases. *Am J Nephrol* **20**, 291–9.

90. Wong, C.K., Ho, C.Y., Li, E.K., and Lam, C.W. (2000) Elevation of proinflammatory cytokine (IL-18, IL-17, IL-12) and Th2 cytokine (IL-4) concentrations in patients with systemic lupus erythematosus. *Lupus* **9**, 589–93.

91. Zhao, X.F., Pan, H.F., Yuan, H., Zhang, W.H., *et al.* (2010) Increased serum interleukin 17 in patients with systemic lupus erythematosus. *Mol Biol Rep* **37**, 81–5.

92. Wong, C.K., Lit, L.C., Tam, L.S., Li, E.K., *et al.* (2008) Hyperproduction of IL-23 and IL-17 in patients with systemic lupus erythematosus: implications for Th17-mediated inflammation in auto-immunity. *Clin Immunol* **127**, 385–93.

93. Crispin, J.C., Oukka, M., Bayliss, G., Cohen, R.A., *et al.* (2008) Expanded double negative T cells in patients with systemic lupus erythematosus produce IL-17 and infiltrate the kidneys. *J Immunol* **181**, 8761–6.

94. Kim, H.S., Kim, I., Kim, J.O., Bae, J.S., *et al.* (2009) No association between interleukin 23 receptor gene polymorphisms and systemic lupus erythematosus. *Rheumatol Int* **30**, 33–8.

95. Sakaguchi, S. (2004) Naturally arising CD4+ regulatory t cells for immunologic self-tolerance and negative control of immune responses. *Annu Rev Immunol* **22**, 531–62.

96. Sakaguchi, S., Sakaguchi, N., Shimizu, J., Yamazaki, S., *et al.* (2001) Immunologic tolerance maintained by CD25+ CD4+ regulatory T cells: their common role in controlling autoimmunity, tumor immunity, and transplantation tolerance. *Immunol Rev* **182**, 18–32.

97. Zhang, X., Izikson, L., Liu, L., and Weiner, H.L. (2001) Activation of CD25(+)CD4(+) regulatory T cells by oral antigen administration. *J Immunol* **167**, 4245–53.

98. Cong, Y., Weaver, C.T., Lazenby, A., and Elson, C.O. (2002) Bacterial-reactive T regulatory cells inhibit pathogenic immune responses to the enteric flora. *J Immunol* **169**, 6112–19.

99. Kang, H.K., and Datta, S.K. (2006) Regulatory T cells in lupus. *Int Rev Immunol* **25**, 5–25.

100. Wolf, D., Hochegger, K., Wolf, A.M., Rumpold, H.F., *et al.* (2005) CD4+CD25+ regulatory T cells inhibit experimental anti-glomerular basement membrane glomerulonephritis in mice. *J Am Soc Nephrol* **16**, 1360–70.

101. Bagavant, H., Thompson, C., Ohno, K., Setiady, Y., *et al.* (2002) Differential effect of neonatal thymectomy on systemic and organ-specific autoimmune disease. *Int Immunol* **14**, 1397–406.

102. Bagavant, H., and Tung, K.S. (2005) Failure of CD25+ T cells from lupus-prone mice to suppress lupus glomerulonephritis and sialoadenitis. *J Immunol* **175**, 944–50.

103. Zheng, J.J., Shi, X.H., Chu, X.Q., Jia, L.M., *et al.* (2004) Clinical features and management of Crohn's disease in Chinese patients. *Chin Med J (Engl)* **117**, 183–8.

104. Scalapino, K.J., Tang, Q., Bluestone, J.A., Bonyhadi, M.L., *et al.* (2006) Suppression of disease in New Zealand Black/New Zealand White lupus-prone mice by adoptive transfer of ex vivo expanded regulatory T cells. *J Immunol* **177**, 1451–9.

105. Crispin, J.C., Martinez, A., and Alcocer-Varela, J. (2003) Quantification of regulatory T cells in patients with systemic lupus erythematosus. *J Autoimmun* **21**, 273–6.

106. Alvarado-Sanchez, B., Hernandez-Castro, B., Portales-Perez, D., Baranda, L., *et al.* (2006) Regulatory T cells in patients with systemic lupus erythematosus. *J Autoimmun* **27**, 110–18.

107. Venigalla, R.K., Tretter, T., Krienke, S., Max, R., *et al.* (2008) Reduced CD4+,CD25- T cell sensitivity to the suppressive function of CD4+,CD25high,CD127 -/low regulatory T cells in patients with active systemic lupus erythematosus. *Arthritis Rheum* **58**, 2120–30.

108. Yan, B., Ye, S., Chen, G., Kuang, M., *et al.* (2008) Dysfunctional CD4+,CD25+ regulatory T cells in untreated active systemic lupus erythematosus secondary to interferon-alpha-producing antigen-presenting cells. *Arthritis Rheum* **58**, 801–12.

109. van Amelsfort, J.M., van Roon, J.A., Noordegraaf, M., Jacobs, K.M., *et al.* (2007) Proinflammatory mediator-induced reversal of CD4+,CD25+ regulatory T cell-mediated suppression in rheumatoid arthritis. *Arthritis Rheum* **56**, 732–42.

110. Wohlfert, E.A., and Clark, R.B. (2007) 'Vive la Resistance!'—the PI3K-Akt pathway can determine target sensitivity to regulatory T cell suppression. *Trends Immunol* **28**, 154–60.

111. Biron, C.A., Nguyen, K.B., Pien, G.C., Cousens, L.P., *et al.* (1999) Natural killer cells in antiviral defense: function and regulation by innate cytokines. *Annu Rev Immunol* **17**, 189–220.

112. Cheent, K., and Khakoo, S.I. (2009) Natural killer cells: integrating diversity with function. *Immunology* **126**, 449–57.

113. Cooper, M.A., Fehniger, T.A., and Caligiuri, M.A. (2001) The biology of human natural killer-cell subsets. *Trends Immunol* **22**, 633–40.

114. Ljunggren, H.G., and Karre, K. (1990) In search of the 'missing self': MHC molecules and NK cell recognition. *Immunol Today* **11**, 237–44.

115. Lanier, L.L. (2008) Up on the tightrope: natural killer cell activation and inhibition. *Nat Immunol* **9**, 495–502.

116. Andoniou, C.E., Coudert, J.D., and Degli-Esposti, M.A. (2008) Killers and beyond: NK-cell-mediated control of immune responses. *Eur J Immunol* **38**, 2938–42.

117. Park, Y.W., Kee, S.J., Cho, Y.N., Lee, E.H., *et al.* (2009) Impaired differentiation and cytotoxicity of natural killer cells in systemic lupus erythematosus. *Arthritis Rheum* **60**, 1753–63.

118. Wither, J., Cai, Y.C., Lim, S., McKenzie, T., *et al.* (2008) Reduced proportions of natural killer T cells are present in the relatives of lupus patients and are associated with autoimmunity. *Arthritis Res Ther* **10**, R108.

119. Green, M.R., Kennell, A.S., Larche, M.J., Seifert, M.H., *et al.* (2005) Natural killer cell activity in families of patients with systemic lupus erythematosus: demonstration of a killing defect in patients. *Clin Exp Immunol* **141**, 165–73.

120. Schepis, D., Gunnarsson, I., Eloranta, M.L., Lampa, J., *et al.* (2009) Increased proportion of CD56bright natural killer cells in active and inactive systemic lupus erythematosus. *Immunology* **126**, 140–6.

121. Bendelac, A., Savage, P.B., and Teyton, L. (2007) The biology of NKT cells. *Annu Rev Immunol* **25**, 297–336.

122. Van Kaer, L. (2007) NKT cells: T lymphocytes with innate effector functions. *Curr Opin Immunol* **19**, 354–64.

123. Yang, J.Q., Singh, A.K., Wilson, M.T., Satoh, M., *et al.* (2003) Immunoregulatory role of CD1d in the hydrocarbon oil-induced model of lupus nephritis. *J Immunol* **171**, 2142–53.

124. Yang, J.Q., Wen, X., Liu, H., Folayan, G., *et al.* (2007) Examining the role of CD1d and natural killer T cells in the development of nephritis in a genetically susceptible lupus model. *Arthritis Rheum* **56**, 1219–33.

125. Yang, S.H., Kim, S.J., Kim, N., Oh, J.E., *et al.* (2008) NKT cells inhibit the development of experimental crescentic glomerulonephritis. *J Am Soc Nephrol* **19**, 1663–71.

126. Zeng, D., Liu, Y., Sidobre, S., Kronenberg, M., *et al.* (2003) Activation of natural killer T cells in NZB/W mice induces Th1-type immune responses exacerbating lupus. *J Clin Invest* **112**, 1211–22.

127. Postol, E., Meyer, A., Cardillo, F., de Alencar, R., *et al.* (2008) Long-term administration of IgG2a anti-NK1.1 monoclonal antibody ameliorates lupus-like disease in NZB/W mice in spite of an early worsening induced by an IgG2a-dependent BAFF/BLyS production. *Immunology* **125**, 184–96.

128. Oishi, Y., Sumida, T., Sakamoto, A., Kita, Y., *et al.* (2001) Selective reduction and recovery of invariant Valpha24JalphaQ T cell receptor T cells in correlation with disease activity in patients with systemic lupus erythematosus. *J Rheumatol* **28**, 275–83.

129. Forestier, C., Molano, A., Im, J.S., Dutronc, Y., *et al.* (2005) Expansion and hyperactivity of CD1d-restricted NKT cells during the progression of systemic lupus erythematosus in (New Zealand Black x New Zealand White)F1 mice. *J Immunol* **175**, 763–70.

130. Sireci, G., Russo, D., Dieli, F., Porcelli, S.A., *et al.* (2007) Immunoregulatory role of Jalpha281 T cells in aged mice developing lupus-like nephritis. *Eur J Immunol* **37**, 425–33.

131. Mesnard, L., Keller, A.C., Michel, M.L., Vandermeersch, S., *et al.* (2009) Invariant natural killer T cells and TGF-beta attenuate anti-GBM glomerulonephritis. *J Am Soc Nephrol* **20**, 1282–92.

132. Hume, D.A. (2006) The mononuclear phagocyte system. *Curr Opin Immunol* **18**, 49–53.

133. Ferenbach, D., and Hughes, J. (2008) Macrophages and dendritic cells: what is the difference? *Kidney Int* **74**, 5–7.

134. Shortman, K., and Liu, Y.J. (2002) Mouse and human dendritic cell subtypes. *Nat Rev Immunol* **2**, 151–61.

135. Witmer-Pack, M.D., Olivier, W., Valinsky, J., Schuler, G., *et al.* (1987) Granulocyte/ macrophage colony-stimulating factor is essential for the viability and function of cultured murine epidermal Langerhans cells. *J Exp Med* **166**, 1484–98.

136. Kruger, T., Benke, D., Eitner, F., Lang, A., *et al.* (2004) Identification and functional characterization of dendritic cells in the healthy murine kidney and in experimental glomerulonephritis. *J Am Soc Nephrol* **15**, 613–21.

137. Hume, D.A., and Gordon, S. (1983) Mononuclear phagocyte system of the mouse defined by immunohistochemical localization of antigen F4/80. Identification of resident macrophages in renal medullary and cortical interstitium and the juxtaglomerular complex. *J Exp Med* **157**, 1704–9.

138. Soos, T.J., Sims, T.N., Barisoni, L., Lin, K., *et al.* (2006) CX3CR1+ interstitial dendritic cells form a contiguous network throughout the entire kidney. *Kidney Int* **70**, 591–6.

139. Fogg, D.K., Sibon, C., Miled, C., Jung, S., *et al.* (2006) A clonogenic bone marrow progenitor specific for macrophages and dendritic cells. *Science* **311**, 83–7.

140. Segerer, S., Hughes, E., Hudkins, K.L., Mack, M., *et al.* (2002) Expression of the fractalkine receptor (CX3CR1) in human kidney diseases. *Kidney Int* **62**, 488–95.

141. Dong, X., Swaminathan, S., Bachman, L.A., Croatt, A.J., *et al.* (2005) Antigen presentation by dendritic cells in renal lymph nodes is linked to systemic and local injury to the kidney. *Kidney Int* **68**, 1096–108.

142. Scholz, J., Lukacs-Kornek, V., Engel, D.R., Specht, S., *et al.* (2008) Renal dendritic cells stimulate IL-10 production and attenuate nephrotoxic nephritis. *J Am Soc Nephrol* **19**, 527–37.

143. Heymann, F., Meyer-Schwesinger, C., Hamilton-Williams, E.E., Hammerich, L., *et al.* (2009) Kidney dendritic cell activation is required for progression of renal disease in a mouse model of glomerular injury. *J Clin Invest* **119**, 1286–97.

144. Iwata, Y., Furuichi, K., Sakai, N., Yamauchi, H., *et al.* (2009) Dendritic cells contribute to autoimmune kidney injury in MRL-Faslpr mice. *J Rheumatol* **36**, 306–14.

145. Woltman, A.M., de Fijter, J.W., Zuidwijk, K., Vlug, A.G., *et al.* (2007) Quantification of dendritic cell subsets in human renal tissue under normal and pathological conditions. *Kidney Int* **71**, 1001–8.

146. Segerer, S., Heller, F., Lindenmeyer, M.T., Schmid, H., *et al.* (2008) Compartment specific expression of dendritic cell markers in human glomerulonephritis. *Kidney Int* **74**, 37–46.

147. Iwasaki, A., and Medzhitov, R. (2004) Toll-like receptor control of the adaptive immune responses. *Nat Immunol* **5**, 987–95.

148. Li, M., Carpio, D.F., Zheng, Y., Bruzzo, P., *et al.* (2001) An essential role of the NF-kappa B/Toll-like receptor pathway in induction of inflammatory and tissue-repair gene expression by necrotic cells. *J Immunol* **166**, 7128–35.

149. Saemann, M.D., Weichhart, T., Zeyda, M., Staffler, G., *et al.* (2005) Tamm-Horsfall glycoprotein links innate immune cell activation with adaptive immunity via a Toll-like receptor-4-dependent mechanism. *J Clin Invest* **115**, 468–75.

150. Bhattacharjee, R.N., and Akira, S. (2006) Modifying toll-like receptor 9 signaling for therapeutic use. *Mini Rev Med Chem* **6**, 287–91.

151. Krieg, A.M., Efler, S.M., Wittpoth, M., Al Adhami, M.J., *et al.* (2004) Induction of systemic TH1-like innate immunity in normal volunteers following subcutaneous but not intravenous administration of CPG 7909, a synthetic B-class CpG oligodeoxynucleotide TLR9 agonist. *J Immunother* **27**, 460–71.

152. Anders, H.J., Vielhauer, V., Eis, V., Linde, Y., *et al.* (2004) Activation of toll-like receptor-9 induces progression of renal disease in MRL-Fas(lpr) mice. *Faseb J* **18**, 534–6.

153. Patole, P.S., Zecher, D., Pawar, R.D., Grone, H.J., *et al.* (2005) G-rich DNA suppresses systemic lupus. *J Am Soc Nephrol* **16**, 3273–80.

154. Wu, X., and Peng, S.L. (2006) Toll-like receptor 9 signaling protects against murine lupus. *Arthritis Rheum* **54**, 336–42.

155. Christensen, S.R., Kashgarian, M., Alexopoulou, L., Flavell, R.A., *et al.* (2005) Toll-like receptor 9 controls anti-DNA autoantibody production in murine lupus. *J Exp Med* **202**, 321–31.

156. Barrat, F.J., and Coffman, R.L. (2008) Development of TLR inhibitors for the treatment of autoimmune diseases. *Immunol Rev* **223**, 271–83.

157. Patole, P.S., Grone, H.J., Segerer, S., Ciubar, R., *et al.* (2005) Viral double-stranded RNA aggravates lupus nephritis through Toll-like receptor 3 on glomerular mesangial cells and antigen-presenting cells. *J Am Soc Nephrol* **16**, 1326–38.

158. Pawar, R.D., Patole, P.S., Zecher, D., Segerer, S., *et al.* (2006) Toll-like receptor-7 modulates immune complex glomerulonephritis. *J Am Soc Nephrol* **17**, 141–9.

159. Barratt, J., Feehally, J., and Smith, A.C. (2004) Pathogenesis of IgA nephropathy. *Semin Nephrol* **24**, 197–217.

160. Fairhurst, A.M., Mathian, A., Connolly, J.E., Wang, A., *et al.* (2008) Systemic IFN-alpha drives kidney nephritis in B6.Sle123 mice. *Eur J Immunol* **38**, 1948–60.

161. Bengtsson, A.A., Sturfelt, G., Truedsson, L., Blomberg, J., *et al.* (2000) Activation of type I interferon system in systemic lupus erythematosus correlates with disease activity but not with antiretroviral antibodies. *Lupus* **9**, 664–71.

162. Ytterberg, S.R., and Schnitzer, T.J. (1983) Serum interferon levels in patients with systemic lupus erythematosus. *Arthritis Rheum* **25**, 401–6.

163. Ronnblom, L., and Alm, G.V. (2002) The natural interferon-alpha producing cells in systemic lupus erythematosus. *Hum Immunol* **63**, 1181–93.

164. Blanco, P., Palucka, A.K., Gill, M., Pascual, V., *et al.* (2001) Induction of dendritic cell differentiation by IFN-alpha in systemic lupus erythematosus. *Science* **294**, 1540–3.

165. Baechler, E.C., Batliwalla, F.M., Karypis, G., Gaffney, P.M., *et al.* (2003) Interferon-inducible gene expression signature in peripheral blood cells of patients with severe lupus. *Proc Natl Acad Sci U S A* **100**, 2610–15.

166. Bennett, L., Palucka, A.K., Arce, E., Cantrell, V., *et al.* (2003) Interferon and granulopoiesis signatures in systemic lupus erythematosus blood. *J Exp Med* **197**, 711–23.

167. Kirou, K.A., Lee, C., George, S., Louca, K., *et al.* (2004) Coordinate overexpression of interferon-alpha-induced genes in systemic lupus erythematosus. *Arthritis Rheum* **50**, 3958–67.

168. Kalkner, K.M., Ronnblom, L., Karlsson Parra, A.K., Bengtsson, M., *et al.* (1998) Antibodies against double-stranded DNA and development of polymyositis during treatment with interferon. *QJM* **91**, 393–9.

169. Gota, C., and Calabrese, L. (2003) Induction of clinical autoimmune disease by therapeutic interferon-alpha. *Autoimmunity* **36**, 511–18.

170. Sledz, C.A., Holko, M., de Veer, M.J., Silverman, R.H., *et al.* (2003) Activation of the interferon system by short-interfering RNAs. *Nat Cell Biol* **5**, 834–9.

171. Bave, U., Magnusson, M., Eloranta, M.L., Perers, A., *et al.* (2003) Fc gamma RIIa is expressed on natural IFN-alpha-producing cells (plasmacytoid dendritic cells) and is required for the IFN-alpha production induced by apoptotic cells combined with lupus IgG. *J Immunol* **171**, 3296–302.

172. Santiago-Raber, M.L., Baccala, R., Haraldsson, K.M., Choubey, D., *et al.* (2003) Type-I interferon receptor deficiency reduces lupus-like disease in NZB mice. *J Exp Med* **197**, 777–88.

173. Dalod, M., Salazar-Mather, T.P., Malmgaard, L., Lewis, C., *et al.* (2002) Interferon alpha/beta and interleukin 12 responses to viral infections: pathways regulating dendritic cell cytokine expression in vivo. *J Exp Med* **195**, 517–28.

174. Nagai, T., Devergne, O., Mueller, T.F., Perkins, D.L., *et al.* (2003) Timing of IFN-beta exposure during human dendritic cell maturation and naive Th cell stimulation has contrasting effects on Th1 subset generation: a role for IFN-beta-mediated regulation of IL-12 family cytokines and IL-18 in naive Th cell differentiation. *J Immunol* **171**, 5233–43.

175. McRae, B.L., Nagai, T., Semnani, R.T., van Seventer, J.M., *et al.* (2000) Interferon-alpha and -beta inhibit the in vitro differentiation of immunocompetent human dendritic cells from CD14(+) precursors. *Blood* **96**, 210–17.

176. Li, S., Kurts, C., Kontgen, F., Holdsworth, S.R., *et al.* (1998) Major histocompatibility complex class II expression by intrinsic renal cells is required for crescentic glomerulonephritis. *J Exp Med* **188**, 597–602.

177. Ruth, A.J., Kitching, A.R., Semple, T.J., Tipping, P.G., *et al.* (2003) Intrinsic renal cell expression of CD40 directs Th1 effectors inducing experimental crescentic glomerulonephritis. *J Am Soc Nephrol* **14**, 2813–22.

178. Norman, M.U., Van De Velde, N.C., Timoshanko, J.R., Issekutz, A., *et al.* (2003) Overlapping roles of endothelial selectins and vascular cell adhesion molecule-1 in immune complex-induced leukocyte recruitment in the cremasteric microvasculature. *Am J Pathol* **163**, 1491–503.

179. Timoshanko, J.R., Kitching, A.R., Iwakura, Y., Holdsworth, S.R., *et al.* (2004) Leukocyte-derived interleukin-1beta interacts with renal interleukin-1 receptor I to promote renal tumor necrosis factor and glomerular injury in murine crescentic glomerulonephritis. *Am J Pathol* **164**, 1967–77.

Chapter 6

Pathology, pathogenesis, and clinical features of severe lupus nephritis

Stephen M. Korbet and Melvin M. Schwartz

The definition of severe lupus nephritis (SLN)

From the beginning of the renal biopsy era, clinicians and pathologists have recognized that some, but not all, patterns of glomerulonephritis (GN) in systemic lupus erythematosus (SLE) lead to progressive renal impairment and require urgent therapeutic consideration.[1,2] In 1957, Muehrcke *et al.*,[1] in the first renal biopsy study of lupus nephritis, reported that patients with SLN that they described as "partial or diffuse glomerular proliferation" (active lupus GN), had a much higher prevalence of progressive renal disease and death than patients whose biopsies showed "no or minor changes" (glomerulitis). In 1964, the same authors,[3] presented a series of 87 patients with SLE, including 47 (54%) patients with active lupus GN that corresponded to SLN as they had previously defined the entity.[1] The patients with active lupus GN presented with renal insufficiency and more severe proteinuria than patients with lupus glomerulitis or membranous lupus. After 8 years of follow-up, death due to end stage renal disease had occurred in 55% of patients with active lupus GN compared to only 7% of patients with glomerulitis or membranous lupus GN. However, as they had observed in an earlier study,[2,4] those patients with SLN who had been treated with high-dose prednisone for an average of 6 months had a better prognosis, with death due to end stage renal disease at 4 years follow-up of only 43%, compared to 92% in patients who had received low-dose prednisone (Figure 6.1). These studies made the important observations that patients with active lupus GN (SLN) presented with more active clinical disease and had a poorer prognosis than patients with less severe inflammatory disease, but the prognosis was significantly improved with aggressive corticosteroid treatment. Although the authors commented on the great variability in the intensity and distribution of the glomerular pathology, these studies did not attempt to subcategorize SLN.

The recognition that SLN could be subclassified into two general histopathological categories was a major development: focal segmental GN (FSGN) was identified as a discrete form of SLN because it involved only a portion of some glomeruli, and it was separated from and contrasted with diffuse global GN (DGGN) that involved the entire tuft of almost all glomeruli. It was also noted that that FSGN could involve a

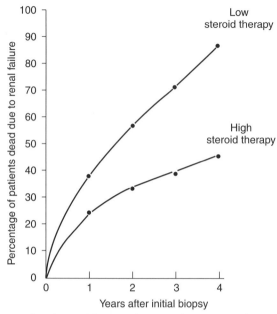

Fig. 6.1 Percentage of patients with severe lupus nephritis dying of renal failure in 4 years. From Pollak VE, Pirani CL, Schwartz FD. The natural history of the renal manifestations of systemic lupus erythematosus. *J Lab Clin Med* 1964; **63**:537–550 with permission from Elsevier.

variable proportion of glomeruli, including instances in which ≥50% of glomeruli were involved.[2,5–7] In a study of 92 cases of lupus nephritis, Baldwin *et al.*[7] defined diffuse proliferative lupus nephritis as global involvement of all or almost all glomeruli. They reported that these patients were more likely to present with hypertension, renal insufficiency, and the nephrotic syndrome, than patients with focal proliferative GN (defined as "sharply delineated segmental proliferation of some tufts, involving from 12% to 55% of the glomeruli") (Table 6.1). Although all patients with diffuse proliferative lupus nephritis were treated with steroids, they had a poorer prognosis, with a 5-year mortality of 71% compared to <30% for other forms of lupus nephritis including focal proliferative GN (Table 6.1).

Other studies reported patients with widespread (≥50%) segmental lesions under the diagnosis of diffuse proliferative lupus nephritis, with the rationale that such a widespread proliferative lesion must be associated with more aggressive disease and a poorer prognosis similar to that of diffuse proliferative lupus nephritis.[8–11] Although insights into lupus nephritis gained from these landmark studies were invaluable, differences in the definitions of the lesions of lupus nephritis, and SLN in particular, caused a lack of consensus concerning the natural history and prognosis of FSGN and DGGN. The need for a well-defined, consensus classification of lupus nephritis was recognized.

In 1975, the World Health Organization (WHO) proposed a classification for lupus nephritis[12] that defined focal proliferative GN as an inflammatory lesion involving <50% of the glomeruli (usually focal and segmental endocapillary proliferation and necrosis), and distinguished it from diffuse proliferative GN that had "changes similar

Table 6.1 The presentation and prognosis of lupus nephritis

	Mesangial	Focal-proliferative	Diffuse-proliferative	Membranous
n	12	12	44	24
Renal insufficiency	17%	17%	82%	25%
Nephrotic syndrome	0	8%	93%	67%
Hypertension	17%	0	55%	33%
Follow-up				
Alive	100%	75%	36%	63%
Renal death	0	0	41%	4%
Nonrenal death	0	25%	23%	33%
5-year mortality	0	30%	71%	30%

Data from Baldwin et al.[7]

to those of focal segmental proliferative GN, but involving more glomerular surface area and greater than 50 percent of glomeruli." By this definition, segmental proliferative GN biopsies with >50% glomerular involvement were included in the category of diffuse proliferative GN. Using the 1975 WHO classification of lupus nephritis, Appel et al.[8,9] reported their experience of 56 patients with SLE renal disease. Although the number of patients was too small to compare the survival of patients with diffuse proliferative (n=9) and focal proliferative (n=14) GN, they found that, despite the use of high-dose steroids, the 4-year survival was worse in patients with diffuse proliferative GN (66%) compared to patients with mesangial (85%) or membranous lupus nephritis (88%). Austin et al.[10] also used the 1975 WHO classification of lupus nephritis, and reported that 72 patients with diffuse proliferative lupus nephritis had a renal survival at 10 years of 75%, compared to 100% for patients with mesangial, focal proliferative (<50% glomerular involvement), or membranous lupus nephritis. These studies clearly demonstrated that diffuse proliferative GN was a severe form of lupus glomerular disease, and although it was shown that aggressive treatment significantly improved the outcomes for patients with diffuse proliferative lupus GN, their prognosis was still inferior to that of patients with other forms of lupus renal disease, including patients with segmental proliferative lupus GN.

In 1980, the Renal Pathology Advisory Group for the International Study of Kidney Disease in Children (Rene Habib, Edmund J. Lewis, Jay Bernstein, Jacob Churg, Lilianne Morel Maroger, Conrad Pirani) proposed a modification of the 1975 WHO classification of lupus GN,[12] and this modified classification was subsequently adopted by the WHO in 1982.[13] The 1982 WHO classification (Table 6.2) defined FSGN as involvement of part of the tuft of some, but not all, glomeruli, and DGGN as involvement of the entire tuft of all, or almost all, glomeruli. The classification did not further define segmental in terms of proportional involvement of the glomerulus because the distinguished pathologists who developed the WHO classification thought that the meaning of "segmental" was self-evident. In addition, their experience with

Table 6.2 The 1982 World Health Organization (WHO) classification of lupus nephritis[13]

I. Normal glomeruli
II. Pure mesangial alterations
III. Focal segmental glomerulonephritis
IV. Diffuse glomerulonephritis
V. Diffuse membranous glomerulonephritis
Va. Pure membranous glomerulonephritis
Vb. Associated with lesions of category II
Vc. Associated with lesions of category III
Vd. Associated with lesions of category IV
IV. Advanced sclerosing glomerulonephritis

lupus GN informed them that segmental lesions could involve >50% of the glomeruli, and they did not use a 50% cut-off to separate FSGN from DGGN. This last point was a major departure from the 1975 WHO classification.

Schwartz et al.[14] specifically addressed the prognostic effect of the proportion of segmental glomerular involvement in SLE: using the 1982 WHO classification, they compared the clinical presentation and course of patients with diffuse global lupus GN to those of patients with segmental proliferative lupus nephritis, who were subcategorized by the proportion of glomeruli with active segmental lesions. They found that compared to patients with mild (1–19%) and moderate (20–49%) involvement, patients with severe segmental proliferative lupus GN (≥50%) presented with higher levels of serum creatinine and proteinuria that were similar to those of patients with diffuse global lupus GN (Table 6.3). More importantly, they found that the 5-year actuarial survival without renal failure in patients with DGGN (53% survival) was almost identical to that of patients with severe segmental (59% survival) and worse than that for patients with mild or moderate segmental involvement (82% survival) (Table 6.3, Figure 6.2). These data supported the notion that the presentation and prognosis of segmental proliferative GN correlated with the extent of glomerular involvement. However, Schwartz et al.[14] suggested that the pathogenic mechanisms may differ between FSGN and diffuse global lupus GN, and although they felt that it was valid on clinical grounds to include patients with segmental proliferative lupus GN involving ≥50% of glomeruli in the category of "severe lupus nephritis," they also believed that it was essential to keep these two discrete forms of lupus GN in separate diagnostic categories because of the pathogenetic implications of the pathology and immunopathology.

The 1982 WHO classification also recognized that patients with membranous lupus GN (1982 WHO Class V) could have coexisting focal segmental (WHO Class Vc) or DGGN (WHO Class Vd). Sloan et al.[15] assessed the impact of coexisting proliferative lesions in 79 patients with membranous lupus GN. They found that patients with membranous lupus GN and either severe segmental GN (≥50% involvement) or DGGN presented with higher levels of serum creatinine and proteinuria (Table 6.4), were less likely to enter a remission despite aggressive immunosuppressive therapy,

Table 6.3 The presentation and prognosis of severe segmental lupus nephritis

	Proportion with segmental lesions			
	1–19%	20–49%	≥50%	DPGN
n	19	9	17	28
Age (years)	31±13	32±10	30±7	29±12
Creatinine (mg/dl)	1.3±0.8	1.5±1.2	1.9±1.5	2.2±2.1
Proteinuria (g/day)	1.3±1.7	1.5±1.3	2.5±2.5	4.4±3.6
Follow-up (months)	48±36	54±51	41±27	29±29
Survival at 5 years	84%	89%	65%	61%

DPGN, diffuse proliferative glomerulonephritis.
Data from Schwartz et al.[14]

and had a poorer prognosis with a 10-year survival without end stage renal disease of 20% compared to 48% in patients with coexisting mild segmental proliferative GN (<50% involvement) and 72% in patients with pure membranous GN (Table 6.4, Figure 6.3). These findings suggested that the prognosis of membranous lupus GN was significantly impacted by the proliferative glomerular lesions, and when these

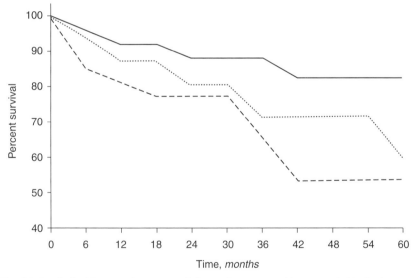

Fig. 6.2 Survival without end stage renal disease in segmental lupus nephritis. Patients with mild and moderate focal segmental glomerulonephritis, <50% of the glomeruli involved (solid line), had the best 5-year actuarial survival (82% survival), and patients with diffuse global glomerulonephritis had the worst survival (53% survival) (interrupted solid line). Patients with severe focal segmental glomerulonephritis ≥50% involvement (dotted line) had a 5-year survival (59% survival) that was not different from patients with diffuse global glomerulonephritis. Reproduced from Schwartz MM, Kawada KS, Corwin HL, Lewis EJ. The prognosis of segmental glomerulonephritis in systemic lupus erythematosus. *Kidney Int* 1987; **32**(2): 274–279, with permission from Macmillan Publishers Ltd.

Table 6.4 The presentation and prognosis of membranous lupus nephritis

	Va+Vb	Vc<50%	Vc≥50%+Vd
n	36	15	28
Creatinine (mg/dl)	0.9±0.03	1.0±0.3	2.1±1.2*
Proteinuria (g/day)	3.3±3.2	3.8±3.2	6.2±4.7*
Follow-up (years)	5.8±5.3	3.6±3.6	2.7±5.4
Remission**	42%	27%	21%
Survival at 5 years	86%	72%	49%*
Survival at 10 years	72%	48%	20%*

Data from Sloan et al.[15]
* $P<0.05$; Vc≥50%+Vd versus Va+Vb.
** Serum creatinine <1.4 mg/dl and proteinuria <1g/day.

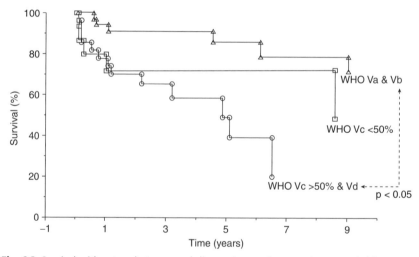

Fig. 6.3 Survival without end stage renal disease in membranous lupus nephritis. Patients with pure membranous glomerulonephritis (MGN) (no or mild mesangial proliferation) (1982 WHO Va and Vb) had the best actuarial 10-year survival (72%), and patients with systemic lupus erythematosus (SLE) MGN and severe focal segmental glomerulonephritis (FSGN) (≥50% involvement) or diffuse global glomerulonephritis (DGGN) had the worst survival (20%). Patients with MGN and mild FSGN (<50% involvement) had a survival (48%) that was not significantly different from that of patients with pure SLE MGN. Reproduced with permission from Sloan RP, Schwartz MM, Korbet SM, Borok RZ (1996). The Lupus Nephritis collaborative Study Group. Long-term outcome in systemic Lupus Erythematosus Membranous Glomerulonephritis. *J Am Soc Nephrol* **7**(2):299-305.[15]

lesions involved ≥50% of the glomeruli, patients with membranous lupus GN had the same poor outcome as patients with proliferative lesions of severe lupus nephritis without coexisting membranous changes.

Based on these observations and the 1982 WHO classification, the Lupus Nephritis Collaborative Study Group[16,17] (see below) defined SLN as active glomerular inflammation involving more than 50% of the nonhyalinized glomeruli, and reported that these widely distributed glomerular lesions included both severe FSGN (WHO III ≥50%) and DGGN (WHO IV), as well as patients with coexisting membranous lesions and severe FSGN (WHO Vc ≥50%) or DGGN (Vd). However, in 1995, the WHO issued an updated classification of lupus nephritis[18] that reinstated the 50% cut-off of the number of glomeruli involved to separate FSGN (<50%) from DGGN(≥50%). Thus, the 1995 WHO classification defined all cases with ≥50% involvement (SLN) as DGGN (WHO IV) irrespective of the segmental or global nature of the lesion.

With the intention of resolving the relationship between severe FSGN and DGGN, among other issues, The International Society of Nephrology and Renal Pathology Society (ISN/RPS), in 2003, proposed its classification of lupus nephritis (Table 6.5).[19] The most significant change was the way in which severe lupus GN was divided into FSGN and DGGN. In the attempt to ensure diagnostic reproducibility and precision, the ISN/RPS classification provided quantitative definitions of segmental and global GN to divide SLN into two categories, diffuse segmental (IV-S) and diffuse global (IV-G) GN. The ISN/RPS division of SLN was intended to avoid the ambiguity of the 1995 WHO classification concerning the definition of a segmental lesion, to be analogous to severe segmental (WHO III ≥50%) and diffuse global (WHO IV) as defined by The Lupus Nephritis Collaborative study group,[16,17] and to use the ISN/RPS classes IV-S and IV-G to test the pathological and outcome differences between severe segmental and DGGN demonstrated by the Lupus Nephritis Collaborative Study Group (Table 6.6).

The way in which severe segmental and DGGN are defined has changed in successive classifications,[1,13,18–20] but the glomerular pathology, seen under the microscope, has remained unchanged. In this chapter, we present the pathological and clinical features of SLN and discuss how the 1982 WHO classification[13] as applied by the Lupus Nephritis Collaborative Study Group and the ISN/RPS[19] classification have affected the pathogenetic and prognostic implications of the diagnosis of SLN.

Table 6.5 The International Society of Nephrology/Renal Pathology Society (2003) classification of lupus nephritis[19]

I. Minimal mesangial lupus nephritis

II. Mesangial proliferative lupus nephritis

III. Focal lupus nephritis (<50% of glomeruli)

IV. Diffuse lupus nephritis (≥50% of glomeruli)

    IV-S. Diffuse segmental lupus nephritis (<50% glomerular surface area)

    IV-G. Diffuse global lupus nephritis (≥50% glomerular surface area)

V. Membranous lupus nephritis

IV. Advanced sclerosing lupus nephritis

Table 6.6 Classifications of severe lupus nephritis: World Health Organization (WHO) (1982) versus International Society of Nephrology/Renal Pathology Society

	Severe segmental glomerulonephritis		Global glomerulonephritis	
	WHO III ≥50%	IV-S	WHO IV	IV-G
Glomerular surface area involved (%)*	<100%	<50%	100%	≥50%
Glomeruli involved (%)†	≥50%	≥50%	100%	≥50%
Glomerular sclerosis‡	No	Yes	No	Yes
Segmental+global lesions§	Yes	Yes	No	Yes

* Percentage surface area involvement of the glomerulus.
† Percentage of glomeruli with lesions.
‡ Glomerular scarring judged to be sequela of lupus glomerulonephritis included in the diagnosis.
§ Mixture of segmental and global lesions as defined in the classification in the diagnostic category.

The glomerular pathology of SLN

Severe lupus nephritis is defined by widespread (≥50%) involvement by either severe FSGN or DGGN. It is imperative that the clinician understand how the definitions of the two forms of SLN affect the presenting features and the outcomes of patients with these discrete forms of lupus GN. Understanding the pathology of these lesions is also critical because it allows the recognition of morphological and immunopathological features that support different pathogenic mechanisms for severe FSGN and DGGN.

Severe FSGN

The intraglomerular distribution of pathology is the singular feature of severe FSGN. A focal distribution means that some, but not all, glomeruli are involved, and within the involved glomeruli, segmental means that the pathology involves only part of the glomerulus (Figure 6.4). Severe FSGN refers to biopsies with segmental lesions[13] involving >50% of the glomeruli, and in the tables, we have designated this category as WHO III ≥50%.[16] Because the features of active segmental inflammation are not dependent upon the proportion of the glomeruli with lesions, there is no rationale for excluding biopsies from this category if 80%, 90%, or even 100% of the glomeruli are involved, as long as glomerular involvement, no matter how extensive, is judged to be segmental in nature. In practice, there are almost always some glomeruli with either normal mesangia or mild mesangial hypercellularity (13±12% of glomeruli in our unpublished observations on the 83 biopsies with SLN reported in Najafi *et al.*[21]), and in the glomeruli with segmental lesions the proportion of glomerular surface area that is involved (that is the two-dimensional projection of the glomerulus on the slide) can vary, with some glomeruli having a segmental lesion involving <50% of the glomerular surface area (34±21% of glomeruli in our experience) and others (35±24% of glomeruli in our experience) where ≥50% of the glomerular surface area is involved (Figure 6.5). However, the glomeruli with the most extensive pathology must have some portion that is relatively uninvolved, and we have defined one glomerular lobule

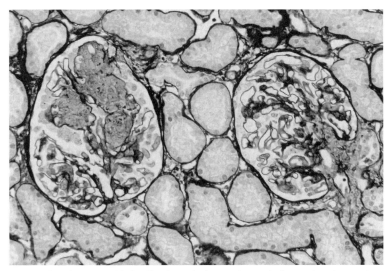

Fig. 6.4 Focal and segmental distribution of glomerular pathology. The glomerulus on the left has an area of endocapillary proliferation and necrosis that involves 25% of the glomerulus (segmental intraglomerular distribution). Because the glomerulus on the right is normal, the pathology involves some but not all glomeruli (focal interglomerular distribution). Methenamine silver periodic acid Schiff stain (Jones), ×33 (see Plate 2).

as the minimum that must be uninvolved to qualify a glomerulus as having a segmental (rather than global) lesion (Figure 6.6).[22]

Light microscopy

The histological manifestations of severe FSGN are varied, and biopsies often include both active segmental glomerular lesions and segmental and global glomerular scars. There are different opinions concerning whether the scarred glomeruli should be included in the definition of FSGN, and in the ISN/RPS classification,[19] the quantitative cut-off between focal and diffuse GN at 50% involvement includes segmental and global scars. In our opinion, the proportion of glomeruli with scars is important data, and along with the extent of interstitial fibrosis, tubular atrophy, and nephrosclerosis, this information concerning chronic, irreversible renal damage is an integral part of the complete renal pathology report. However, we also believe that the proportion of morphologically viable glomeruli with active lesions is the key diagnostic feature because glomeruli with active inflammation are the appropriate, potentially responsive targets for current therapy. The most common histological finding in severe FSGN is endocapillary proliferation of glomerular cells and infiltration of leukocytes,[21] but any of the features of active glomerular inflammation, first described by Pirani[23] and included in the WHO classifications of lupus GN (Table 6.7),[13,18] qualify a glomerulus if the distribution is focal and segmental.

Severe FSGN often has histopathological evidence of glomerular necrosis, including karyorrhexis, fibrinoid necrosis, fibrin exudates, and destruction of the glomerular

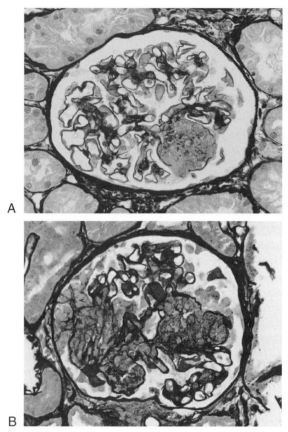

Fig. 6.5 Variable glomerular involvement in focal segmental glomerulonephritis within the same biopsy. (A) One glomerular lobule, comprising 5–10% of the glomerular surface area has a necrotizing lesion with karyorrhexis and rupture of the glomerular basement membrane. The remainder of the glomerulus is normal. (B) More than 50% of the glomerular surface area shows endocapillary proliferation, but the uninvolved capillaries are relatively normal. Methenamine silver periodic acid Schiff stain (Jones), (A) and (B), ×66 (see Plate 3).

capillary wall with ruptures of the glomerular basement membrane. These findings are rarely all present in the same glomerulus, but any one is evidence of glomerular necrosis. In addition, cellular crescents may be used as a surrogate for glomerular necrosis[24] because their pathogenesis requires necrosis with rupture of the glomerular capillary wall and leakage of plasma proteins and formed elements into Bowman's space.

Fluorescence microscopy

There are two characteristic patterns of immune aggregate deposition in severe FSGN: mesangial and pauci-immune.[21,25–28] In the mesangial pattern (Figure 6.7), most of the deposits are confined to the mesangium with no or negligible, small, weakly staining deposits in the peripheral capillary walls. The deposits are immunoglobulin

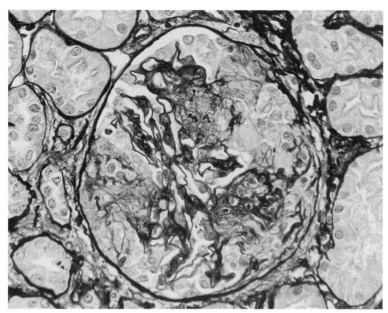

Fig. 6.6 Glomerulus with focal segmental glomerulonephritis involving more than 80% of the tuft. There is endocapillary proliferation and necrosis in more than 80% of the glomerular surface area with destruction of the architecture and multiple foci with ruptures of glomerular basement membrane. The uninvolved capillaries in the center of the glomerulus comprise two lobules with relatively normal appearance. Methenamine silver periodic acid Schiff stain (Jones), ×66 (see Plate 4).

(IgG)-dominant, although IgA and IgM can be co-deposited along with C3 and other complement components. The pauci-immune pattern (Figure 6.8) has deposits confined to segmental areas that correspond to sites of glomerular necrosis and are often associated with fibrin and nonimmune proteins such as albumin and α-2-macroglobulin. When severe FSGN coexists with membranous GN, there are widespread, granular, glomerular basement membrane immune deposits. In general, severe FSGN is not associated with large subendothelial deposits.

Table 6.7 Active lesions in lupus glomerulonephritis[13]

Cellular proliferation
Disruption of capillary walls
Polymorphs and karyorrhexis
Hematoxylin bodies
Crescents, cellular or fibrocellular
"Wire-loops" (by light microscopy)
Hyaline thrombi
Fibrin thrombi
Segmental fibrin deposition

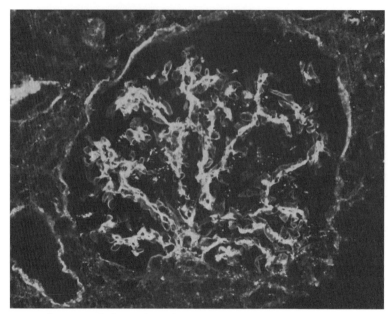

Fig. 6.7 Focal segmental glomerulonephritis with a mesangial pattern of immunofluorescence. Immunoglobulin (Ig)G is strongly stained in the mesangium and focally in Bowman's capsule and the tubular basement membrane, but the peripheral glomerular capillary walls are almost completely void of deposits. Fluorescein isothiocyanate rabbit anti-human IgG, ×100 (see Plate 5).

Electron microscopy

The ultrastructure correlates with the immune aggregates seen by immunofluorescence microscopy: there are either mesangial electron-dense deposits (Figure 6.9) or a pauci-immune pattern with no or few deposits. Despite the association between subendothelial deposits and proliferative GN,[29–31] subendothelial deposits are either completely absent or only very focal and small.

In our opinion, severe FSGN can involve less than or greater than 50% of the glomerular surface area because the pathological features are similar, and we do not find that the greater amount of segmental involvement is associated with a qualitative difference in the pathology. This impression is supported by immunopathological and ultrastructural findings that suggest a common pathogenesis, regardless of the proportion of the glomerular surface area that is involved (see below, Pathogenesis of FSGN).[22,26] In this discussion, we do not address FSGN involving <50% of the glomeruli, because these cases do not meet the definition of severe lupus GN. However, segmental GN biopsies with <50% involvement have the same pathological features as severe FSGN. Renal physicians should be aware that a classification based on the proportion of glomerular involvement is subject to misclassification errors solely as the result of the statistical rules that govern sampling, and these errors are accentuated in the small glomerular sample typically seen in renal biopsies. In other words, a significant number of biopsies with a good prognosis (<50% glomerular involvement)

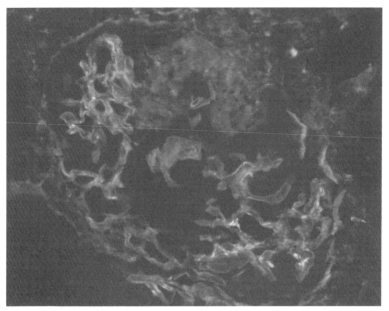

Fig. 6.8 Focal segmental glomerulonephritis with a pauci-immune pattern of immunofluorescence. There is no significant glomerular staining for immunoglobulin (Ig)G either in the mesangium or the peripheral capillary walls. Fluorescein isothiocyanate rabbit anti-human IgG, ×100 (see Plate 6).

and a poor prognosis (≥50% involvement) will be misclassified because the biopsy sample is not truly representative of the glomerular population in the whole kidney (Table 6.8).[32] Although patients with segmental lesions involving <50% of glomeruli may have a more favorable response to therapy,[5–7,14] the lesions are no less destructive and share a similar pathogenic mechanism to biopsies with more widespread lesions (≥50% of the glomeruli). Because of the similar glomerular pathology and the statistical overlap created by the 50% cut-off, patients with FSGN involving <50% of the glomeruli should receive the same therapeutic considerations as those with severe FSGN.

Diffuse global glomerulonephritis

Diffuse global glomerulonephritis is identified by both the diffuse and global distribution of pathology (Figure 6.10): diffuse means that all or almost all glomeruli are involved (94% of glomeruli in our unpublished observations on the 83 biopsies with SLN reported by Najafi *et al.*[21]), and within the involved glomeruli, global means that acute inflammation involves the entire glomerulus. The 1982 WHO classification[13] calls this category IV or diffuse glomerulonephritis (WHO IV), and the classification implies and we have inferred that DGGN does not include severe segmental GN. Global and segmental glomerular scarring (11% in our experience) and chronic tubular and interstitial lesions are seen in biopsies with DGGN,[21,26] but these chronic changes do not play a role in its definition or diagnosis. However, glomerular scarring

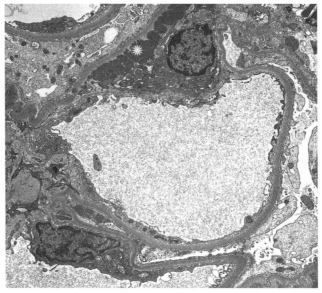

Fig. 6.9 Electron microscopy in focal segmental glomerulonephritis with a mesangial immunofluorescence pattern. The biopsy had 50% glomerular involvement by focal segmental necrotizing glomerulonephritis. The one complete and two partial capillary loops seen in this photomicrograph have no electron-dense deposits, but there is a large mesangial deposit at the top of the picture (asterisk). Uranyl acetate and lead citrate, ×4000.

Table 6.8 Sample size requirements in glomerulonephritis: minimum number of abnormal glomeruli necessary in a biopsy to assume a 50% involvement

Number of glomeruli in biopsy specimen	Abnormal glomeruli that must be present to be certain of ≥50% involvement	
	Number	% of glomeruli
8	7	87.5%
15	11	73.3%
20	14	70%
30	20	66.6%
40	27	67.5%

According to the binomial distribution, the estimation of the proportion of abnormal glomeruli can be subject to considerable variability when a small sample size is used. This table illustrates the number and percent of glomeruli that must be abnormal per sample size, to give 95% assurance that 50% of glomeruli in the kidney are abnormal. Data from Corwin et al.[32]

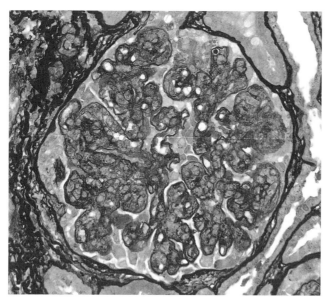

Fig. 6.10 Diffuse global distribution of glomerular pathology. The glomerulus shows endocapillary proliferation involving almost every capillary (global). There is also widespread glomerular basement thickening and double contours consistent with subendothelial deposits. All the glomeruli in the biopsy showed similar pathology (diffuse). Methenamine silver periodic acid Schiff stain, ×66 (see Plate 7).

should receive the same consideration in the biopsy report as described above in severe FSGN.

Light microscopy

Glomerular histopathology may have several discrete patterns. Diffuse endocapillary proliferation is the most common, with global glomerular hypercellularity caused by proliferation of mesangial and endothelial cells and infiltration of leukocytes. The membranoproliferative pattern combines lobulation, hypercellularity, and thickening of the glomerular capillary walls with duplication of the glomerular basement membrane on periodic acid Schiff (PAS) and methenamine silver PAS (Jones) stains, and it should be recognized and classified separately from the combination of DGGN and membranous GN. Crescentic GN has cellular crescents of proliferating epithelial cells and leukocytes in Bowman's space. However, the diffuse global distribution of any of the features of active glomerular disease, for example wire-loops (Table 6.7), qualifies as DGGN. Glomerular necrosis may occur in DGGN, but the histopathological features of necrosis (karyorrhexis, fibrinoid necrosis, and glomerular basement membrane rupture) are inconstant and are often difficult to detect against the background of intense global inflammation. When present, epithelial crescents that are readily identified in DGGN may be used as surrogates for glomerular necrosis.[24] Diffuse global glomerulonephritis frequently has wire-loops (Figure 6.11A) and hyaline thrombi (Figure 6.11B), histological features that correlate with massive

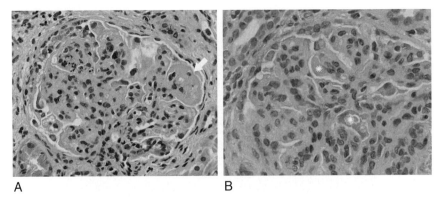

A   B

Fig. 6.11 Wire-loops and hyaline thrombi are histological features that correspond to massive glomerular immune aggregate deposition. (A) Diffuse global glomerulonephritis (DGGN) with proliferation, neutrophilic exudates, and a wire-loop at 1–2 o'clock (arrow). The wire-loop comprises hyalin, eosinophilic thickening of the capillary wall, and, although they can be widespread, they often involve only one or two capillaries. (B) DGGN with hyaline thrombi in two capillaries (asterisks). The thrombus in the center of the picture is within a capillary with a wire-loop. Hematoxylin and eosin, (A) ×66, (B) ×132 (see Plate 8).

immune complex deposition, and this is in contrast with severe FSGN which infrequently shows these histological features.[21,22,26]

Fluorescence microscopy

There are diffuse (all glomeruli) large, mesangial, and capillary wall deposits of immunoglobulins and complement components (Figure 6.12). Immunoglobulin G is usually dominant, but immunoglobulins A and M frequently co-localize in the deposits. The capillary wall deposits often have a smooth outer border because they are located beneath the endothelium and are limited by the basement membrane. Focal or global, granular deposits may indicate a concomitant membranous GN, and a complex picture with both granular and subendothelial deposits is a frequent finding in DGGN. Immunoglobulin thrombi in the glomerular capillaries correspond to the hyalin/nonfibrin thrombi seen by light microscopy. The immunofluorescence pattern is in contrast with the sparse deposits seen in severe FSGN.

Electron microscopy

The ultrastructure reflects and reinforces the histopathology and immunopathology. Electron-dense deposits correspond to immune deposits seen by fluorescence microscopy and wire-loops and hyalin thrombi seen by light microscopy. Electron-dense deposits may be seen in the mesangium and on both sides and within the glomerular basement membrane, but massive subendothelial deposits involving the entire circumference of the capillary and capillary thrombi are characteristic of WHO IV (Figure 6.13).[21,22,29,30]

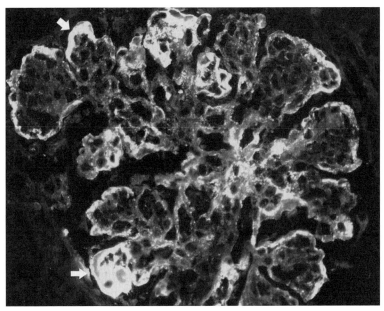

Fig. 6.12 Immunofluorescence pattern in diffuse global glomerulonephritis. The peripheral capillary walls contain massive discontinuous linear deposits of immunoglobulin (Ig)G. The deposits have a characteristic smooth outer contour (arrows) because they are located in the subendothelial space, and their outer extent is limited and formed by the glomerular basement membrane (GBM). There are also focally intense mesangial deposits. Fluorescein isothiocyanate rabbit anti-human IgG, ×40 (see Plate 9).

The ISN/RPS classification of SLN

The International Society of Nephrology/Renal Pathology Society Class IV (diffuse lupus nephritis)[19] corresponds to SLN, because it is defined as any combination of segmental or global glomerular lesions (active and chronic) that involve ≥50% of the glomeruli. However, the definitions of segmental and global lesions in the ISN/RPS classification are different from those in the 1982 WHO classification, and the 1982 WHO classification as interpreted by the Lupus Nephritis Collaborative Study Group (Table 6.6).[13,16,17] As a result, the ISN/RPS definitions of diffuse segmental (IV-S) and diffuse global (IV-G) GN significantly change the distinction between the segmental and global forms of SLN. The first difference is the inclusion of therapeutically unresponsive scars in the definition of SLN that changes the diagnostic focus from active, potentially responsive lesions to the proportion of glomeruli with any lesion. Even though ISN/RPS classes IV-S and IV-G are designated active (A), chronic (C), or mixed active and chronic (A/C), the proportion of glomeruli with active lesions in contrast to scars is missing from the diagnostic line. The blurring of the distinction between active and chronic glomerular pathology means cases will be included in ISN/RPS Class IV with no, or only a few, active lesions.

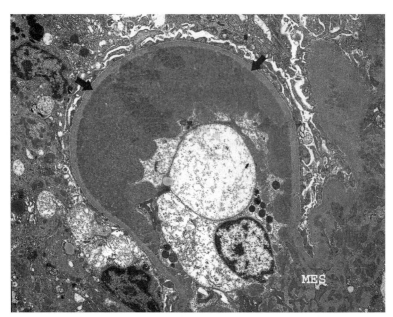

Fig. 6.13 Electron microscopy of diffuse global glomerulonephritis. The glomerular capillary contains a massive subendothelial electron-dense deposit that involves the entire peripheral capillary wall. Notice that the subendothelial deposit is limited by the glomerular basal lamina (arrows) and that it has a smooth outer contour. The mesangium (MES) contains scattered electron-dense deposits. Uranyl acetate and lead citrate, ×4000.

The ISN/RPS definitions that separate segmental and global glomerular lesions on the basis of the proportion of glomerular surface area involvement (the two-dimensional projection of the glomerulus on the slide) are significantly different from the 1982 WHO definitions of severe FSGN and DGGN, and they change the way in which severe segmental lesions are distributed between the segmental and global classes, change the prognosis of the segmental and global lesions, and lead to problems in the reproducibility and classification of SLN. Severe segmental GN in the 1982 WHO classification (WHO III ≥50%) includes biopsies with segmental lesions irrespective of the extent of glomerular surface area involved (i.e. < and ≥50% of the glomerular surface area), but in the ISN/RPS classification, severe segmental GN (ISN/RPS Class IV-S) includes only patients with <50% glomerular surface involvement. Thus, the ISN/RPS classification transfers the most extensively involved segmental lesions (those with ≥50% involvement of the glomerular surface area) from the category of severe FSGN, the category that most accurately describes their pathology and in which they are associated with other cases that have similar, but less extensive, glomerular lesions, to ISN/RPS Class IV-G (diffuse global GN), in which they form a substantial, morphologically discrete minority grouped with a majority of cases of DGGN (Figure 6.14). In our experience,[22] SLN is equally divided between segmental (WHO Class III ≥50%, 39 cases) and global (WHO Class IV, 44 cases) lesions, but when we reclassified the cases using the ISN/RPS criteria, the ratio of diffuse segmental and DGGN (ISN/RPS Class IV-S/Class IV-G) was

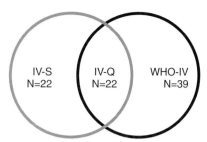

Fig. 6.14 This Venn diagram demonstrates the shifts that occur between biopsies classified as segmental and global according to the definitions in the 1982 World Health Organization (WHO)[13] and the International Society of Nephrology/Renal Pathology Society (ISN/RPS) classification.[19] The circle on the left represents WHO III ≥50% and the overlap, labeled IV-Q, represents the cases of segmental GN that transfer to ISN/RPS IV-G when the ISN/RPS definitions are applied. IV-S is the Class of diffuse segmental in the ISN/RPS classification, less the cases (IV-Q) that combine with the WHO IV cases to produce ISN/RPS IV-G. In our cases of severe lupus nephritis,[22] the ISN/RPS classification transfers 50% (22/44) of WHO III ≥50% to ISN/RPS IV-G to produce a ratio of IV-S/IV-G=22/61 (0.32). Reproduced with permission from Schwartz MM, Korbet SM, Lewis EJ (2008). The prognosis and pathogenesis of Severe Lupus Glomerulonephritis. *Nephrol Dial Transplant*; **23**: 1298-1306.

22/61,[22] similar to that observed by others who have reported the classification of SLN using ISN/RPS criteria.[33] We found that the ratio favoring DGGN in the ISN/RPS classification results from reclassifying and transferring of cases of severe FSGN (SSGN) with ≥50% glomerular surface area involvement (a group we refer to as IV-Q, Figure 6.14) from SSGN into the Diffuse Global category (ISN/RPS Class IV-G).[22] Furness *et al.*[34] found the same relative increase in IV-G, and they ascribed it to transfers from WHO Class III (≥50%) and Class V. We conclude that the ISN/RPS Classes IV-S and IV-G[19] are constituted differently from severe FSGN (WHO Class III ≥50%) and DGGN in the 1982 WHO classification.[13,16,17] These substantial differences invalidate comparisons between clinical outcomes for patients whose renal biopsies are classified in the ISN/RPS classification and the 1982 WHO classification, as reported by the Lupus Nephritis Collaborative Study Group,[13,16,17] and they obviate the goal of the ISN/RPS classification of testing the significance differences in outcome observed between severe FSGN and DGGN.[22]

The ISN/RPS was developed to ensure diagnostic reproducibility. Two studies have looked at the reproducibility of the distinction between ISN/RPS classes IV-S and IV-G. Thirty-six renal pathologists enrolled in the United Kingdom National Renal Pathology External Quality Assessment Scheme examined the histopathology and the fluorescence microscopy reports from 20 consecutive patients with the biopsy coded as SLE.[34] As part of a comparison of the reproducibility of the ISN/RPS and the 1995 WHO classifications, the same pathologists were asked to subclassify the biopsies in Class IV into either IV-S or IV-G using only the published descriptions of the classification, and for this distinction, the level of interobserver agreement was low (kappa 0.35). In the second study,[35] three renal pathologists classified 10 renal biopsies from patients with proliferative lupus nephritis, included in the first Dutch lupus nephritis study, according to the published criteria of the 1995 WHO[18] and the ISN/RPS[19] classifications. The intraclass correlation coefficients (ICC) were low for both the WHO and the ISN/RPS classifications (ICC<0.02), and even when the subclasses were removed and the ISN/RPS classification was simplified to classes II, III, IV-S, IV-G, V and VI, the ICC only increased from 0.181 to 0.405. The difficulties experienced by these two groups of pathologists may be explained by the heterogeneous glomerular involvement that characterizes ISN/RPS Class IV with a mixture of normal glomeruli and glomeruli with < and ≥50% surface area involvement by inflammation or scarring. In addition, the semiquantitative distinction between diffuse segmental (IV-S) and DGGN (IV-G) requires that a pathologist estimate the proportion of glomerular surface area in every glomerulus in the biopsy, and because the errors in serial estimates are additive, this is another source of interobserver variation. In addition, the ISN/RPS quantitative definitions themselves may cause overlap of the diagnostic categories because the small glomerular sample in the biopsies and the statistical rules that govern sampling will lead to misclassification of a significant number of biopsies because the biopsy sample is not representative of the glomerular pathology in the whole kidney (Table 6.8).[22,32]

The pathogenesis of SLN

The pathogenesis of SLN is multi-factorial, but in this chapter we will focus on the pathological features of severe FSGN and DGGN that support different pathogenetic mechanisms for these two lesions. In general, the serological features seen in patients with SLN[16,21,26] support an immune complex pathogenesis, and, in our experience, almost all patients with SLN have active serologies with elevated anti-native DNA titers and low serum complement components.[16,21] Although the serum complement C3 tends to be more depressed in DGGN than in severe FSGN,[16,21,26] we have not found any presenting serological features useful in predicting whether the biopsy will show one pattern or the other.[16] One interpretation of the relationship between the lesions is that FSGN and DGGN represent progression of the same pathogenic mechanism.[6,8,9,12,20] However, other pathogenic mechanisms, in addition to classic, circulating immune complex injury, have been implicated in SLE GN, including coagulopathies, anti-endothelial antibodies, in situ immune complex formation, and pauci-immune necrotizing GN. These diverse processes, acting alone or in concert, provide an alternative explanation for the diverse histopathology and morphological patterns that characterize severe lupus GN, and this diversity supports the hypothesis that pathology in lupus GN can be caused by more than one mechanism. The possibility of diverse pathogenetic mechanisms also highlights the need for a classification based on morphological findings that reflect pathogenesis[13,16] rather than one that simply enumerates the proportion of glomerular involvement.[19] In the case of the two lesions that comprise SLN, there are clear differences in the pathology when SLN is dichotomized into severe FSGN and DGGN using the 1982 WHO classification,[16,21,22] and the different pathologies and immunopathologies of the severe FSGN and DGGN imply that they are caused by different mechanisms of injury.

Diffuse global glomerulonephritis

Diffuse global glomerulonephritis is the form of SLN that corresponds most closely to an immune complex-mediated mechanism of glomerular injury, and its pathology reflects peripheral glomerular capillary wall, subendothelial immune complex deposits, and the inflammatory reaction that these deposits incites. In pathology studies, the diffuse global pattern of glomerulonephritis has correlated with the presence of subendothelial deposits. Baldwin et al.[7] reported 24 biopsies showing diffuse proliferative lupus nephritis (DGGN) that had prominent subendothelial and mesangial immune deposits. Hill et al.[29] reported 34 cases of diffuse proliferative or membranoproliferative GN (DGGN) and all had mesangial and diffuse subendothelial capillary deposits. Schwartz et al. and the Lupus Nephritis Collaborative Study Group[16,17] reported that peripheral capillary wall deposits evidenced by wire-loops ($41\pm35\%$ versus $14\pm21\%$, $P<0.01$) and massive subendothelial deposits ($34\pm27\%$ versus $9\pm15\%$, $P<0.001$) were seen significantly more often in 35 biopsies showing DGGN than in 24 biopsies showing severe FSGN (Figure 6.15). In a retrospective study of patients from their practice with SLN, using the pathological criteria developed by the Lupus Nephritis Collaborative Study Group,[16,17] Behara et al.[36] also showed significantly more histological and ultrastructural evidence of immune aggregate deposition in DGGN than in severe FSGN. They extended these observations by grading the intensity of peripheral capillary IgG deposits (0–3+) in 39 patients with SLN without mem-

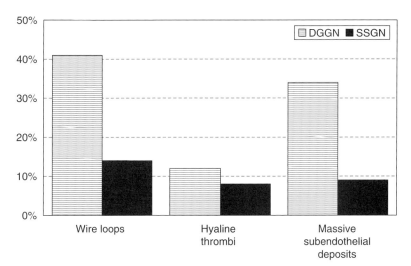

Fig. 6.15 Baseline histological feature comparing diffuse global glomerulonephritis (DGGN) and severe focal segmental glomerulonephritis (SSGN) classified using modified 1982 World Health Organization (WHO) criteria. There is significantly more evidence of immune aggregate deposition in biopsies showing DGGN than severe FSGN: wire-loops, $P<0.01$; hyaline thrombi, $P<0.05$; massive subendothelial deposits, $P<0.001$. Data from Najafi et al.[21]

branous GN (severe FSGN 25 patients and DGGN 14), and they showed that DGGN had significantly more peripheral capillary wall immune deposits than severe FSGN (intensity of IgG was 1.9±1.2 versus 0.9±1.2, P=0.03) (Figure 6.16). The widespread glomerular immune deposits that are characteristic of DGGN localize to the peripheral capillary wall and correspond to wire-loops, large, peripheral capillary immune aggregates, and massive subendothelial deposits (Figure 6.15).[6,7,16,21,22,26,29,30] Diffuse global glomerulonephritis is considered to be a disease in which immune aggregates, formed in the circulation, are deposited in the glomeruli, where they incite an endocapillary proliferative and exudative inflammatory reaction.[26] The morphological evidence of glomerular immune aggregate deposition in the glomerular capillaries in DGGN is in contrast to the paucity of immune deposits seen in severe FSGN (Figure 6.15).

Focal segmental glomerulonephritis

The distribution of glomerular lesions in severe FSGN is different from that in DGGN, and the paucity of glomerular immune aggregates and the virtual absence of subendothelial deposits constitute the strongest evidence that severe FSGN is not mediated by the same classic immune complex mediated mechanism as DGGN. Jacob Churg wrote "It is uncertain whether focal lupus nephritis as defined, is produced by the same immunological mechanisms as mesangial and diffuse forms, because in some instances immune deposits are absent from the focal lesion though present elsewhere in the glomerulus."[13] Specifically, Grishman and Churg found essentially no immune deposits in 6/10 focal segmental lesions studied by electron microscopy, and

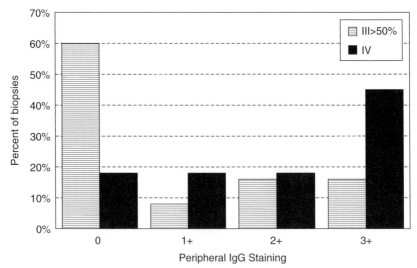

Fig. 6.16 Morphological evidence of glomerular immune complex deposition in severe lupus nephritis subclassified as severe focal segmental glomerulonephritis (SSGN) and diffuse global glomerulonephritis (DGGN), using the criteria developed by the Lupus Nephritis Collaborative Study Group (Schwartz, 1989; Lewis, 1992). Data from Behara V, Whittier W, Korbet S, Schwartz M, Martens M, Lewis E. (2007). Severe segmental lupus nephritis: A pauci-immune glomerulonephritis. *J Am Soc Nephrol*; **18**: 217A.

the uninvolved portions of the glomeruli and glomeruli without segmental GN had either no pathological changes or isolated mesangial deposits.[28] This observation was confirmed in our study of SLN, which analyzed the morphological evidence of capillary immune aggregates in severe FSGN and DGGN. Najafi et al.[21] found significantly fewer glomeruli with wire-loops (14±21% versus 41±35%, P<0.01), hyaline thrombi (4±9% versus 14±17%, P<0.05) and massive subendothelial deposits (9±15% versus 34±27%, P<0.001) in severe segmental GN than in diffuse global GN (Figure 6.15). Additional evidence of the pauci-immune nature of severe FSGN was provided by Behara et al.,[36] who reported that the intensity of peripheral glomerular deposits of IgG, with glomerular fluorescence graded from 0–3+, was less in 25 patients with severe FSGN compared to 14 patients with DGGN (0.9±1.2 versus 1.9± 1.2, P=0.03), and the proportion with no deposits was greatest among those with severe FSGN (Figure 6.16). In studies that utilize the ISN/RPS classification for severe lupus nephritis, it is not surprising that the immunological differences are less striking because many examples of severe FSGN, with a paucity of peripheral immune deposits, are categorized as diffuse global GN (ISN/RPS IV-G), diluting the evidence of immune deposits. When severe segmental GN is divided into those with <50% and ≥50% glomerular surface area involvement, the histological and ultrastructural evidence of immune aggregate deposition, wire-loops, hyaline thrombi, and massive subendothelial deposits, is similar, and severe segmental GN with ≥50% glomerular surface area involvement has significantly less evidence of immune aggregate deposition than the cases of diffuse global GN with which they are classified in the ISN/RPS classification (Figure 6.17). Mittal et al.[37] classified 33 cases as ISN/RPS classes IV-S (n=11) and IV-G (n=22), and they found that although the proportion of glomeruli with wire-loops (68% versus 27%, P=0.06) and subendothelial deposits (81% versus 55%, P=0.21) was greater in biopsies with IV-G than IV-S, the differences were not significant. Hill et al.[26] classified biopsies with SLN using the ISN/RPS system. Patients with diffuse segmental GN (IV-S) had lower scores for histological features related to subendothelial immune aggregate deposition, including glomerular macrophage/monocytes (0.86±0.77 versus 1.77±0.92, P=0.001), glomerular capillary immune deposits (9.0±3.2 versus 12.8±3.5, P=0.001), and subendothelial deposits (1.8±1.1 versus 2.9±09, P <0.002). Interestingly, when the authors studied relatively pure forms of segmental and global GN (those in which 80% of the glomeruli had either segmental or global GN, using ISN/RPS criteria, respectively) the relative paucity of immune deposits in 'pure' segmental GN over 'pure' global GN increased. Thus, the pathogenesis of FSGN does not appear to be related to circulating immune complexes deposited in the glomerular capillary wall.

The focal segmental distribution of the inflammatory lesion that is the basis for the morphological classification of FSGN is also characteristic of glomerular involvement in the systemic small vessel vasculitides, and this pathological congruence implies that the pathogenesis of FSGN in SLE is similar to that of the systemic vasculitides. Segmental glomerular inflammation in the systemic vasculitides is also often necrotizing in nature with glomerular fibrinoid necrosis, karyorrhexis, rupture of the capillary walls, and cellular crescents. These histological features of necrosis may be seen in both FSGN and DGGN, and their presence does not always distinguish the two lesions.[21,22,24,37]

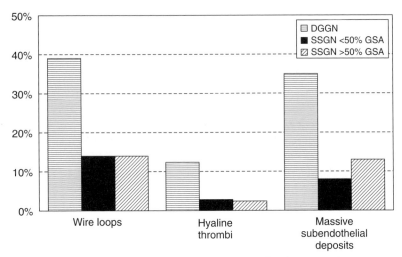

Fig. 6.17 Baseline histological features comparing severe focal segmental glomerulonephritis with <50% and ≥50% glomerular surface area involvement and diffuse global glomerulonephritis (DGGN) classified using modified 1982 World Health Organization (WHO) criteria. The amount of immune aggregate deposition is similar in biopsies showing <50% and ≥50% glomerular surface area (GSA) involvement, and there is significantly more evidence of immune aggregate deposition in biopsies showing DGGN. Wire-loops, P=0.001; hyaline thrombi, P=0.002; massive subendothelial deposits, P<0.0001. Data from Schwartz et al.[22]

However, Hill[26] reported that the percentage of affected glomeruli with fibrinoid necrosis was much higher in ISN/RPS Class IV-S than IV-G (13.3±15.3 versus 5.6±8.0, P=0.03). A significant additional finding was fibrinoid necrosis in the absence of endocapillary proliferation, suggesting necrosis in the absence of immune aggregate-mediated glomerular proliferation, in one-third of the involved glomeruli in IV-S and in none of the involved glomeruli in IV-G (P=0.0015). Antineutrophil cytoplasmic antibody (ANCA) is the best-characterized mechanism of pauci-immune necrotizing GN,[38] and there are a few reports of associations between ANCA and lupus GN.[27,39–41] Although the majority of patients with SLN do not have an ANCA with specificity for the common cytoplasm antibodies proteinase 3 or myeloperoxidase,[42] anti-endothelial cell antibodies[43,44] and other neutrophil cytoplasmic antibodies[45,46] have been reported. Therefore, the pathology suggests a pauci-immune, vasculitic process in severe lupus FSGN, but the precise mechanism is unknown in most cases.

Implications of the pathological classification of SLN

It is clear that the categories of segmental and global GN in SLN are constituted differently in the ISN/RPS and the WHO classifications, but the clinician needs to ask whether the differences in how SLN is subclassified in these two systems are clinically relevant. Based on the data, the answer, in our opinion, is a resounding yes. In the first part of this chapter, we have shown that the 1982 WHO classification[13,16,47,48] dichotomizes SLN into segmental (severe FSGN) and global (DGGN) forms of glomerulonephritis that appear to have different pathogeneses. Diffuse global glomerulonephritis is apparently mediated by the abundant immune deposits that are demonstrated in the biopsy. In contrast, severe FSGN lacks similar pathological evidence of immune aggregate deposition, and we and others[21,22,26] have postulated that the typical glomerular lesion seen in severe FSGN occurs by a vasculitic mechanism analogous to that of the pauci-immune forms of necrotizing glomerulonephritis. Furthermore, we have shown that when the same cases are classified using the ISN/RPS definitions, these important pathological findings and their pathogenic and therapeutic implications are lost.[22] In the following section, we will consider the effect that the two classifications have on the clinical presentation, response to therapy, and prognosis of patients with SLN.

Clinical features and prognosis of SLN

During the past 20 years clinicopathological studies have provided important insights into the presentation and prognosis in patients with SLN,[10,11,49–54] and they have advanced our understanding of the benefits and risks of various immunosuppressive regimens in the treatment of SLN and the importance of inducing a remission and preventing relapses with the use of maintenance immunosuppressive therapy.[55–58] Unfortunately, many of these studies did not differentiate severe FSGN from DGGN and also included patients who did not have SLN. As a result, in many studies it is difficult to specifically evaluate differences in presentation and outcome of severe FSGN and DGGN. However, studies conducted by the Lupus Nephritis Collaborative Study Group (LNCSG) and those utilizing the ISN/RPS classification allow one to clearly compare and contrast the clinical features and prognosis of patients with severe FSGN and DGGN lupus nephritis.

Insights from the Lupus Nephritis Collaborative Study Group

In 1981 the LNCSG initiated a prospective randomized trial assessing the value of plasmapheresis in 86 patients with SLN. The trial was initially conducted from April 1981 to December 1988[17] and only patients with a histological diagnosis of SLN, defined using a modification of the 1982 WHO classification of lupus nephritis[13,16,48] as described above, were included. Severe FSGN (WHO category III ≥50%) was present in 24 patients, DGGN (WHO category IV) was present in 35 patients and the remaining patients had membranous glomerulonephritis with superimposed severe FSGN (category Vc ≥50%; 20 patients) or DGGN GN (category Vd; six patients) and one patient was not classifiable. Patients were randomized to receive either plasmapheresis plus "standard therapy" with steroids and oral cyclophosphamide or standard therapy alone and treated according to a defined protocol.[17,59]

The plasmapheresis study demonstrated no added benefit of plasmapheresis to "standard therapy"[17] and was formally terminated in March of 1986, but clinical follow-up was obtained for 10 years. This extended follow-up allowed the LNCSG to further examine the impact of various clinical and histological features on long-term outcomes in patients with SLN.

Table 6.9 The presentation of severe lupus nephritis

	III≥50%	IV	Vc≥50%+Vd
n	24	35	26
Age (years)	36±16	29±8	31±13
Race			
White	63%	66%	58%
Black	29%	14%	35%
Creatinine (mg/dl)	1.6±1.0	1.8±1.1	2.1±1.5
Proteinuria (g/day)	4.4±2.9	6.3±4.1	6.8±4.3
Serology			
Low C3	96%	100%	96%
Low C4	58%	67%	54%
Elevated dsDNA	92%	97%	100%

Data from Najafi et al.[21]

In 2001, Najafi et al.,[21] reporting for the LNCSG, found that the presenting clinical and serological features were indistinguishable among the three histological groups of patients with severe lupus nephritis (Table 6.9). Contrary to the expectation that patients with the more widely distributed glomerular lesion of DGGN would experience the worst clinical outcome, they observed that patients with severe FSGN had a significantly worse prognosis than patients with DGGN (Table 6.10 and Figure 6.18). Patients with severe FSGN were significantly less likely to enter a remission or have stable renal function at last follow-up compared to those with DGGN. Additionally, patients with severe FSGN were almost three times as likely to progress to end stage renal disease as patients with DGGN despite receiving the same aggressive therapy, whereas patients with DGGN were over eight times more likely to enter a complete remission (serum creatinine ≤1.4 mg/dl and proteinuria ≤0.33 g/day). Furthermore, Najafi et al.[21] made the important observation that patients with SLN and coexisting membranous lesions have a clinical course and prognosis that is essentially identical to

Table 6.10 The follow-up of severe lupus nephritis

	III≥50%	IV	Vc≥50%+Vd
n	24	35	26
Follow-up (months)	124±61	126±64	108±70
Complete remission	38%	60%*	27%
Stable renal function	38%	63%*	35%
ESRD or death	62%	37%	65%

* P<0.05
ESRD, end stage renal disease.
Data from Najafi et al.[21]

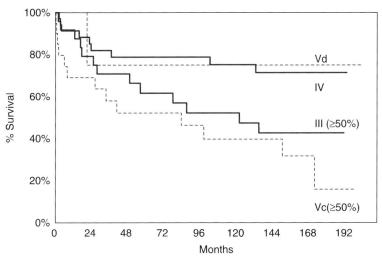

Fig. 6.18 Renal survival is based on histological categorization. Patients with severe lupus nephritis and coexisting membranous lesions have a clinical course that is essentially identical to that of patients with severe focal segmental glomerulonephritis (World Health Organization, WHO, III ≥50%) or diffuse global glomerulonephritis (WHO IV) without membranous lesions. P=0.01, overall; P=0.05, IV versus III ≥50%; P=0.002, IV versus Vc ≥50%. Reproduced from Najafi CC, Korbet SM, Lewis EJ, Schwartz MM, Reichlin M, Evans J (2001). Significance of histologic patterns of glomerular injury upon long-term prognosis in severe lupus glomerularnephritis. *Kidney Int*; **59**(6):2156-2163, with permission from Macmillan Publishers Ltd.

that of patients with severe FSGN or DGGN without membranous lesions (Figure 6.18). The 10-year renal survival for severe FSGN or DGGN without membranous lesions was 52% and 75%, respectively, and with membranous lesions it was 40% and 75% respectively (Figure 6.18). Thus, in patients with membranous lupus nephritis, the proliferative component predicts outcome. As a result, in subsequent publications by the LNCSG the patients with membranous lesions were often combined and evaluated under their proliferative component rather than independently.

Risk factors for progression in SLN

Risk factors for progression to end stage renal disease (ESRD) in patients with SLN identified in studies done by the LNCSG include, in addition to the glomerular lesion of severe FSGN, an elevated serum creatinine at biopsy, non-White race, and failure to attain a remission.[21,60–62] In a study of the racial difference in SLN performed by the LNCSG, Korbet et al.[62] found that Black patients were over twice as likely to progress to ESRD as White patients, whereas White patients were 2.6 times more likely to enter a remission. The poorer outcome in Black patients with SLN has been observed in other studies.[56,63,64] In 1995, Austin et al.,[63] reporting their experience in 166 patients, 77% of whom had diffuse proliferative lupus nephritis, found that 41% of Black patients had doubled their serum creatinine at 5 years compared to 18% of White patients (P=0.0006). Dooley et al.,[64] in a study of 89 patients (51 Black and 38 White) with SLN, also demonstrated that, despite similar baseline clinical, laboratory and pathological features, and the use of aggressive treatment, Black patients had a poorer renal outcome. Progression to ESRD occurred in 16% of Black patients compared to 5% of White patients, and the renal survival at 5 years was 58% for Black patients and 95% for White patients (P=0.007). By multivariate analysis, Black patients had a relative risk of progressing to ESRD that was 11 times that of White patients (P=0.03). The different outcomes may, in part, be related to the different types of glomerular pathology experienced by White and Black patients with severe lupus nephritis. Austin et al.[63] suggested that the poorer renal prognosis in Black patients with SLN resulted from the fact that they were over twice as likely to have "high-risk" histology (presence of cellular crescents and interstitial fibrosis), as White patients (29% versus 13%, P<0.05). A similar observation was made in the study by Korbet et al.[62] for the LNCSG, where Black patients were significantly more likely to have severe FSGN, a lesion associated with a higher risk of progression, compared to White patients (76% versus 44%, P<0.05). Thus, the racial differences in prognosis observed among patients with SLN may result from the fact that Black patients tend to have a necrotizing glomerular lesion that is less likely to respond to "standard" therapy for SLN and is more likely to progress.

The value of a remission in SLN

The LNCSG provided a number of insights regarding the favorable prognosis associated with attaining a remission.[60,61] Patients with SLN attaining a complete remission (defined by a serum creatinine of ≤1.4 mg/dl and proteinuria ≤0.33 g/day) with aggressive therapy had significantly better outcomes than patients not attaining a remission. The patient and renal survival at 10 years was 95% and 94%, respectively, in those patients attaining a remission compared to 60% and 31%, respectively, in nonremitters. Even patients attaining a partial remission (defined by ≤25% increase in baseline serum creatinine and ≥50% reduction in baseline proteinuria to ≤1.5 g/day) had an improved prognosis compared to patients who never entered a remission (Figure 6.19). A number of features at baseline have been found to be predictive of a complete remission, including race, level of serum creatinine, level of proteinuria, and chronicity index.[61,65] In the patients with SLN studied by Chen et al.,[60] patients entering a complete remission had less advanced renal disease compared to those with partial or no remission. The average serum creatinine at the time of biopsy in patients attaining a complete remission was 1.2±0.5 mg/dl compared to 2.1±0.9 mg/dl and 2.6 mg/dl (P<0.0001) for patients with partial or no remission respectively. This finding is consistent with that reported by Baldwin et al.,[7] who, over 30 years ago, recognized that patients with a serum creatinine <2 mg/dl at the time of treatment had a higher remission rate. Ioannidis et al.[58] have found that one of the most significant predictors of a failure to attain a remission is the delay in the time from diagnosis of nephritis to the initiation of therapy. A delay in treatment of >3 months resulted in a 42% reduction in likelihood of attaining a remission in proteinuria (defined by a ≥30% reduction in proteinuria to <3 g/day). These observations emphasize the importance of early diagnosis and treatment.

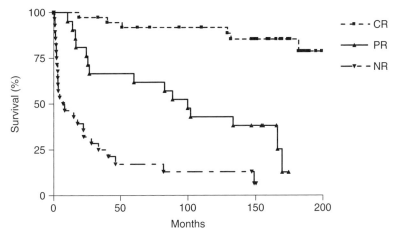

Fig. 6.19 Patient survival without end stage renal disease in severe lupus nephritis based on remission status. CR, complete remission; PR, partial remission; NR, no remission. P<0.0001, overall; P<0.0001, CR versus NR; P<0.0001, CR versus PR; P=0.0005, PR versus NR. From Chen YE, Korbet SM, Katz RS, Schwartz MM, Lewis EJ. Value of a complete or partial remission in severe lupus nephritis. *Clin J Am Soc Nephrol* 2008; **3**(1): 46–53.

Insights from the International Society of Nephrology and Renal Pathology Society classification

Since the publication of the ISN/RPS classification in 2004, six retrospective studies have been published, of which two assess the value of the classification in general[66,67] and four focus specifically on the subcategories of Class IV.[26,35,37,68] A comparison of the presenting clinical and serological characteristics of patients with Class IV-S and IV-G lesions observed in these studies is presented in Table 6.11. The level of serum creatinine and proteinuria at presentation was not significantly different in the majority of studies. However, when differences did occur they tended to be worse in Class IV-G patients. Compared to Class IV-S patients, Class IV-G patients had a significantly higher serum creatinine in one study[35] and higher level of proteinuria in two studies.[26,68] The serological parameters were also similar among the two groups, with both having hypocomplementemia and elevated dsDNA titers. Thus, consistent with the observations of Najafi *et al.*,[21,26] patients with IV-S and IV-G have similar clinical and serological features at presentation in general.

The outcomes reported for patients with IV-S and IV-G are presented in Table 6.12. The remission rate was similar in the four studies where it was assessed, with the exception of that reported by Kim *et al.*,[68] who found that patients with IV-S had a higher complete remission rate than patients with IV-G (67% versus 33%, P<0.05). However, the overall complete and partial remission rate was similar for the two groups (92% versus 88%). The determinant of renal outcome varied among studies and was assessed based on level of glomerular filtration rate,[68] proportion reaching, or time to, end stage renal disease,[67] proportion doubling baseline serum creatinine,[26,35,66]

Table 6.11 Presentation of severe lupus nephritis using International Society of Nephrology/Renal Pathology Society classification: retrospective studies

	Mittal et al.[37]		Yokoyama et al.[67]		Hill et al.[26]		Kim et al.[68]		Hiramatsu et al.[66]		Grootscholten et al.[35]	
Country	USA		Japan		France		Korea		Japan		Netherlands	
	IV-S	IV-G	IV-S	IV-G	IV-S	IV-G	IV-S	IV-G	IV-S	IV-G	IV-S	IV-G
n	11	22	6	17	15	31	12	30	14	41	15	57
Age (years)	31	36	31	36	35 (overall)		33	32			37	31
Race												
White	36%	36%			63% (overall)						87%	70%
Black	36%	27%			17% (overall)							
HTN					20%	42%	33%	37%			27%	61%*
SCr (mg/dl)	0.9	1.4	1.3	1.3	1.2	1.7	0.9	1.0	0.6	0.8	1.1	1.3*
UPro (g/day)			3.9	3.7	2.7	6.3*	2.3	5.1*	2.1	5.4	3.5	4.2
UPro ≥3.5g/day	80%	89%	67%	59%					43%	81%		
C3 (mg/dl)	53	57			59	50	48	51			54	43*
Low C3	88%	60%										
C4 (mg/dl)	8	13*					11	10			12	10*
Low C4	88%	62%										
CH50	43	112	22	18	42	30*			11	12		
Low CH50 (U/ml)	86%	73%										
dsDNA (IU/ml)	94	23			409	656	1205	804*			141	166
High dsDNA	78%	43%										

* P<0.05.
CH50, total hemolytic complement; HTN, hypertension; SCr, serum creatinine; UPro, urine protein.

or a combination of proportion doubling serum creatinine or reaching end stage renal disease.[37] Based on these evaluations, patients with IV-S tended to do worse than IV-G in two studies,[37,67] but no significant differences in outcome were found between patients with IV-S or IV-G in any of the studies (Table 6.12). Yokoyama et al.[67] found that 67% of IV-S patients progressed to end stage renal disease, compared to 29% of IV-G patients, and the median renal survival was 95 and 214 months respectively. Additionally, Mittal et al.[37] found that 30% of IV-S patients doubled their serum creatinine or progressed to end stage renal disease compared to only 9% of IV-G patients. The observation from these studies that patients with severe SLN, as defined by the ISN/RPS classification (IV-S), did no worse than patients with diffuse global lupus nephritis (ISN/RPS Class IV-G), was clearly in conflict with the observations of the LNCSG.[21,61]

Why do the clinical observations differ?

It is unclear exactly why the clinical outcomes of patients with SLN reported by the LNCSG and subsequent reports using the ISN/RPS classification are so different, but there are several possibilities. The first relates to study design. The LNCSG study was prospective, and it utilized a large group of patients with SLN, a very specific treatment protocol,[59] and had long-term follow-up. In contrast, all of the studies utilizing the ISN/RPS classification were retrospective and did not use standardized treatment protocols. Additionally, the majority of studies using the ISN/RPS classification consist of comparatively small numbers of patients with short-term follow-up (Table 6.12). The difference in follow-up may have a major impact on outcome because it has been clearly demonstrated that long-term follow-up is required in patients with lupus nephritis to clearly establish the impact of treatment and assess outcomes.[69] A second consideration is the vasculitic nature of the segmental lesion, suggesting that patients in the LNCSG have done worse as they were systematically undertreated given the reliance on prednisone, the short-term course of cyclophosphamide, and the proven ineffectiveness of plasmapheresis. Finally, and equally important to study design, there are differences in the way in which the subgroups of SLN are defined in the two classifications. As previously discussed, compared to the classification used by the LNCSG, the ISN/RPS classification relegates biopsies with segmental lesions that involve ≥50% of the glomerular surface area to Class IV-G. As a result of this practice, the ISN/RPS classification could easily conceal differences in outcomes between patients with Class IV-S and IV-G. All of these issues help to account for the differences in outcome observed between these studies and point out the difficulty in even trying to compare results. The impact on clinical outcomes that is created by the differences in the two classifications is extremely important to understand.

In order to evaluate the clinical impact of the ISN/RPS classification relative to the modified 1982 WHO classification for SLN, Schwartz et al.[22] reclassified the biopsies from patients in the LNCSG using the ISN/RPS criteria. Because the ISN/RPS classification uses 50% glomerular surface area involvement to separate the cases of severe segmental GN classified as diffuse segmental GN (IV-S) from cases of severe segmental GN classified as DGGN (IV-G), biopsies with severe FSGN with < and ≥ 50%

Table 6.12 Prognosis of severe lupus nephritis using International Society of Nephrology/Renal Pathology Society classification: retrospective studies

	Mittal et al.[37] USA		Yokoyama et al.[67] Japan		Hill et al.[26] France		Kim et al.[68] Korea		Hiramatsu et al.[66] Japan		Grootscholten et al.[35] Netherlands	
	IV-S	IV-G	IV-S	IV-G	IV-S	IV-G	IV-S	IV-G	IV-S	IV-G	IV-S	IV-G
n	11	22	6	17	15	31	12	30	14	41	15	57
FU (months)	38	55	187 (overall)		120 (overall)		60 (overall)		84 (overall)		78	76
CR	0	5%	33%	65%			67%*	33%			53%	56%
PR	20%	9%					25%	50%				
GFR(ml/min)							86	73				
SCrx2	20%	0			35%	40%					0	9%
ESRD	10%	9%	67%	29%								
Renal survival												
-10 years**					65%	60%			90%	80%		
Median time to ESRD (months)			95	214								

* P<0.05.

** End-point of doubling of SCr.

CR, complete remission; ERSD, end stage renal disease; FU, follow-up; GFR, glomerular filtration rate; PR, partial remission; SCr, serum creatinine.

glomerular surface area involvement were separately evaluated and compared to the patients in IV-G whose glomeruli showed DGGN. The histological features for biopsies with SSGN remained similar and pauci-immune in nature irrespective of the glomerular surface area involved (Figure 6.17), and this was in contrast to DGGN where evidence of immune-complex deposition dominated. Although baseline clinical and serological features were not significantly different among the three groups, there was a significant difference in outcomes. The remission rates were significantly different among the three groups, with those patients with SSGN having ≥50% glomerular surface area involvement having the poorest response to treatment, those with DGGN the best remission rate, and patients with SSGN having lesions with <50% glomerular surface area involvement having a remission rate that was intermediate (23% versus 56% versus 41%, P=0.03). As a result, it is not unexpected that patients with SSGN having ≥50% glomerular surface area involvement had a significantly worse prognosis for renal survival, (Figure 6.20A). Although patients with DGGN had the best prognosis, the prognosis for those with SSGN and <50% glomerular surface area involvement was intermediate. Thus, if the patients with SSGN are included together, irrespective of the extent of glomerular surface area involvement, as was done by the LNCSG, patients with severe FSGN (WHO III ≥50%) have a significantly worse prognosis than patients with DGGN (WHO IV) (Figure 6.20A, B). However, if, as was done in the ISN/RPS classification, the SSGN patients with ≥50% glomerular surface area involvement are included in the diffuse global nephritis group (IV-G) the difference in outcome between the two groups is lost (Figure 6.20A, C). By relegating patients with the most severe segmental involvement to the category of DGGN (IV-G), the ISN/RPS classification conceals important differences that were seen in patients with severe segmental disease. This ultimately has important therapeutic implications given the putative differences in the pathogenesis of these two lesions.

Conclusion

Severe lupus nephritis is a pathological diagnosis that refers to biopsies with glomerulonephritis involving ≥50% of the glomeruli that have either a segmental or global intraglomerular distribution. Patients with SLN have a more aggressive form of the disease with a poorer prognosis, but early diagnosis and treatment with prednisone and immunosuppressive regimens can lead to a remission and improved overall prognosis. It is important to note that different criteria used to distinguish segmental from global GN in the 1982 WHO and ISN/RPS classifications lead to significant redistribution of cases between the two categories and this is reflected in differences in the pathogenic and prognostic implications of the biopsy. Using the 1982 WHO classification, the histopathology and immunopathology suggest that severe FSGN and DGGN have different pathogenic mechanisms: DGGN appears to be caused by the subendothelial deposition of circulating immune complexes, and severe FSGN has pauci-immune pathological features suggesting a vasculitic mechanism. In the outcome analysis using 1982 WHO classification, severe FSGN had fewer therapeutic remissions, more rapid progression of renal disease, and progressed more frequently to end

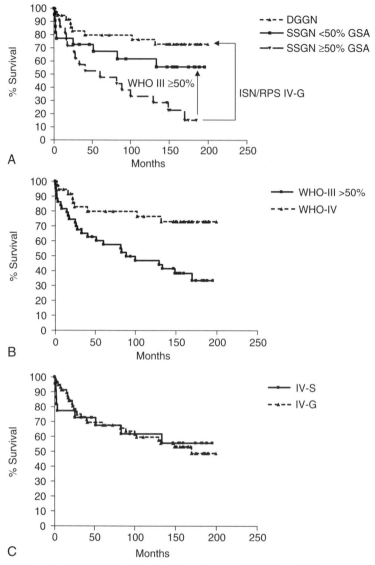

Fig. 6.20 Renal survival. (A) Renal survival in patients with diffuse global glomerulonephritis (DGGN) and those with severe focal segmental glomerulonephritis (SSGN) subcategorized by the extent of glomerular surface area (GSA) involved by a segmental lesion (< or ≥50% GSA). Renal survival for patients with SSGN ≥50% GSA was significantly worse than for DGGN (P=0.001) and those with SSGN <50% GSA had an intermediate outcome. (B) Patients classified by the World Health Organization (WHO) classification (SSGN ≥50% GSA included in the WHO III ≥50% category). The renal survival was significantly worse for patients with SSGN (WHO Class III ≥50%) than for patients with WHO Class IV (WHO-IV, P=0.0028). (C) Patients classified by the International Society of Nephrology/Renal Pathology Society (ISN/RPS) classification (SSGN ≥50% GSA included in the DGGN category). There is no difference in outcome between patients with diffuse segmental (IV-S) and DGGN (IV-G). From Schwartz MM, Korbet SM, Lewis EJ. The prognosis and pathogenesis of Severe Lupus Glomerulonephritis. *Nephrol Dial Transplant* 2008; **23**: 1298–1306.

stage renal disease. In contrast, when SLN is dichotomized using the ISN/RPS classification, these important pathogenic and prognostic findings are lost.

These observations have implications for the renal physician. The possibility of using the renal pathology to guide the treatment of patients with SLN may have the greatest impact, and this implies therapeutic approaches guided by the underlying pathogenetic mechanism rather than a "one size fits all" approach. Based on the clinicopathological information available, we believe patients with severe segmental GN should be treated with cytotoxic regimens designed for vasculitic lesions, whereas patients with the immune complex-mediated lesion of DGGN may be treated equally effectively with regimens requiring less intense cytotoxic approaches. Ideally, this approach would avoid undertreating one lesion and overtreating the other, and would avoid or minimize side effects. In analyzing the literature, it is important that the reader understand how the focal segmental and diffuse global forms of SLN are defined. If the pathological division does not reflect homogeneous pathogenesis, the results will be compromised by including potentially unresponsive patients in the treatment groups. For example, it may be futile to treat patients with pauci-immune, vasculitis-like severe FSGN with agents designed to reduce antibody production. Finally, as new agents are developed to treat SLN, the design of therapeutic trials must be cognizant of the pathogenic implications of the renal pathology and must use this information to develop pathogenetically homogeneous treatment groups that allow targeting of specific mechanisms of glomerular injury and to avoid masking a therapeutic effect by including responsive and unresponsive lesions in the study group. It must also be recognized that more than one pathogenetic process may coexist in a given patient with lupus nephritis. Patients with immune complex-mediated membranous lupus nephritis[15,21,70,71] or DGGN[24] can have a coexisting pauci-immune process. In therapeutic trials targeting these complex lesions, treatment of both the humoral and pauci-immune processes needs to be considered.[70,72]

References

1. Muehrcke, R.C., Kark, R.M., Pirani, C.L., and Pollak, V.E. (1957) Lupus nephritis: A clinical and pathologic study based on renal biopsies. *Medicine* **36**, 1–146.
2. Pollak, V.E., Pirani, C.L., Kark, and R.M. (1961) Effect of large doses of prednisone on the renal lesions and life span of patients with lupus glomerulonephritis. *J Lab Clin Med* **57**, 495–511.
3. Pollak, V.E., Pirani, C.L., and Schwartz, F.D. (1964) The natural history of the renal manifestations of systemic lupus erythematosus. *J Lab Clin Med* **63**, 537–50.
4. Pollak, V.E., Kark, R.M., and Pirani, C.L. (1961) Corticosteroid therapy in lupus nephritis. Importance of adequate dosage. *Bull Rheum Dis* **11**, 249–50.
5. Pollak, V.E., Pirani, C.L., Dujovne, I., and Dillard, M.G. (1973) The Clinical Course of Lupus Nephritis: Relationship to the Renal Histologic Findings. In: *Glomerulonephritis* (Kincaid-Smith, P., Mathew, T.H., Becker, E.L., eds), pp. 1167–82. John Wiley and Sons, New York.
6. Baldwin, D.S., Lowenstein, J., Rothfield, N.F., Gallo, G., and McCluskey, R.T. (1970) The clinical course of the proliferative and membranous forms of lupus nephritis. *Ann Intern Med* **73**(6), 929–42.

7. Baldwin, D.S., Gluck, M.C., Lowenstein, J., and Gallo, G.R. (1977) Lupus nephritis. Clinical course as related to morphologic forms and their transitions. *Am J Med* **62**(1), 12–30.

8. Appel, G.B., Silva, F.G., Pirani, C.L., Meltzer, J.I., and Estes, D. (1978) Renal involvement in systemic lupus erythematosus (SLE): A study of fifty-six patients emphasizing histologic classification. *Medicine* **57**, 371–410.

9. Appel, G.B., Cohen, D.J., Pirani, C.L., Meltzer, J.I., and Estes, D. (1987) Long-term follow-up of patients with lupus nephritis. A study based on the classification of the World Health Organization. *Am J Med* **83**, 877–85.

10. Austin, H.A., III, Muenz, L.R., Joyce, K.M., Antonovych, T.T., and Balow, J.E. (1984) Diffuse proliferative lupus nephritis: identification of specific pathologic features affecting renal outcome. *Kidney Int* **25**(4), 689–95.

11. Austin, H.A., III, Boumpas, D.T., Vaughan, E.M., and Balow, J.E. (1994) Predicting renal outcomes in severe lupus nephritis: contributions of clinical and histologic data. *Kidney Int* **45**, 544–50.

12. McCluskey, R.T. (1975) Lupus nephritis. In: *Kidney pathology: Decennial* (Summers, S.C., ed.), pp. 456–9. Appleton & Lange, New York.

13. Churg, J., and Sobin, L.H. (1982) *Renal Disease: Classification and Atlas of Glomerular Disease*. Igaku-Shoin, Tokyo.

14. Schwartz, M.M., Kawala, K.S., Corwin, H.L., and Lewis, E.J. (1987) The prognosis of segmental glomerulonephritis in systemic lupus erythematosus. *Kidney Int* **32**(2), 274–9.

15. Sloan, R.P., Schwartz, M.M., Korbet, S.M., Borok, R.Z., for the Lupus Nephritis Collaborative Study Group. (1996) Long-Term Outcome in Systemic Lupus Erythematosus Membranous Glomerulonephritis. *J Am Soc Nephrol* **7**, 299–305.

16. Schwartz, M.M., Lan, S.P., Bonsib, S.M., Gephardt, G.N., Sharma, H.M., for the Lupus Nephritis Collaborative Study Group. (1989) Clinical outcome of three discrete histologic patterns of injury in severe lupus glomerulonephritis. *Am J Kidney Dis* **13**, 273–83.

17. Lewis, E.J., Hunsicker, L.G., Rohde, R.D., Lachin, J.M., for the Lupus Nephritis Collaborative Study Group. (1992) A controlled trial of plasmapheresis therapy in severe lupus nephritis. The Lupus Nephritis Collaborative Study Group. *N Engl J Med* **326**, 1373–9.

18. Churg, J., Bernstein, J., and Glassock, R.J. (1985) Lupus Nephritis. Renal Disease. *Classification and Atlas of Glomerular Diseases*, pp. 151–80. Igaku-Shoin, New York.

19. Weening, J.J., D'Agati, V.D., Schwartz, M.M., Seshan, S.V., Alpers, C.E., Appel, G.B., *et al.* (2004) The classification of glomerulonephritis in systemic lupus erythematosus revisited. *Kidney Int* **65**(2), 521–30.

20. McCluskey, R.T. (1970) Lupus nephritis. *Pathol Annu* **5**, 125–44.

21. Najafi, C.C., Korbet, S.M., Lewis, E.J., Schwartz, M.M., Reichlin, M., and Evans, J. (2001) Significance of histologic patterns of glomerular injury upon long-term prognosis in severe lupus glomerulonephritis. *Kidney Int* **59**(6), 2156–63.

22. Schwartz, M.M., Korbet, S.M., and Lewis, E.J. (2008) The Prognosis and Pathogenesis of Severe Lupus Glomerulonephritis. *Nephrol Dial Transplant* **23**, 1298–306.

23. Pirani, C.L., Pollak, V.E., and Schwartz, F.D. (1964) The reproducibility of semiquantitative analyses of renal histology. *Nephron* **1**, 230–7.

24. Schwartz, M.M., Korbet, S.M., Katz, R.S., and Lewis, E.J. (2009) Evidence of concurrent immunopathological mechanisms determining the pathology of severe lupus nephritis. *Lupus* **18**(2), 149–58.

25. Schwartz, M.M., Roberts, J.L., and Lewis, E.J. (1983) Necrotizing glomerulitis of systemic lupus erythematosus. *Hum Pathol* **14**(2), 158–67.

26. Hill, G.S., Delahousse, M., Nochy, D., and Bariety, J. (2005) Class IV-S versus class IV-G lupus nephritis: clinical and morphologic differences suggesting different pathogenesis. *Kidney Int* **68**(5), 2288–97.

27. Charney, D.A., Nassar, G., Truong, L., and Nadasdy, T. (2000) 'Pauci-Immune' proliferative and necrotizing glomerulonephritis with thrombotic microangiopathy in patients with systemic lupus erythematosus and lupus-like syndrome. *Am J Kidney Dis* **35**(6), 1193–206.

28. Grishman, E., and Churg, J. (1982) Focal segmental lupus nephritis. *Clin Nephrol* **17**(1), 5–13.

29. Hill, G.S., Hinglais, N., Tron, F., and Bach, J.F. (1978) Systemic lupus erythematosus. Morphologic correlations with immunologic and clinical data at the time of biopsy. *Am J Med* **64**(1), 61–79.

30. Dujovne, I., Pollak, V.E., Pirani, C.L., and Dillard, M.G. (1972) The distribution and character of glomerular deposits in systemic lupus erythematosus. *Kidney Int* **2**(1), 33–50.

31. Dillard, M.G., Tillman, R.L., and Sampson, C.C. (1975) Lupus Nephritis. Correlations between the clinical course and presence of electron-dense deposits. *Lab Invest* **32**(3), 261–9.

32. Corwin, H.L., Schwartz, M.M., and Lewis, E.J. (1988) The importance of sample size in the interpretation of renal biopsy. *Am J Nephrol* **8**, 85–9.

33. Markowitz, G.S., and D'Agati, V.D. (2007) The ISN/RPS 2003 classification of lupus nephritis: An assessment at 3 years. *Kidney Int* **71**(6), 491–5.

34. Furness, P.N., and Taub, N. (2006) Interobserver reproducibility and application of the ISN/RPS classification of lupus nephritis-a UK-wide study. *Am J Surg Pathol* **30**(8), 1030–5.

35. Grootscholten, C., Bajema, I.M., Florquin, S., Steenbergen, E.J., Peutz-Kootstra, C.J., Goldschmeding, R. *et al.* (2008) Interobserver agreement of scoring of histopathological characteristics and classification of lupus nephritis. *Nephrol Dial Transplant* **23**(1), 223–30.

36. Behara, V., Whittier, W., Korbet, S., Schwartz, M., Martens, M., and Lewis, E. (2010) Pathogenetic features of severe segmental lupus nephritis. *Nephrol Dial Transplant* **25**, 153–9.

37. Mittal, B., Hurwitz, S., Rennke, H., and Singh, A.K. (2004) New subcategories of class IV lupus nephritis: are there clinical, histologic, and outcome differences? *Am J Kidney Dis* **44**(6), 1050–9.

38. Jennette, J.C., and Thomas, D.B. (2007) Pauci-immune and antineutrophil cytoplasmic autoantibody-mediated crescentic glomerulonephritis and vasculitis. In: *Heptinstall's Pathology of the Kidney* (Jennette, J.C., Olson, J.M., Schwartz, M.M., Silva, F.G., eds), pp. 643–74. Lippincott Williams &Wilkins, Philadelphia.

39. Arahata, H., Migita, K., Izumoto, H., Miyashita, T., Munakata, H., Nakamura, H., *et al.* (1999) Successful treatment of rapidly progressive lupus nephritis associated with anti-MPO antibodies by intravenous immunoglobulins. *Clin Rheumatol* **18**(1), 77–81.

40. Marshall, S., Dressler, R., and D'Agati, V. (1997) Membranous lupus nephritis with antineutrophil cytoplasmic antibody- associated segmental necrotizing and crescentic glomerulonephritis. *Am J Kidney Dis* **29**(1), 119–24.

41. Nasr, S.H., D'Agati, V.D., Park, H.R., Sterman, P.L., Goyzueta, J.D., Dressler, R.M., *et al.* (2008) Necrotizing and crescentic lupus nephritis with antineutrophil cytoplasmic antibody seropositivity. *Clin J Am Soc Nephrol* **3**(3), 682–90.

42. Sen, D., and Isenberg, D.A. (2003) Antineutrophil cytoplasmic autoantibodies in systemic lupus erythematosus. *Lupus* **12**(9), 651–8.

43. Del Papa, N., Conforti, G., Gambini, D., La Rosa, L., Tincani, A., D'Cruz, D., *et al.* (1994) Characterization of the endothelial surface proteins recognized by anti-endothelial antibodies in primary and secondary autoimmune vasculitis. *Clin Immunol Immunopathol* **70**, 211–6.

44. Renaudineau, Y., Dugue, C., Dueymes, M., and Youinou, P. (2002) Antiendothelial cell antibodies in systemic lupus erythematosus. *Autoimmun Rev* **1**(6), 365–72.

45. Chin, H.J., Ahn, C., Lim, C.S., Chung, H.K., Lee, J.G., Song, Y.W., *et al.* (2000) Clinical implications of antineutrophil cytoplasmic antibody test in lupus nephritis. *Am J Nephrol* **20**(1), 57–63.

46. Pradhan, V.D., Badakere, S.S., Bichile, L.S., and Almeida, A.F. (2004) Anti-neutrophil cytoplasmic antibodies (ANCA) in systemic lupus erythematosus: prevalence, clinical associations and correlation with other autoantibodies. *J Assoc Physicians India* **52**, 533–7.

47. Anderson, L., Sinsakul, M., Korbet, S., and Schwartz, M. (2002) Membranous glomerulonephritis with segmental necrosis and/or crescents (Abstract). *J Am Soc Nephrol* **13**, 660A.

48. Schwartz, M.M., Bernstein, J., Hill, G.S., Holley, K., Phillips, E.A., for the Lupus Nephritis Collaborative Study Group (1989) Predictive value of renal pathology in diffuse proliferative lupus glomerulonephritis. *Kidney Int* **36**, 891–6.

49. Chan, T.M., Li, F.K., Tang, C.S., Wong, R.W., Fang, G.X., Ji, Y.L., *et al.* (2000) Efficacy of mycophenolate mofetil in patients with diffuse proliferative lupus nephritis. Hong Kong-Guangzhou Nephrology Study Group. *N Engl J Med* **343**(16), 1156–62.

50. Chan, T.M., Tse, K.C., Tang, C.S., Lai, K.N., and Li, F.K. (2005) Long-term outcome of patients with diffuse proliferative lupus nephritis treated with prednisolone and oral cyclophosphamide followed by azathioprine. *Lupus* **14**(4), 265–72.

51. Chan, T.M., Tse, K.C., Tang, C.S., Mok, M.Y., and Li, F.K. (2005) Long-term study of mycophenolate mofetil as continuous induction and maintenance treatment for diffuse proliferative lupus nephritis. *J Am Soc Nephrol* **16**(4), 1076–84.

52. Ginzler, E.M., Dooley, M.A., Aranow, C., Kim, M.Y., Buyon, J., Merrill, J.T., *et al.* (2005) Mycophenolate mofetil or intravenous cyclophosphamide for lupus nephritis. *N Engl J Med* **353**(21), 2219–28.

53. Gourley, M.F., Austin, H.A., III, Scott, D., Yarboro, C.H., Vaughan, E.M., Muir, J., *et al.* (1996) Methylprednisolone and cyclophosphamide, alone or in combination, in patients with lupus nephritis. A randomized, controlled trial. *Ann Intern Med* **125**(7), 549–57.

54. Mok, C.C., Ying, K.Y., Ng, W.L., Lee, K.W., To, C.H., Lau, C.S., *et al.* (2006) Long-term outcome of diffuse proliferative lupus glomerulonephritis treated with cyclophosphamide. *Am J Med* **119**(4), 355–33.

55. Balow, J.E. (2005) Clinical presentation and monitoring of lupus nephritis. *Lupus* **14**(1), 25–30.

56. Contreras, G., Lenz, O., Pardo, V., Borja, E., Cely, C., Iqbal, K., *et al.* (2006) Outcomes in African Americans and Hispanics with lupus nephritis. *Kidney Int* **69**(10), 1846–51.

57. Illei, G.G., Takada, K., Parkin, D., Austin, H.A., Crane, M., Yarboro, C.H., *et al.* (2002) Renal flares are common in patients with severe proliferative lupus nephritis treated with pulse immunosuppressive therapy: long-term followup of a cohort of 145 patients participating in randomized controlled studies. *Arthritis Rheum* **46**(4), 995–1002.

58. Ioannidis, J.P., Boki, K.A., Katsorida, M.E., Drosos, A.A., Skopouli, F.N., Boletis, J.N., *et al.* (2000) Remission, relapse, and re-remission of proliferative lupus nephritis treated with cyclophosphamide. *Kidney Int* **57**(1), 258–64.

59. Clough, J.D., Lewis, E.J., and Lachin, J.M. (1990) Treatment protocols of the lupus nephritis collaborative study of plasmapheresis in severe lupus nephritis. The Lupus Nephritis Collaborative Study Group. *Prog Clin Biol Res* **337**, 301–7.

60. Chen, Y.E., Korbet, S.M., Katz, R.S., Schwartz, M.M., and Lewis, E.J. (2008) Value of a complete or partial remission in severe lupus nephritis. *Clin J Am Soc Nephrol* **3**(1), 46–53.

61. Korbet, S.M., Lewis, E.J., Schwartz, M.M., Reichlin, M., Evans, J., and Rohde, R.D. (2000) Factors predictive of outcome in severe lupus nephritis. Lupus Nephritis Collaborative Study Group. *Am J Kidney Dis* **35**(5), 904–14.

62. Korbet, S.M., Schwartz, M.M., Evans, J., and Lewis, E.J. (2007) Severe lupus nephritis: racial differences in presentation and outcome. *J Am Soc Nephrol* **18**(1), 244–54.

63. Austin, H.A.,III, Boumpas, D.T., Vaughan, E.M., and Balow, J.E. (1995) High-risk features of lupus nephritis: importance of race and clinical and histological factors in 166 patients. *Nephrol Dial Trans* **10**(9), 1620–8.

64. Dooley, M.A., Hogan, S., Jennette, C., and Falk, R. (1997) Cyclophosphamide therapy for lupus nephritis: poor renal survival in black Americans. Glomerular Disease Collaborative Network. *Kidney Int* **51**(4), 1188–95.

65. Mok, C.C. (2005) Prognostic factors in lupus nephritis. *Lupus* **14**(1), 39–44.

66. Hiramatsu, N., Kuroiwa, T., Ikeuchi, H., Maeshima, A., Kaneko, Y., Hiromura, K., *et al.* (2008) Revised classification of lupus nephritis is valuable in predicting renal outcome with an indication of the proportion of glomeruli affected by chronic lesions. *Rheumatology (Oxford)* **47**(5), 702–7.

67. Yokoyama, H., Wada, T., Hara, A., Yamahana, J., Nakaya, I., Kobayashi, M., *et al.* (2004) The outcome and a new ISN/RPS 2003 classification of lupus nephritis in Japanese. *Kidney Int* **66**(6), 2382–8.

68. Kim, Y.G., Kim, H.W., Cho, Y.M., Oh, J.S., Nah, S.S., Lee, C.K. *et al.* (2008) The difference between lupus nephritis class IV-G and IV-S in Koreans: focus on the response to cyclophosphamide induction treatment. *Rheumatology (Oxford)* **47**(3), 311–14.

69. Austin, H.A.,III, Klippel, J.H., Balow, J.E., le Riche, N.G., Steinberg, A.D., Plotz, P.H., *et al.* (1986) Therapy of lupus nephritis. Controlled trial of prednisone and cytotoxic drugs. *New Engl J Med* **314**(10), 614–19.

70. Bao, H., Liu, Z.H., Xie, H.L., Hu, W.X., Zhang, H.T., and Li, L.S. (2008) Successful treatment of class V+IV lupus nephritis with multitarget therapy. *J Am Soc Nephrol* **19**(10), 2001–10.

71. Nasr, S.H., Said, S.M., Valeri, A.M., Stokes, M.B., Masani, N.N., D'Agati, V.D., *et al.* (2009) Membranous glomerulonephritis with ANCA-associated necrotizing and crescentic glomerulonephritis. *Clin J Am Soc Nephrol* **4**(2), 299–308.

72. Glassock, R.J. (2008) Multitarget therapy of lupus nephritis: base hit or home run? *J Am Soc Nephrol* **19**(10), 1842–4.

Chapter 7

Lupus membranous nephropathy[*]

Howard A. Austin III, Gabor G. Illei, and
James E. Balow

Introduction

Lupus membranous nephropathy (LMN) is characterized by widespread subepithelial and/or intramembranous immune deposits, diffuse glomerular capillary wall thickening, and, frequently, mesangial expansion. These morphological attributes are observed in approximately 10–20% of lupus patients who develop clinically significant renal involvement during the course of their disease.[1] Furthermore, LMN is one of the most common causes of secondary membranous nephropathy, accounting for approximately 20% of those patients.[2] Comparable to people with idiopathic membranous nephropathy, individuals with LMN are at increased long-term risk for end stage renal disease (ESRD) and complications of the nephrotic syndrome.

Historical perspective on lupus membranous nephropathy

In the pre-electron microscopy era, it was common to use the term "membranous" to describe capillary wall thickening in essentially any form of glomerular disease. Pathologists recognized differences in staining properties between "membranous" lesions, but considered these differences to be mostly related to the age of the capillary wall lesions rather than to any unique pathogenesis. In the first textbook of renal pathology published in 1950, Bell noted that, although there were several types of glomerular lesions in lupus erythematosus, the most frequent form was patchy thickening of the capillary loops, which he described as "membranous" change.[3] In lupus nephritis, "membranous" subsequently was commonly used to describe irregular capillary wall thickenings, including wire-loop lesions, lesions that were integral features of lupus glomerulonephritis. In the original Dubois textbook devoted to lupus erythematosus published in 1966, Pollak and Pirani modified this perspective somewhat, suggesting that the bulk of membranous lesions represented an inactive form of lupus glomerulonephritis.[4]

The advent of immunofluorescence microscopy allowed the detection of immune deposits in glomerular lesions and electron microscopy offered the tools to distinguish different patterns and locations of depositions of antibodies and other immune reactants. Capillary wall thickening appreciated by light microscopy was further resolved and nomenclature refined. Some thickenings were due to deposition of subendothelial immune complexes and/or fibrin as elements of proliferative lupus nephritis. Others were due to mesangial interposition beneath the endothelium, defining the membranoproliferative or mesangiocapillary variant of diffuse proliferative lupus nephritis. Still others were explained by widespread and essentially uniform deposition of antibody and complement components along the external (subepithelial) aspect of the glomerular basement membrane (GBM), a process that evoked reactive thickening of the substance of the basement membrane. By the late 1960s, consensus had developed that the term, membranous nephropathy, should be reserved for the latter cases. Some cases of membranous nephropathy were easily recognized by light microscopy when there was nearly uniform thickening of glomerular capillary loops, epimembranous deposits on trichrome stains, and basement membrane spikes on silver stains. However, the key criterion for diagnosis of LMN was the presence of nearly uniform subepithelial and/or intramembranous electron-dense deposits.

The first international effort to standardize the classification of lupus nephritis occurred in 1974 under the auspices of the World Health Organization (WHO).[5] Lupus membranous nephropathy was assigned as Class V lupus nephritis, with no subdivisions. However, a revision of the WHO classification system in 1982 expanded the definition of Class V LMN to include subsets of patients with pure membranous nephropathy (Class Va), mixed membranous and mesangial nephropathy (Class Vb), mixed membranous and focal (Class Vc), and diffuse (Class Vd) endocapillary proliferation.[6] The latter subclasses of patients were deemed much more likely to experience renal functional deterioration than patients with LMN who did not have concurrent endocapillary proliferation.[7] Consequently, some studies that used this expanded definition of LMN showed that LMN had the worst prognosis among all classes of lupus nephritis.[8] The 1995 revision of the WHO classification scheme[9] and the 2003 International Society of Nephrology/Renal Pathology Society (ISN/RPS) classification of lupus nephritis[10] avoided this issue by eliminating subclasses Vc and Vd and returning to the original WHO classification approach to LMN. This chapter will focus on patients whose renal biopsies manifest LMN without substantive endocapillary proliferation (see Figures 7.1–7.4). Patients who have mixed membranous and proliferative forms of lupus nephritis should be treated according to recommendations for the proliferative component (see Figure 7.5).

Pathogenesis

Lupus membranous nephropathy is characterized by subepithelial (epimembranous) immune deposits along the peripheral capillary loops, leading to uniform glomerular capillary wall thickening. There are very few data about the pathogenesis of LMN, but the subepithelial distribution of immune complex deposits suggests a mechanism more similar to idiopathic membranous nephropathy (IMN) than proliferative lupus nephritis, which is characterized by subendothelial deposits. Both animal models[11,12] and observations in idiopathic[13] and neonatal membranous nephropathy (MN)[14] suggest that immune complexes form *in situ* when an antibody binds specifically to

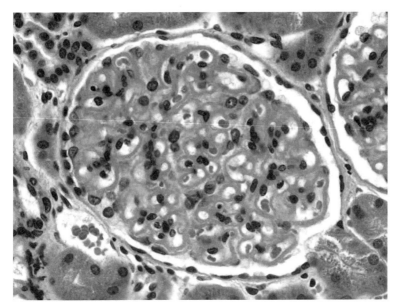

Fig. 7.1 Lupus membranous nephropathy. Global thickening of glomerular capillary loops. Moderate increase of mesangial cellularity characteristic of secondary membranous nephropathy. H&E, 400x (see Plate 10).

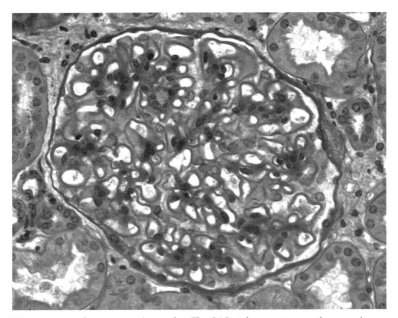

Fig. 7.2 Lupus membranous nephropathy. The PAS stain accentuates the prominence and stiffening of the capillary loops. PAS, 400x (see Plate 11).

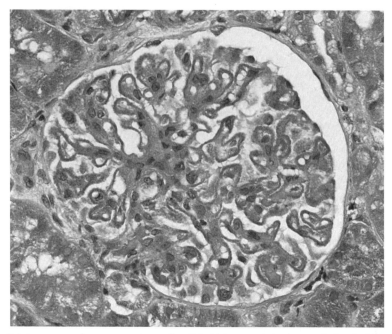

Fig. 7.3 Lupus membranous nephropathy. This trichrome stain demonstrates that the thickening of capillary loops is due to combination of aggregates of immune deposits and reactive glomerular basement thickening. Note the magenta-staining granular deposits along the external (subepithelial) aspect of the blue-staining glomerular basement membranes. Masson trichrome, 400x (see Plate 12).

an antigen constitutively expressed by the GBM or to soluble antigens that become localized on the glomerular capillary wall.

The target antigens in both neonatal MN (neutral endopeptidase) and IMN (M-type phospholipase A2 receptor) are expressed by podocytes on the outside of the GBM. Podocytes are also the main site of injury in LMN, and although the target antigen in lupus has not yet been identified, it is reasonable to assume that podocytes have a pivotal role in the development of LMN by providing antigenic targets for circulating antibodies for *in situ* formation of glomerular deposits. Subepithelial immune complex deposition triggers a complex cascade of events leading to podocyte injury, such as podocyte flattening and effacement. The subsequent development of proteinuria is complement dependent and involves the formation of C5b-C9, the membrane attack complex (MAC). The importance of MAC was demonstrated in animal models of MN, where depletion of C6 prevented proteinuria without affecting the formation of subepithelial deposits.[15] Similar to animal models of MN, urinary excretion of C5b-C9 is higher in patients with both IMN or LMN compared to other kidney diseases, suggesting that the same mechanism is important in humans.[16] In contrast to mesangial and endothelial cells, podocytes hypertrophy but do not proliferate in response to immunological injury. With time, there is thickening of the GBM due to an increase

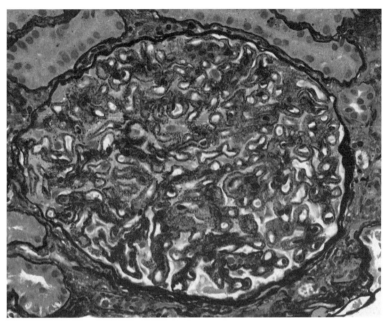

Fig. 7.4 Lupus membranous nephropathy. This silver stain accentuates the typical pattern of basement membrane thickening. The immune aggregates attached to and embedded within the basement membrane are unstained, causing spikes and moth-eaten appearance of the capillary loops. Jones silver stain, 400x (see Plate 13).

in the accumulation of extracellular matrix protein synthesis by the hypertrophied podocytes.[17] The exact mechanism of how C5b-C9 induces podocyte injury is not known, but the accumulation of reactive oxygen species,[18,19] increased expression of matrix metalloproteinases,[20,21] and changes in cytoskeleton due to loss of nephrin[22,23] may play an important role.

T and B lymphocytes are central to the initiation and maintenance of autoimmunity. In addition to autoantibody production, they contribute to glomerular injury by the production of chemokines, cytokines, and other inflammatory mediators in the kidney. Differential activation of CD4+ T helper cells in Th1 or Th2 cells has been proposed as a potential explanation for the variety of glomerular injuries in animal models.[24] T helper 1 and Th2 cells can be distinguished by their cytokine profiles and their abilities to generate different types of immune effector responses. Models of proliferative glomerulonephritides are associated with a predominantly Th1 response, whereas nonproliferative diseases, including membranous nephropathies, show a Th2 dominance. Recently, it was shown in the MRL/*lpr* mouse model of proliferative lupus nephritis that shifting the usual Th1 to a Th2 dominance converted diffuse proliferative to membranous nephritis.[25,26] Whether this distinction can be applied to human disease is unclear, especially in systemic lupus erythematosus, which cannot be clearly defined as a Th1 or Th2 disease and where proliferative and membranous nephritis frequently coexist.

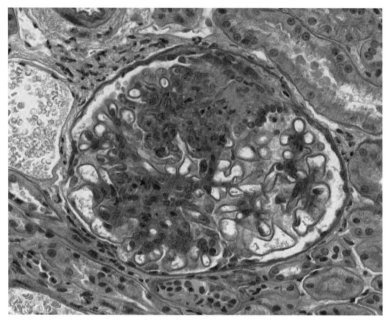

Fig. 7.5 Mixed lupus membranous and proliferative nephropathy. This glomerulus demonstrates the irregular pattern observed with mixed histology. In this single glomerular tuft, there are segments with simple capillary loop thickening (lower right), with superimposed marked mesangial expansion (lower left), and with loss of patency of capillary loops due to highly active endocapillary proliferation, karyorrhexis and early crescent formation (top). PAS, 400x (see Plate 14).

Renal biopsy features and classification

As noted previously, the inconstant criteria for diagnosis among various historical series of patients has made it difficult to define the characteristic clinical and pathological features of LMN. The 2003 ISN/RPS classification scheme should improve understanding of the natural history of LMN based on its precise criteria for diagnosis, i.e. glomerular capillary deposition of continuous granular subepithelial immune deposits. However, it is clear that under the rubric of LMN there remains a range of appearances and distributions of particular lesions. Mesangial deposits are almost always present in association with variable mesangial cell and matrix expansion (often considered to represent the "lowest common denominator" for all forms of lupus nephritis). When LMN and focal or diffuse proliferative lupus nephritis coexist in the same biopsy, both classes should be specified in the diagnostic line. Some investigators recommend staging the GBM reaction to the immune deposits (as originally applied to idiopathic membranous nephropathy), although this is not a formal component of the ISN/RPS schema. Stage 1 is defined by subepithelial deposits without substantive thickening of the GBM; stage 2, by subepithelial deposits with outward projections (spikes) of expanding GBM; stage 3, by incorporation of deposits within the GBM; and stage 4, by

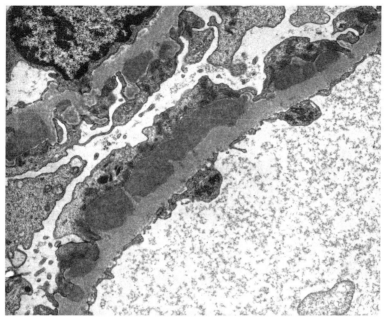

Fig. 7.6 Ultrastructure of glomerular capillaries in lupus membranous nephropathy. Electron dense deposits along the external surface (subepithelial) of two glomerular capillary loops. This case represents relatively early stage nephropathy in that basement membranes are near normal thickness with only minor external surface irregularities and spikes. Podocyte foot process fusion is seen overlying the electron dense deposits. Uranyl acetate and lead citrate, 18900x.

extremely thickened GBM with vacant spaces left by resorbed intramembranous deposits.[27] Stages 3 and 4 are usually associated with substantial loss of nephron integrity due to segmental or global glomerulosclerosis, tubular atrophy, and interstitial fibrosis (see Figures 7.6–7.8). Finally, a rare acute crescentic lesion may be seen in LMN, presumably due to rupture of a highly disordered and damaged GBM.

Mixed membranous and proliferative forms of lupus nephritis and their dire prognostic implications are relatively easily appreciated. However, many cases initially comprising pure proliferative lupus nephritis (predominantly subendothelial deposits with no or a few scattered subepithelial deposits) rather commonly evolve features that superficially resemble LMN during the course of treatment. Thus, although subendothelial deposits may regress, subepithelial deposits may increase in number, but they tend to differ from those of true LMN by their irregularity in size, shape, and distribution.[28]

Patients with LMN may express sudden worsening in proteinuria, urinary sediment, and/or renal function. Superimposed proliferative lupus nephritis, crescentic glomerulonephritis, thrombotic microangiopathy, and renal vein thrombosis should be considered and documented, where feasible, by renal biopsy.

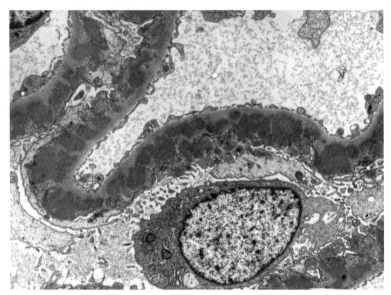

Fig. 7.7 Ultrastructure of an advanced stage lupus membranous nephropathy. Heavy electron dense deposits, basement membrane thickening with spikes, and epithelial cell foot process fusion. Uranyl acetate and lead citrate, 11250x.

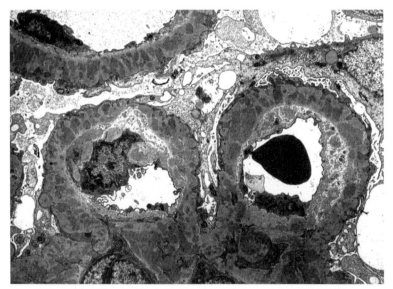

Fig. 7.8 Ultrastructure of a case with mixed membranous and proliferative lupus nephropathy in three glomerular capillaries. The membranous component is apparent with heavy intramembranous electron dense deposits. Heavy mesangial electron dense deposits are seen (bottom). Electron dense subendothelial deposits of varying stages of deposition and resorption separate the endothelium from the basement membrane. Uranyl acetate and lead citrate, 5000x.

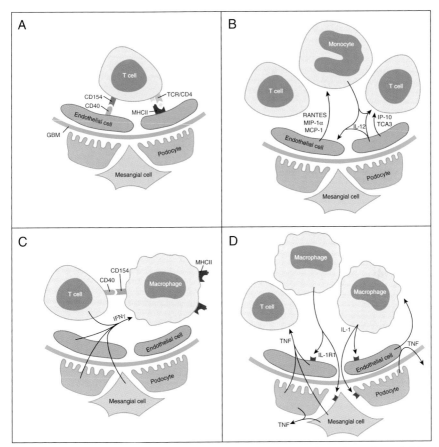

Plate 1 Mechanisms of effector T cell-directed injury in crescentic nephrotoxic nephritis (NTN) have been demonstrated using chimeric mice with selective leukocyte or intrinsic renal cell deletions of major histocompatibility complex (MHC)II,[176] CD40,[177] interleukin (IL)12,[29] interferon (IFN)γ,[44] tumor necrosis factor (TNF),[178] IL1β and IL1 receptor I.[179] Effector T cells require MHCII and CD40 expression by intrinsic renal cells to recognize nephritogenic antigens and initiate injury (A). Intrinsic renal cell production of monocyte and T cell chemoattractant chemokines and IL12 directs further leukocyte influx (B). T cell expression of CD40 and IFNγ from T cells and intrinsic renal cells activates monocytes to macrophages (C). Macrophages produce IL1, which acts via IL1 receptor I on intrinsic renal cells to induce TNF production and crescentic injury (D) (see Fig. 5.2).

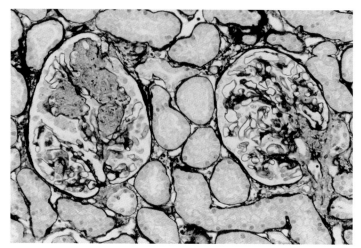

Plate 2 Focal and segmental distribution of glomerular pathology. The glomerulus on the left has an area of endocapillary proliferation and necrosis that involves 25% of the glomerulus (segmental intraglomerular distribution). Because the glomerulus on the right is normal, the pathology involves some but not all glomeruli (focal interglomerular distribution). Methenamine silver periodic acid Schiff stain (Jones), ×33 (see Fig. 6.4).

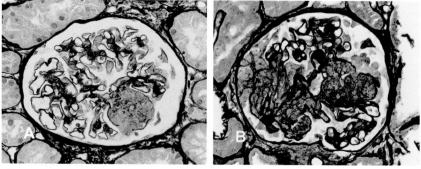

Plate 3 Variable glomerular involvement in focal segmental glomerulonephritis within the same biopsy. (A) One glomerular lobule, comprising 5–10% of the glomerular surface area has a necrotizing lesion with karyorrhexis and rupture of the glomerular basement membrane. The remainder of the glomerulus is normal. (B) More than 50% of the glomerular surface area shows endocapillary proliferation, but the uninvolved capillaries are relatively normal. Methenamine silver periodic acid Schiff stain (Jones), (A) and (B), ×66 (see Fig. 6.5).

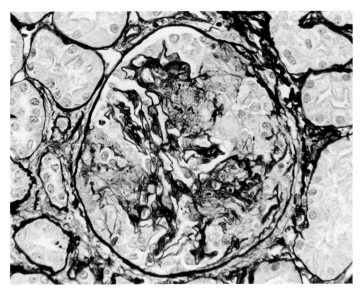

Plate 4 Glomerulus with focal segmental glomerulonephritis involving more than 80% of the tuft. There is endocapillary proliferation and necrosis in more than 80% of the glomerular surface area with destruction of the architecture and multiple foci with ruptures of glomerular basement membrane. The uninvolved capillaries in the center of the glomerulus comprise two lobules with relatively normal appearance. Methenamine silver periodic acid Schiff stain (Jones), ×66 (see Fig. 6.6).

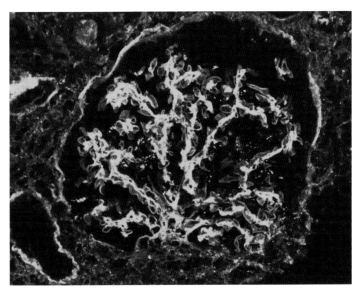

Plate 5 Focal segmental glomerulonephritis with a mesangial pattern of immunofluorescence. Immunoglobulin (Ig)G is strongly stained in the mesangium and focally in Bowman's capsule and the tubular basement membrane, but the peripheral glomerular capillary walls are almost completely void of deposits. Fluorescein isothiocyanate rabbit anti-human IgG, ×100 (see Fig. 6.7).

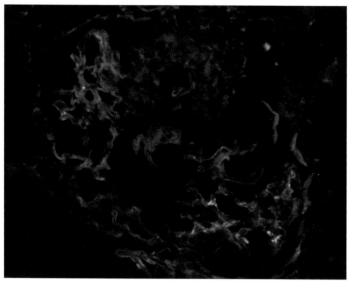

Plate 6 Focal segmental glomerulonephritis with a pauci-immune pattern of immunofluorescence. There is no significant glomerular staining for immunoglobulin (Ig)G either in the mesangium or the peripheral capillary walls. Fluorescein isothiocyanate rabbit anti-human IgG, ×100 (see Fig. 6.8).

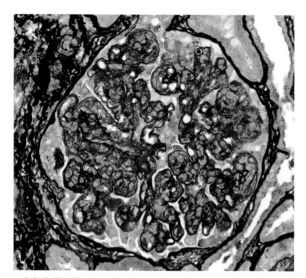

Plate 7 Diffuse global distribution of glomerular pathology. The glomerulus shows endocapillary proliferation involving almost every capillary (global). There is also widespread glomerular basement thickening and double contours consistent with subendothelial deposits. All the glomeruli in the biopsy showed similar pathology (diffuse). Methenamine silver periodic acid Schiff stain, ×66 (see Fig. 6.10).

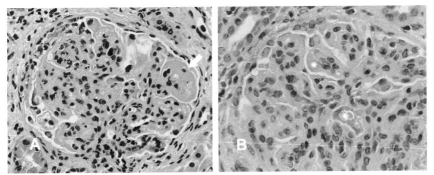

Plate 8 Wire-loops and hyaline thrombi are histological features that correspond to massive glomerular immune aggregate deposition. (A) Diffuse global glomerulonephritis (DGGN) with proliferation, neutrophilic exudates, and a wire-loop at 1–2 o'clock (arrow). The wire-loop comprises hyalin, eosinophilic thickening of the capillary wall, and, although they can be widespread, they often involve only one or two capillaries. (B) DGGN with hyaline thrombi in two capillaries (asterisks). The thrombus in the center of the picture is within a capillary with a wire-loop. Hematoxylin and eosin, (A) ×66, (B) ×132 (see Fig. 6.11).

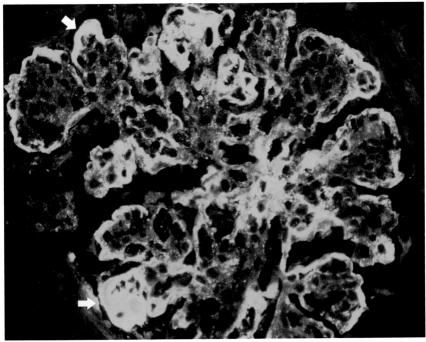

Plate 9 Immunofluorescence pattern in diffuse global glomerulonephritis. The peripheral capillary walls contain massive discontinuous linear deposits of immunoglobulin (Ig)G. The deposits have a characteristic smooth outer contour (arrows) because they are located in the subendothelial space, and their outer extent is limited and formed by the glomerular basal membrane (GBM). There are also focally intense mesangial deposits. Fluorescein isothiocyanate rabbit anti-human IgG, ×40 (see Fig. 6.12).

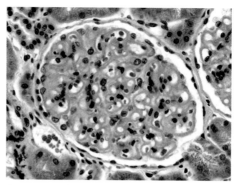

Plate 10 Lupus membranous nephropathy. Global thickening of glomerular capillary loops. Moderate increase of mesangial cellularity characteristic of secondary membranous nephropathy. H&E, 400x (see Fig. 7.1).

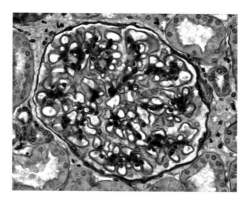

Plate 11 Lupus membranous nephropathy. The PAS stain accentuates the prominence and stiffening of the capillary loops. PAS, 400x (see Fig. 7.2).

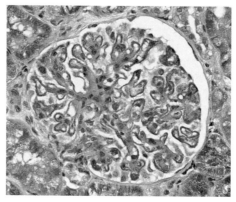

Plate 12 Lupus membranous nephropathy. This trichrome stain demonstrates that the thickening of capillary loops is due to combination of aggregates of immune deposits and reactive glomerular basement thickening. Note the magenta-staining granular deposits along the external (subepithelial) aspect of the blue-staining glomerular basement membranes. Masson trichrome, 400x (see Fig. 7.3).

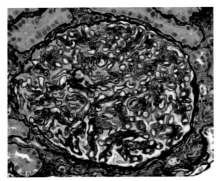

Plate 13 Lupus membranous nephropathy. This silver stain accentuates the typical pattern of basement membrane thickening. The immune aggregates attached to and embedded within the basement membrane are unstained, causing spikes and moth-eaten appearance of the capillary loops. Jones silver stain, 400x (see Fig. 7.4)

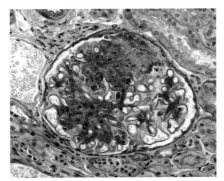

Plate 14 Mixed lupus membranous and proliferative nephropathy. This glomerulus demonstrates the irregular pattern observed with mixed histology. In this single glomerular tuft, there are segments with simple capillary loop thickening (lower right), with superimposed marked mesangial expansion (lower left), and with loss of patency of capillary loops due to highly active endocapillary proliferation, karyorrhexis and early crescent formation (top). PAS, 400x (see Fig. 7.5).

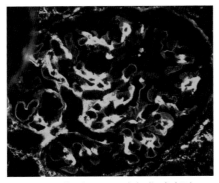

Plate 15 Fluorescence microscopy for immunoglobulin (Ig)G in a renal glomerulus in a patient who has the nephrotic syndrome due to lupus podocytopathy There are no IgG deposits in the peripheral capillary loops and all deposits are confined to the glomerular mesangium. Magnification, 40× (see Fig. 8.1).

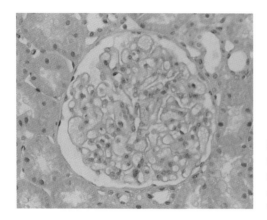

Plate 16 Lupus podocytopathy with minimal change lesion by light microscopy. There are no morphological abnormalities noted. Hematoxylin and eosin, magnification 66× (see Fig. 8.3).

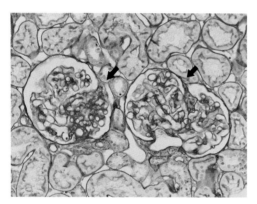

Plate 17 Lupus podocytopathy with focal segmental glomerular sclerosis by light microscopy. There are small segmental glomerular scars with adhesions (arrows) that do not involve the glomerular hilum, in two glomeruli. In some cases this can be accompanied by increased numbers of visceral epithelial cells in the area of the scar and increased mesangial cellularity. Neither of these abnormalities is noted in this example. Periodic acid Schiff stain, magnification 50× (see Fig. 8.4).

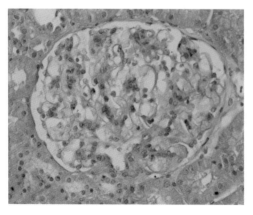

Plate 18 Lupus podocytopathy with increased numbers of cells in the glomerular mesangium. Increased connective tissue components in the mesangium can accompany this abnormality. Otherwise the glomerular histological structure is normal. In lupus, this structural abnormality is usually associated with some mesangial immune deposits, which contain IgG, but may also contain other immunoglobulins and complement components. Hematoxylin and eosin, magnification 66×(see Fig. 8.5).

Clinical presentation

Patients with systemic lupus erythematosus (SLE) should be followed closely for the development of lupus kidney disease. The importance of this caveat is underscored by the results of a retrospective study of 773 SLE patients reported by the University of California, San Francisco.[29] The investigators analyzed the time from the diagnosis of SLE to the first manifestations of renal disease to identify predictors of new onset lupus nephritis. They found that approximately 50% of men, 20% of women, 40% of Asian Americans, 30% of African Americans, 30% of Hispanic Americans, and 15% of European Americans developed lupus nephritis within 1 year of the diagnosis of SLE. The early clinical signs of LMN can be particularly subtle. Essentially, all patients with LMN present with proteinuria. However, the majority of the patients in some studies of LMN did not have the nephrotic syndrome when first recognized.[30–33] Furthermore, patients with LMN may appear to have quiescent SLE with few extrarenal manifestations, absent anti-DNA antibodies, and normal or near normal serum complement values.[7,34–36] Consequently, early detection of LMN may require vigilant monitoring of urinary protein excretion.

On presentation, patients with LMN often complain of features of the nephrotic syndrome, including nocturia, weight gain, and edema, which can be severe in some cases, leading to anasarca. In published series of LMN, the proportion of patients that present with the nephrotic syndrome varies widely, reflecting in large part, the heterogeneous inclusion criteria for these studies.[37–40] On average, more than 50% of patients with LMN have presented with the nephrotic syndrome and others have developed the nephrotic syndrome during the course of their disease.[1,41]

Different from patients with proliferative lupus nephritis, it is unusual for patients with LMN to present with renal insufficiency or hypertension,[32,40] but these features may evolve slowly over time. The urinary sediment is typically dominated by features of the nephrotic syndrome (including oval fat bodies and fatty casts). Microscopic hematuria is frequently observed in patients with LMN, but the presence of large numbers of red cell or white cell casts strongly suggests the presence of proliferative or mixed membranous and proliferative lupus nephritis.[34,40,42] Serological measures of lupus activity also tend to distinguish patients with LMN from those with proliferative lupus kidney disease.[32,34,35,40] In contrast to patients with proliferative lupus nephritis, those with LMN frequently, but not invariably, have normal (or near-normal) serum complement and anti-dsDNA levels. Despite these differences in the clinical presentation of proliferative and membranous lupus nephritis, the clinical characteristics of these types of lupus kidney disease overlap. A renal biopsy is needed to determine the exact histological type, as well as the severity of lupus nephritis; this information may help to clarify the prognosis and may facilitate deliberations regarding therapeutic options for the patient.

Small numbers of patients have been reported who were considered to have idiopathic membranous nephropathy for several months to years before they developed a compelling syndrome of other clinical and laboratory features that justified a diagnosis of SLE.[43–45] These patients often presented with serological and/or renal biopsy abnormalities that were suggestive, but not diagnostic, of lupus nephritis, including a positive antinuclear antibody (ANA), hypocomplementemia, C1q deposition, tubulo-reticular inclusions, as well as mesangial and small subendothelial electron-dense deposits. Patients with these features (particularly those with combinations of these abnormalities) should be followed especially closely for the development of other, potentially serious manifestations of SLE that may have an impact on prognosis and treatment recommendations.[46]

Prognosis of lupus membranous nephropathy

Table 7.1 shows 10-year patient and renal function survival data from different centers around the world. Although the average 10-year patient and renal survival estimates are each approximately 80%, the results from individual studies range widely from about 45% to 95%.[7,8,33,36,40,47–55] This diversity in the clinical course of patients with LMN underscores the need to consider the impact of potentially important demographic, clinical, and histological features that may affect the outcomes of patients with LMN. To date, the analyses of prognostic factors in patients with LMN have been limited by relatively small study populations compared to the studies of IMN that resulted in a robust predictive model for that disease. Consequently, we lack convincing and consistent information about potentially important prognostic factors among patients with LMN.

This concern is illustrated by the inconsistent information that has emerged about the predictive value of nephrotic-range proteinuria. Sloan, Mok, and Mercadal and their respective colleagues found that nephrotic proteinuria at baseline did not predict

Table 7.1 Ten-year cumulative survival estimates*

Author	Year	Location	Number of patients	Renal survival	Patient survival	Patient +/or renal survival
Tateno et al.[40]	1983	Japan	14			85%
Wang and Looi[55]	1984	Malaysia	13		75%	
Austin et al.[49]	1986	NIH	16	65%	74%	
Appel et al.[48]	1987	New York	10	47%	45%	
Leaker et al.[53]	1987	Australia	20		84%	
GISNEL[47]	1992	Italy	91	90%		
Pasquali et al.[36]	1993	Italy	42			92%
Bakir et al.[50]	1994	Chicago	22			90%
Donadio et al.[8]	1995	Rochester	67	63%		
Sloan et al.[7]	1996	Chicago	36			72%
Bono et al.[51]	1999	England	21		55%	
Huong et al.[52]	1999	France	32	77%	90%	
Mercadal et al.[54]	2002	France	66	88%		
Sun et al.[33]	2008	China	100	93%	98%	

* Updated and modified from reference.[119]

subsequent renal function deterioration in three separate studies of LMN.[7,54,56] On the other hand, Sun and colleagues recently showed that baseline nephrotic proteinuria was an independent predictor of end stage renal failure in a study of 100 Chinese patients with LMN.[33] In the context of a prospective study of treatment for LMN, we analyzed the predictive value of relatively severe baseline proteinuria (>5 g/day), comparable to the approach that has been used in several studies of IMN.[57,58] We found (by univariate and multivariate survival analysis) that this level of high-grade proteinuria at study entry was independently associated with a decreased probability of complete or partial remission of proteinuria during the first year of treatment.[59]

Of interest, Mercadal and colleagues found that patients who developed nephrotic syndrome at any time during follow-up were at increased risk for progressive renal failure.[54] This observation is potentially quite important as it is not uncommon for patients with LMN to progress from low-grade proteinuria on presentation to nephrotic-range proteinuria during follow-up. However, by multivariate analysis, the presence of nephrotic syndrome during follow-up was not an independent predictor of renal function deterioration. Transition to proliferative lupus nephritis was a stronger predictor of doubling serum creatinine in this study.[54]

Troyanov and colleagues have shown that both complete and partial remissions of nephrotic proteinuria are independently associated with a slower rate of renal function deterioration and a decreased risk of renal failure in a large study of IMN.[60] Sun and colleagues have provided comparable observations in their study of LMN.[33] They found that failure to achieve a complete or partial remission of proteinuria despite treatment was an independent predictor of end stage renal failure.

Sloan and colleagues showed that the initial serum creatinine was the only independent clinical risk factor that predicted death and/or end stage renal failure in their study that included patients with "pure" LMN and those with mixed membranous and proliferative lupus nephritis.[7] However, when the analysis was restricted to patients with "pure" LMN (i.e. the subject of this chapter), the initial serum creatinine was no longer an independent predictor of death and/or renal failure. This may reflect the observation that relatively few patients with "pure" LMN present with an elevated serum creatinine.

Although race, ethnicity, and socioeconomic factors have emerged as significant predictors of renal outcomes in studies of predominantly proliferative lupus nephritis, it is unclear to what degree these demographic factors influence the variability in the prognosis of LMN reported from various centers around the world (Table 7.1). Barr and colleagues have shown that poverty is an important independent predictor of renal function deterioration among patients with proliferative lupus nephritis.[61] Furthermore, compared to non-Hispanic White patients, Black and Hispanic patients with proliferative lupus nephritis are more likely to manifest high-risk renal biopsy features and to develop end stage renal failure.[61–68] On the other hand, Bakir and colleagues concluded that the prognosis of Black patients with LMN in their study was comparable to that observed among White patients.[50] Before adjusting for the effect of other prognostic factors, we found that Black and Hispanic patients appeared to have a relatively poor prognosis in our treatment trial of LMN; they were less likely than non-Hispanic White patients to achieve a complete or partial remission of proteinuria.[59] However, after statistical adjustment for the impact of severe baseline proteinuria, the predictive value of race and ethnicity appeared to diminish. Although this result seems to support Bakir's observation, it is clear that much larger studies are needed to determine the impact of race, ethnicity, and socioeconomic factors on the prognosis of patients with LMN.

Finally, the prognosis of patients with LMN appears to have improved over the past several decades as our therapeutic armamentarium has grown to provide more effective supportive care for the myriad of medical problems that these patients tend to develop.[48] This is an important consideration when evaluating the safety and efficacy of immunosuppressive drug treatments for LMN. Comparisons to "historical controls" are likely to be complicated by changes in supportive care that may confound interpretation of the results.

Supportive therapies

Nephrotic syndrome

Patients with LMN are at high risk for cardiovascular and cerebrovascular events because of an unfortunate constellation of risk factors associated with SLE and the nephrotic syndrome. Michael Ward has estimated that acute myocardial infarction and cerebrovascular accidents occur eight times more often among young women with SLE (18–44 years old) than among young women without SLE.[69] Although traditional risk factors for coronary artery disease have been identified in a high proportion of patients with SLE (even among those not on corticosteroids),[70] Rahman and Esdaille and their respective colleagues have shown that the high incidence of coronary artery disease and stroke in SLE patients cannot be fully explained by these traditional risk factors alone.[71,72] Factors related to chronic lupus activity, including systemic inflammation, antiphospholipid antibodies, and vasculitis, are likely also to be contributory.

For many patients with LMN, the risk of cardiovascular and cerebrovascular events is further exacerbated by the nephrotic syndrome. Ordonez and colleagues have shown that patients with the nephrotic syndrome are 5.5 times more likely to experience a myocardial infarction and 2.8 times more likely to die from a coronary event compared to age- and sex-matched non-nephrotic patients followed in the same health plan.[73] Consequently, it is not surprising that during extended follow-up, approximately 50% of deaths among patients with lupus nephritis have been due to cardiovascular and cerebrovascular events.[8,51,74]

As hyperlipidemia is a common complication of membranous nephropathy that is likely to contribute to the risk of progressive renal disease, as well as the risk of cardiovascular disease, a comprehensive lipid-lowering strategy should be employed.[75,76] This should include appropriate dietary recommendations, exercise, and weight reduction (when indicated). Lipid-lowering agents are also frequently necessary. Twenty to 40% reductions in total cholesterol and low-density lipoprotein (LDL) cholesterol are often achieved with 3-hydroxy-3-methylglutaryl-coenzyme A (HMG Co-A) reductase inhibitors. Cautious follow-up is recommended if a statin is combined with a fibric acid derivative or a calcineurin inhibitor.

Blockade of the renin–angiotensin system with an angiotensin converting enzyme (ACE) inhibitor or an angiotensin receptor blocker (ARB) is frequently recommended for patients with LMN. In addition to lowering blood pressure and reducing proteinuria, there is substantial evidence that these agents slow the progression of diabetic and nondiabetic kidney diseases. Jafar and colleagues showed by meta-analysis that ACE inhibitors are renoprotective in nondiabetic patients with more than 0.5 g/day of proteinuria.[77] Limited experience suggests that patients with MN may achieve a further reduction in proteinuria from the addition of a renin inhibitor (aliskiren) if they have modest levels of persistent proteinuria (1–3 g/day) after a 6-month trial of an ACE inhibitor or an ARB.[78] On the other hand, patients with persistent nephrotic-range proteinuria despite a reasonable trial of an ACE inhibitor or an ARB, should be considered for one of the immunosuppressive regimens that will be described later in this chapter, in an effort to induce a remission of the immune-mediated kidney disease.

Thromboembolic diathesis

Patients with LMN are at increased risk for both arterial and venous thromboembolic events attributable to a number of factors, including persistent nephrotic syndrome and antiphospholipid antibodies. In recent studies, the incidence of thrombotic complications has ranged from 3 to 28% (Table 7.2).[33,36,54,56,59,79] Chi Chiu Mok reported that the cumulative risk of an arterial thrombosis in patients with LMN was 8.4% after 5 years and 16.7% after 10 years of follow-up.[41] Pasquali[36] and Mok[56] observed that thrombotic events in patients with LMN were associated with the presence of antiphospholipid antibodies. On the other hand, Mercadal and colleagues[54] found that clinically significant thromboses were associated with the occurrence of nephrotic syndrome at any time during follow-up, but were not associated with nephrotic syndrome at baseline or with antiphospholipid antibodies. It has been argued, based on decision analyses, that the benefits of prophylactic anticoagulation for patients with MN and the nephrotic syndrome outweigh the risks.[80,81] However, as far as the authors are aware, no prospective controlled trials have been done to define the risks/benefits of this approach. Based on currently available information, it is reasonable to consider prophylactic anticoagulation for patients with a protracted course of severe nephrotic syndrome associated with marked hypoalbuminaemia.

Table 7.2 Incidence of thromboembolic complications in lupus membranous nephropathy

Author	Year	Location	Follow-up (years)	Nephrotic/total pts	Incidence of thromboses
Pasquali[36]	1993	Italy	6.1	13/26	23%
Radhakrishnan[79]	1993	New York	6.2	32/50	28%
Mercadal[54]	2002	France	6.9	42/66	23%
Mok[56]	2004	China	7.5	22/38	13%
Sun[33]	2008	China	6.5	31/100	3%
Austin[59]	2009	NIH	5.0	37/42	17%

Immunosuppressive therapies

As we lack solid, evidenced-based guidelines for identifying the patients with LMN who should receive immunosuppressive drug regimens, treatment recommendations are based, in part, on extrapolations of information derived from large studies of the natural history of IMN.[41,82] Persistent nephrotic syndrome (despite nonimmunosuppressive interventions) puts patients with IMN and LMN at increased risk for progressive renal failure and thromboembolic complications, as well as cardiovascular and cerebrovascular events, and is a widely accepted indication for immunosuppressive therapy. Factors related to SLE activity appear to exacerbate the risk for thrombotic and vascular events among patients with LMN, further strengthening the justification for immunosuppressive treatments in these patients. Deteriorating renal function is certainly an important indication for immunosuppressive therapy among patients with both IMN and LMN. For patients with a history of LMN, it is important to consider whether declining renal function is due to transformation from membranous to proliferative lupus nephritis. Depending on the clinical presentation, a repeat renal biopsy may be indicated to clarify the diagnosis and guide therapy. Patients with LMN often develop other (extrarenal) manifestations of SLE that may also require immunosuppressive treatments.

Corticosteroids

Placebo controlled randomized trials have not been performed to determine whether corticosteroids lead to improved renal outcomes among patients with LMN. Donadio and colleagues found no difference in renal outcomes in a retrospective study of 28 patients treated with high-dose, low-dose, or no corticosteroids.[83] Five of seven patients had persistent nephrotic syndrome after high-dose steroids. Likewise, Gonzalez-Dettoni and Tron observed comparable outcomes in 12 patients treated with high-dose corticosteroids and four patients who received no steroid therapy; they concluded that high-dose corticosteroids alone are not indicated for LMN.[35] Several uncontrolled studies (to be reviewed below) have observed more favorable renal outcomes following interventions with alternative immunosuppressive treatments (azathioprine, alkylating agents, calcineurin inhibitors, or mycophenolate mofetil), usually combined with corticosteroids. In our randomized controlled trial of treatment for LMN, we found that regimens that included alternate day prednisone plus an adjunctive immunosuppressive agent (either pulse cyclophosphamide or cyclosporine) were more effective than prednisone alone in inducing remissions of proteinuria.[59] Consequently, if LMN patients with persistent nephrotic proteinuria and/or declining renal function are offered an empiric trial of high-dose alternate day prednisone alone, the trial should be brief (no more than 2 months, followed by tapering) to minimize the risk of insidious toxicities from a therapy that is relatively ineffective for LMN.

Azathioprine

In an uncontrolled, prospective study, Mok and colleagues evaluated the effect of azathioprine (up to 2 mg/kg per day) and prednisone (0.8–1.0 mg/kg per day for 6–8 weeks, then tapered) in 38 Chinese LMN patients.[56] Fifty-eight per cent of the patients were nephrotic. Two patients withdrew shortly after starting treatment because of idiosyncratic reactions to azathioprine (hypersensitivity in one and agranulocytosis in the other). Twelve months after starting treatment, 67% of the patients had achieved a complete remission (proteinuria <1 g/day, stable or improved serum creatinine and normal C3 for ≥6 months) and 21% had a partial remission (≥50% reduction in proteinuria to <3 g/day and stable or improved serum creatinine). Patients who achieved a remission were maintained on low-dose prednisone and azathioprine. Over a mean follow-up of 12 years, 19 renal flares (15 proteinuric and four nephritic) were observed in 13 (34%) patients.[84] Repeat renal biopsy during 10 of these renal flares revealed LMN in four, diffuse proliferative lupus nephritis in two, and mixed membranous and proliferative lupus nephritis in four. Renal flares were treated with increased doses of corticosteroids and/or alternative immunosuppressive regimens including cyclophosphamide, mycophenolate mofetil, and tacrolimus; most patients achieved another remission. Subsequently, azathioprine could be resumed for maintenance therapy; 66% of the patients were still on azathioprine at their last follow-up visit. There were 11 infections in seven patients; five episodes required hospitalization. Although azathioprine treatment of LMN was generally associated with favorable outcomes in this study, it should be noted that 42% of the patients had less than nephrotic proteinuria at baseline, 34% experienced renal flares and none of the patients were from potentially high-risk demographic (Hispanic or African American) groups.

Alkylating agents

In 19 nephrotic LMN patients, Moroni and colleagues retrospectively evaluated the effect of the alternate month cytotoxic drug regimen that they had previously shown to be effective in patients with IMN.[38] Most of the patients with less than 5 g/day of proteinuria received corticosteroids alone, whereas most of those who excreted more than 5 g/day of urinary protein were treated with a 6-month regimen of alternate month corticosteroids and chlorambucil. Four patients (two in each treatment group) had mixed membranous and focal proliferative lupus nephritis. Even though most patients in the chlorambucil group were at increased risk for an unfavorable outcome (because of relatively high-grade proteinuria), patients treated with chlorambucil and corticosteroids were significantly more likely to be in complete or partial remission at the last follow-up visit compared to those who were treated with corticosteroids alone. Whereas Moroni and colleagues observed reversible leukopenia in one of their LMN patients treated with alternate month chlorambucil and corticosteroids, Wang et al. described six Chinese patients with LMN who developed severe pancytopenia associated with this regimen.[85] The authors expressed concern that Chinese SLE patients may be particularly susceptible to this adverse outcome.

Chan and colleagues evaluated the safety and efficacy of sequential immunosuppression in an uncontrolled study of 20 nephrotic patients with LMN.[37] Patients received cyclophosphamide (2–2.5 mg/kg/day) for 6 months, followed by azathioprine (2 mg/kg/day). Prednisolone was initiated at 0.8 mg/kg/day and then gradually tapered to a maintenance dose of 10 mg/day by 6 months. Within the first year, 55% achieved a complete remission (urine protein <0.3 g/day) and 35% had a partial remission (urine protein 0.3–3.0 g/day). Serum albumin was significantly lower among those who failed to respond compared to those who achieved a complete remission. Four renal and four extrarenal relapses were observed at 4 years, on average. Three of the four renal relapses were associated with transformation to mixed proliferative and membranous lupus nephritis. Complications included herpes zoster in 40% and pulmonary tuberculosis in 20% of the patients. Hemorrhagic cystitis, premature ovarian failure, and malignancy were not observed in this cohort. Nonetheless, there is appropriate concern about the potential toxicity of extended courses of daily oral cyclophosphamide for LMN.

In an effort to minimize the toxicity of cyclophosphamide therapy for lupus nephritis, investigators have evaluated the safety and efficacy of relatively short courses of daily oral cyclophosphamide (used by the Lupus Nephritis Collaborative Study Group),[86] an alternate month regimen (reported by Moroni and colleagues),[38] sequential immunosuppression (described by Chan and colleagues),[37] and intermittent pulse cyclophosphamide.[59] We studied the latter approach in a randomized, controlled trial of immunosuppressive regimens for LMN to be described in another section of this chapter.

Calcineurin inhibitors

The antiproteinuric effect of calcineurin inhibitors in membranous nephropathy is likely to be multi-factorial, related to its immunosuppressive action on T cells, to a direct effect on the actin cytoskeleton of podocytes, and, to a lesser extent, changes in renal hemodynamics.[87–89] Several pilot studies have explored the efficacy and toxicity of calcineurin inhibitors in LMN.[90–96] Radhakrishnan and colleagues treated 10 nephrotic LMN patients with cyclosporine (up to 4–6 mg/kg/day) and prednisone (in eight patients) for 6–43 months (mean, 21 months).[93] Proteinuria decreased to <1 g/day in six patients and to 1–2 g/day in another two patients. The three patients who had mixed membranous and proliferative renal histology at baseline experienced renal and extrarenal flares of SLE while on cyclosporine that called for additional immunosuppressive therapy. Side effects included new or worsening hypertension in six patients and transient elevations of serum creatinine in two patients. Follow-up renal biopsies in five patients (after 10–21 months of therapy) showed progression from predominantly Stage 2 to Stage 3 membranous nephropathy. There was a reduction in the number of relatively recently formed electron-dense deposits at or near the subepithelial surface of the GBM.

Hallegua and colleagues also studied the effect of cyclosporine (2–6 mg/kg/day for an average of 2 years) in 10 patients with LMN.[90] Proteinuria decreased from an average of 5.6 g/day at baseline to 1.4 g/day at last follow-up. Frequently observed increases in serum creatinine and blood pressure responded to reductions in cyclosporine doses and reinforcement of antihypertension regimens.

Hu and colleagues treated 23 LMN patients (baseline proteinuria >2.5 g/day) for a mean of 17 months with cyclosporine (starting dose 3.5–5.5 mg/kg/day) and prednisone (mean starting dose 24 mg/day).[91] They observed complete remissions (proteinuria <0.5 g/day) in 12 patients (52%), and partial remissions (>50% reduction in proteinuria) in another 10 patients (43%). Relapse of proteinuria occurred in a third of the responders after withdrawing cyclosporine for 4–24 months. The authors suggest that maintenance cyclosporine (CSA) therapy may be needed to reduce the risk of relapse and may be appropriate in patients lacking clinical or histological evidence of CSA nephrotoxicity.

Comparable recommendations have been offered for patients with IMN because of the high incidence of relapse (up to 48%) following discontinuation of a calcineurin inhibitor.[97] Cattran and colleagues suggested that CSA could be tapered off over 3–4 months in patients with IMN who achieve a complete remission.[98] On the other hand, they recommended much more gradual tapering of CSA (over several years) for patients with IMN who achieve a partial remission. Because of concerns about the chronic toxicities of calcineurin inhibitors, it will be important to identify alternative approaches to reduce the risk of relapse after stopping these agents. Preliminary evidence from small uncontrolled studies suggests that the addition of another immunosuppressive drug (for example, rituximab in IMN and azathioprine in LMN) may lead to sustained remissions and facilitate earlier withdrawal of the calcineurin inhibitor.[94,95,99]

Controlled trial of cyclophosphamide and cyclosporine

Forty-two patients with LMN (median baseline proteinuria 5.4 g/day, range 2.7–15.4 g/day) participated in a randomized, controlled trial to evaluate the effects of adding adjunctive immunosuppressive agents to prednisone alone.[59] All patients received conventional high-dosage alternate-day prednisone (initiated at 40 mg/m^2 body surface area, approximately 1 mg/kg body weight). The adjunctive regimens consisted of alternate month intravenous pulse cyclophosphamide (IVCY, ranging from 0.5 to 1.0 g/m^2 body surface area) for six doses or cyclosporine (CSA, initiated at 200 mg/m^2/day, approximately 5 mg/kg/day) for 11 months. At 1 year, remission of proteinuria was significantly more likely among patients treated with IVCY (60%) and among those treated with CSA (83%), compared to those treated with prednisone alone (27%). By multivariate survival analysis, treatment with prednisone alone and high-grade proteinuria (>5 g/day) were each independently associated with a decreased probability of remission. Within 5 years after stopping the adjunctive immunosuppressive regimen, the cumulative probability of a relapse of nephrotic syndrome was significantly higher among patients treated with CSA (60%) compared to those treated with IVCY (17%). Cyclosporine was stopped abruptly after completing 11 months of therapy; we can only speculate whether gradual tapering of CSA would have led to fewer relapses. Ten patients who had failed to respond to prednisone alone, or CSA, or who had relapsed after responding to CSA were treated with IVCY for a median duration of 2 years (every 2 months for the first year, then quarterly). Nine of these patients were Black or Hispanic; the median protein excretion rate was 6.8 g/day. The probability of remission was 70% at 18 months and 80% at 36 months in this high-risk group of patients, but only two of eight responders achieved a complete remission of proteinuria (<0.3 g/day), raising the concern that less satisfactory results may be obtained when an immunosuppressive agent is started relatively late in the clinical course, after chronic irreversible renal histological changes have developed. Adverse events included insulin-requiring diabetes (three cases), pneumonia (one on prednisone alone, two on CSA, and one on an extended course of IVCY) and localized herpes zoster (two cases on IVCY).

Mycophenolate mofetil

Several investigators have described their experience using mycophenolate mofetil (MMF) as treatment for patients with LMN.[31,100–104] Kasitanon and colleagues treated 10 patients with "pure" LMN (Group 1) and 19 patients with mixed membranous and proliferative lupus nephritis (Group 2) using MMF (up to 3 g/day), prednisone (titrated for extrarenal features of SLE), and an ACE inhibitor or an ARB (if tolerated).[31] Only 11% of the patients with nephrotic proteinuria achieved a complete remission (proteinuria <0.5 g/day). Three patients in Group 1 had nephrotic-range proteinuria (>3 g/day) at baseline; one achieved a partial remission (≥50% reduction in proteinuria). Six patients in Group 2 presented with nephrotic proteinuria; one had a complete remission at 12 months. On the other hand, about 50% of the patients who had less than nephrotic-range proteinuria on presentation experienced a complete remission. There was no apparent difference in the remission rates among patients with or without superimposed endocapillary proliferative lesions.

Kapitsinou and colleagues have reported a somewhat different experience.[101] They have observed relatively unfavorable outcomes among patients with mixed membranous and proliferative renal histology. Although two of three patients with "pure" LMN achieved a complete or partial remission on MMF (2 g/day) and corticosteroids, all three patients with mixed membranous and proliferative lupus nephritis failed to respond to this regimen.

Spetie and colleagues described 13 treatment-naïve LMN patients who received MMF (mostly, 1–2 g/day) and prednisone (titrated to control extrarenal manifestations of SLE), as well as an ACE inhibitor and/or an ARB.[104] Ten patients had nephrotic proteinuria and one had mixed membranous and focal proliferative histology. After a mean follow-up of 16 months, nine patients were in complete remission (urine protein to creatinine ratio (p/c) < 0.5) and two patients had a partial remission (≥50% reduction in the urine p/c to <3).

Radhakrishnan and colleagues have reported a pooled analysis of 84 patients with LMN who participated in two multi-center randomized controlled trials that compared MMF and IVCY as induction therapies in 510 patients with lupus nephritis; most had proliferative lupus kidney disease.[103,105–107] After 24 weeks, the 65 (77%) patients with LMN who completed the 24 weeks of therapy specified in the protocol (33 patients on MMF and 32 on IVCY) showed similar responses to MMF and IVCY. Both treatment groups manifested similar and significant reductions in proteinuria, and essentially stable renal function. Nineteen LMN patients were withdrawn from these studies (nine from MMF and 10 from IVCY) because of adverse events, treatment failure, or patient preference. There was one death in each group; similar numbers of infections and gastrointestinal symptoms were observed on the two regimens. Based on these observations, it appears that the short-term renal outcomes of patients with LMN are comparable following induction therapy with either MMF or IVCY, but the authors indicate that their pooled analysis may lack sufficient statistical power to detect differences between the regimens. At present, many favor MMF because of ease of administration and concerns about the toxicity of IVCY. On the other hand, it is important to emphasize that both regimens are associated with potentially significant toxicities and that information about long-term outcomes (including risk of relapse) is not available for MMF. We need data from controlled trials that include larger numbers of patients with LMN followed for longer periods of time to clarify the risk/benefit profile of immunosuppressive regimens for LMN.

Experimental therapies

Rituximab

Rituximab is a monoclonal chimeric anti-CD20 antibody, which induces profound and lasting B cell depletion. It was initially developed as a treatment for B cell lymphomas, but over the past decade it has emerged as an effective treatment for various autoimmune diseases. Several small studies in IMN showed promising effects (recently reviewed),[97,108] and early uncontrolled reports suggested efficacy in proliferative lupus nephritis. However, in a randomized controlled Phase 3 study, the combination of rituximab and mycophenolate was not more effective than mycophenolate alone.[109] There have been no formal studies evaluating rituximab in LMN, and data from case reports and small case series are mixed. Two case reports showed remission in refractory LMN with rituximab,[110,111] whereas in a small series, three of five patients with LMN did not respond to rituximab.[112]

Future therapies

The optimal treatment for LMN, as for any other disease, would maximize therapeutic efficacy while minimizing toxicity by targeting specific step(s) in the pathogenesis. Although this should remain our ultimate goal, given our limited understanding of the etiology and pathophysiology of LMN, it is more likely that in the near term, novel treatment studies will be based on analogies with IMN, and, to a lesser degree, proliferative lupus nephritis. As described earlier, podocyte damage in LMN is caused by the subepithelial deposition of autoantibody-containing immune complexes in the basement membrane leading to complement activation and the accumulation of inflammatory mediators. Interfering with this process is a reasonable approach.

Antigen-specific T-cell activation requires a two-stage signaling process. If T lymphocytes are activated through their antigen-specific T cell receptor in the absence of a co-stimulatory "second" signal mediated by co-stimulatory receptor–ligand pairs, the T cell receptor–antigen/major histocompatibility complex (MHC) interaction induces apoptosis, clonal deletion of antigen-specific T cells, and, ultimately, anergy or even tolerance. Blocking co-stimulatory pathways, such as CD28 or its ligands, or interfering with several co-stimulatory pathways simultaneously may increase efficacy. Abatacept (cytotoxic T lymphocyte antigen (CTLA)4-immunoglobulin(Ig)) is a fusion protein derived from the extracellular domain of CTLA4 and the Fc portion of IgG1 that blocks B7/CD28 interaction and inhibits T cell activation. Cytotoxic T lymphocyte antigen 4-Ig prevents the progression of renal disease and prolongs survival in NZB/W mice.[113] Abatacept has been approved by the US Food and Drug Administration (FDA) for use in moderate to severe rheumatoid arthritis. A Phase 2 study, presented as a late-breaking abstract at the 2008 Annual Scientific Meeting of the American College of Rheumatology, failed to show clinical efficacy in nonrenal lupus. A clinical trial in proliferative lupus nephritis is still ongoing (www.clinicaltrials.gov).

B cells are not only producers of autoantibodies; they are also effective antigen presenting cells and remain reasonable targets of therapy despite the conflicting results between clinical studies in proliferative lupus nephritis and IMN. CD20 is an attractive target for B cell-depleting therapy, and in addition to rituximab, there are several humanized anti-CD20 monoclonal antibodies and small molecules targeting CD20 under development. The expression of CD22 on B cells is very similar to CD20 and epratuzumab, a humanized anti-CD22 monoclonal antibody, is currently in Phase 3 studies in SLE (www.clinicaltrials.gov).

Complement activation and the formation of C5b-C9 are essential for the progression of LMN. Eculizumab is a recombinant humanized monoclonal antibody that binds specifically to complement protein C5 and inhibits cleavage to C5a and C5b, preventing the formation of MAC. It has been approved for the treatment of paroxysmal nocturnal hematuria. In a study of 200 patients with IMN, eculizumab was no different from placebo at reducing proteinuria at 4 months. As complement activity was not completely inhibited in most patients, it is not clear if the result of this study reflects true inefficacy or suboptimal dosing.[114] Therefore, evaluating eculizumab in SLE and LMN would be reasonable.

Cytokines are important mediators of autoimmunity and inflammation, and, although their exact role in LMN is not yet defined, some are attractive therapeutic targets. B lymphocyte stimulator (BLyS) is a recently described stimulator of B cells. In murine models of SLE serum levels of BLyS are increased, and BLyS transgenic mice develop lupus-like disease. Treatment with soluble BLyS receptors significantly decreased proteinuria and increased survival of NZB/W mice.[115] Belimumab is a fully human anti-BlyS monoclonal antibody. Phase III studies have shown modest statistically significant efficacy over standard of care in nonrenal lupus[116] (Human Genome Sciences press release: www.hgsi.com/latest/human-genome-sciences-and-glaxosmithkline-announce-positive-results-in-second-of-two-phase-3-trials-of-benlysta-in-systemic-lupus-erythema-3.html). There is no experience to date with the use of belimumab in lupus nephritis. Other anti-BlyS monoclonal antibodies and alternative approaches to inhibit BLyS, such as soluble receptors, are in various phases of development.

Type I interferons serve as a link between the innate and adaptive immune system. Recognition of the importance of the increased expression of interferon-regulated genes in SLE (the so-called interferon signature), along with data showing beneficial effects of blocking interferon in animal models of lupus, makes them an attractive target. The first studies to assess the safety of interferon α blockade have been completed and showed biological suppression of the interferon signature.[117] Efficacy trials are under way.

Tumor necrosis factor (TNF) has both inflammatory and anti-inflammatory properties, and its overall effect on SLE is still controversial. In a small open-label safety trial, infliximab (a humanized anti-TNF monoclonal antibody) was well tolerated and patients had improvement in their inflammatory organ involvement. Interestingly, anti-dsDNA levels increased, but this was not associated with any obvious clinical consequences. Proteinuria decreased by more than 50% in the four patients with nephritis (including one with refractory LMN) and remained low for at least 1 year.[118] Further studies are under way to define the role of TNF inhibition in the treatment of lupus nephritis.

The development of clinically effective novel agents for LMN will take many years and requires a significant increase in research focusing on the pathogenesis of LMN, as well as designed, appropriately powered clinical trials. An alternative and parallel approach is to improve the use of existing treatments by using them in combination or sequentially. As many existing treatments are effective for subsets of patients, it is equally important to identify biomarkers that can predict who will or will not respond to a particular treatment.

Current treatment recommendations

Table 7.3 summarizes several treatment options for patients with LMN who are not participating in a clinical trial. All patients should be offered nonimmunosuppressive strategies (including angiotensin antagonists) for renoprotection, minimization of proteinuria, and optimization of blood pressure control (<130/80 mmHg). Other interventions (diet, exercise, weight loss, cessation of smoking, and lipid-lowering medications) are frequently needed to address common cardiovascular risk factors. Prophylactic aspirin or anticoagulant therapy may be indicated if high-titer anticardiolipin antibodies or persistent severe nephrotic syndrome are present. Immunosuppressive therapy for patients with non-nephrotic proteinuria is directed toward extrarenal manifestations of SLE. Patients with persistent nephrotic or near nephrotic proteinuria are candidates for immunosuppressive treatments with the goals of inducing a remission of proteinuria and reducing the risk of slowly progressive renal failure. As data from controlled and uncontrolled studies indicate that corticosteroids alone are relatively ineffective therapy for LMN, combination immunosuppressive drug regimens should be considered for first line therapy, especially for patients with high-risk clinical, histological or demographic prognostic indicators. At present, published studies support the use of moderate-dose corticosteroids plus a calcineurin inhibitor, MMF, or azathioprine as first line immunosuppressive therapy for LMN. The approach should be individualized based on the patient's co-morbid conditions and preferences. We frequently recommend treatment with a calcineurin inhibitor because of the high remission rates observed in patients with LMN. After a remission has been achieved, we gradually taper to the lowest dose that will sustain the remission, and then repeatedly attempt to taper off the calcineurin inhibitor following guidelines that have been described for patients with IMN.[98] In general, we recommend reserving cytotoxic drug regimens for high-risk patients who have failed to respond to or who have relapsed after treatment with one of the first line immunosuppressive regimens. Although progress has been made, it is clear that none of these regimens is optimal. Better understanding of basic pathogenetic mechanisms and continued investigations of innovative treatments are needed to refine our approach to the treatment of LMN.

Table 7.3 Options and recommendations for treatment of lupus membranous nephropathy

---

A. Supportive therapies

- ◆ Angiotensin antagonists for renoprotection and to reduce proteinuria
- ◆ Optimize blood pressure control (<130/80) starting with an ACE inhibitor and/or ARB, as tolerated
- ◆ Diuretics to help control edema, blood pressure and potassium, if needed
- ◆ Low-sodium, low-fat, and moderate protein diet plus exercise
- ◆ Weight reduction and cessation of smoking when indicated to address these cardiovascular risk factors
- ◆ Lipid-lowering medications, starting with HMG Co-A reductase inhibitors, as needed
- ◆ Prophylactic aspirin or anticoagulation if high titer anticardiolipin antibodies or severe persistent nephrotic syndrome are present

B. Immunosuppressive therapy for patients with low-grade proteinuria

- ◆ Directed to treat extrarenal manifestations of SLE

C. Immunosuppressive therapy for nephrotic or near-nephrotic proteinuria

1 First line: moderate-dose alternate day prednisone (e.g. 0.5–1.0 mg/kg for up to 2 months, followed by tapering to ~0.25 mg/kg alternate days, combined with:

- ◆ Cyclosporine, ≤5 mg/kg/day
- ◆ Mycophenolate mofetil, ≤3 g/day
- ◆ Azathioprine, 2 mg/kg/day (limited experience)[56]

2 Cytotoxic drug regimens for high-risk patients who have failed to respond to or who have relapsed after responding to a first line regimen:

- ◆ Pulse cyclophosphamide, ≤1 g/m^2 every 2 months for 1 year plus moderate dose alternate day prednisone
- ◆ Alternate month regimen: pulse methylprednisolone, 1 g/day for 3 days, followed by prednisone (0.5 mg/kg/day) for 27 days during months 1, 3, and 5 alternating with cyclophosphamide (2 mg/kg/day) or chlorambucil (0.2 mg/kg/day) for 30 days during months 2, 4, and 6
- ◆ Sequential immunosuppressive regimen: daily oral cyclophosphamide (2 mg/kg/day) for ≤6 months followed by azathioprine (2 mg/kg/day) plus moderate dose alternate day prednisone

---

ACE, angiotensin converting enzyme; ARB, angiotensin receptor blocker; HMG Co-A, 3-hydroxy-3-methylglutaryl-coenzyme A; SLE, systemic lupus erythematosus.

Acknowledgement

This work was supported by the Intramural Research Program of the National Institute of Diabetes and Digestive and Kidney Diseases, National Institutes of Health.

References

1. Korbet, S.M. (1999) Membranous lupus glomerulonephritis. In: *Lupus nephritis* (Lewis, E.J., Schwartz, M.M., and Korbet, S.M., eds), pp. 219–40. Oxford University Press, Oxford.

2. Glassock, R.J. (1992) Secondary membranous glomerulonephritis. *Nephrol Dial Transplant* **7** Suppl 1, 64–71.

3. Bell, E.T. (1950) *Renal Diseases*, pp. 326–8. Lea and Febiger, Philadelphia.

4. Pollak, V.E., and Pirani, C.L. (1966) Pathology of the kidney in SLE: serial renal biopsy studies of the effects of therapy. In: *Lupus Erythematosus* (Dubois, E.L., ed.), pp. 54–65. McGraw-Hill, New York.

5. McCluskey, R.T. (1975) Lupus nephritis. In: *Kidney Pathology Decennial* (Sommers, S.C., ed.), pp. 435–50. Appleton-Century-Crofts, East Norwalk, CT.

6. Churg, J., and Sobin, L.H. (1982) Lupus nephritis. In: *Renal Disease: Classification and Atlas of Glomerular Disease*, pp. 127–49. Igaku-Shoin, Tokyo.

7. Sloan, R.P., Schwartz, M.M., Korbet, S.M., and Borok, R.Z. (1996) Long-term outcome in systemic lupus erythematosus membranous glomerulonephritis. Lupus Nephritis Collaborative Study Group. *J Am Soc Nephrol* **7**, 299–305.

8. Donadio, J.V., Jr., Hart, G.M., Bergstralh, E.J., and Holley, K.E. (1995) Prognostic determinants in lupus nephritis: a long-term clinicopathologic study. *Lupus* **4**, 109–15.

9. Churg, J., Bernstein, J., and Glassock, R.J. (1995) Lupus nephritis. In: *Renal Disease: Classification and Atlas of Glomerular Diseases*, pp. 151–79. Igaku-Shoin, Tokyo.

10. Weening, J.J., D'Agati, V.D., Schwartz, M.M., Seshan, S.V., Alpers, C.E., Appel, G.B., *et al.* (2004) The classification of glomerulonephritis in systemic lupus erythematosus revisited. *J Am Soc Nephrol* **15**, 241–50.

11. Nangaku, M., and Couser, W.G. (2005) Mechanisms of immune-deposit formation and the mediation of immune renal injury. *Clin Exp Nephrol* **9**, 183–91.

12. Ronco, P., and Debiec, H. (2007) Target antigens and nephritogenic antibodies in membranous nephropathy: of rats and men. *Semin Immunopathol* **29**, 445–58.

13. Beck, L.H., Jr., Bonegio, R.G., Lambeau, G., Beck, D.M., Powell, D.W., Cummins T.D., *et al.* (2009) M-type phospholipase A2 receptor as target antigen in idiopathic membranous nephropathy. *N Engl J Med* **361**, 11–21.

14. Debiec, H., Guigonis, V., Mougenot, B., Decobert, F., Haymann, J.P., Bensman, A., *et al.* (2002) Antenatal membranous glomerulonephritis due to anti-neutral endopeptidase antibodies. *N Engl J Med* **346**, 2053–60.

15. Baker, P.J., Ochi, R.F., Schulze, M., Johnson, R.J., Campbell, C., and Couser, W.G. (1989) Depletion of C6 prevents development of proteinuria in experimental membranous nephropathy in rats. *Am J Pathol* **135**, 185–94.

16. Schulze, M., Donadio, J.V., Jr., Pruchno, C.J., Baker, P.J., Johnson, R.J., Stahl, R.A., *et al.* (1991) Elevated urinary excretion of the C5b-9 complex in membranous nephropathy. *Kidney Int* **40**, 533–8.

17. Shankland, S.J., Eitner, F., Hudkins, K.L., Goodpaster, T., D'Agati, V., and Alpers, C.E. (2000) Differential expression of cyclin-dependent kinase inhibitors in human glomerular disease: role in podocyte proliferation and maturation. *Kidney Int* **58**, 674–83.

18. Danilewicz, M., and Wagrowska-Danilewicz, M. (2007) Analysis of renal immunoexpression of cyclooxygenase-1 and cyclooxygenase-2 in lupus and nonlupus membranous glomerulopathy. *Pol J Pathol* **58**, 221–6.

19. Neale, T.J., Ullrich, R., Ojha, P., Poczewski, H., Verhoeven, A.J., and Kerjaschki, D. (1993) Reactive oxygen species and neutrophil respiratory burst cytochrome b558 are produced by kidney glomerular cells in passive Heymann nephritis. *Proc Natl Acad Sci U S A* **90**, 3645–9.

20. McMillan, J.I., Riordan, J.W., Couser, W.G., Pollock, A.S., and Lovett, D.H. (1996) Characterization of a glomerular epithelial cell metalloproteinase as matrix

metalloproteinase-9 with enhanced expression in a model of membranous nephropathy. *J Clin Invest* **97**, 1094–101.

21. Tveita, A., Rekvig, O.P., and Zykova, S.N. (2008) Glomerular matrix metalloproteinases and their regulators in the pathogenesis of lupus nephritis. *Arthritis Res Ther* **10**, 229.

22. Doublier, S., Ruotsalainen, V., Salvidio, G., Lupia, E., Biancone, L., Conaldi, P.G., *et al.* (2001) Nephrin redistribution on podocytes is a potential mechanism for proteinuria in patients with primary acquired nephrotic syndrome. *Am J Pathol* **158**, 1723–31.

23. Saran, A.M., Yuan, H., Takeuchi, E., McLaughlin, M., Salant, D.J. (2003) Complement mediates nephrin redistribution and actin dissociation in experimental membranous nephropathy. *Kidney Int* **64**, 2072–8.

24. Tipping, P.G., and Kitching, A.R. (2005) Glomerulonephritis, Th1 and Th2: what's new? *Clin Exp Immunol* **142**, 207–15.

25. Igawa, T., Nakashima, H., Sadanaga, A., Masutani, K., Miyake, K., Shimizu, S., *et al.* (2009) Deficiency in EBV-induced gene 3 (EBI3) in MRL/lpr mice results in pathological alteration of autoimmune glomerulonephritis and sialadenitis. *Mod Rheumatol* **19**, 33–41.

26. Shimizu, S., Sugiyama, N., Masutani, K., Sadanaga, A., Miyazaki, Y., Inoue, Y., *et al.* (2005) Membranous glomerulonephritis development with Th2-type immune deviations in MRL/lpr mice deficient for IL-27 receptor (WSX-1). *J Immunol* **175**, 7185–92.

27. Ehrenreich, T., and Churg, J. (1968) Pathology of membranous nephropathy. In: *Pathology Annual* (Sommers, S.C., ed.). Appleton-Century-Crofts, New York.

28. Hecht, B., Siegel, N., Adler, M., Kashgarian, M., and Hayslett, J.P. (1976) Prognostic indices in lupus nephritis. *Medicine (Baltimore)* **55**, 163–81.

29. Seligman, V.A., Lum, R.F., Olson, J.L., Li, H., and Criswell, L.A. (2002) Demographic differences in the development of lupus nephritis: a retrospective analysis. *Am J Med* **112**, 726–9.

30. Chen, Q., Liu, Z., Hu, W., Chen, H., Zeng, C., and Li, L. (2003) Class V lupus nephritis: a clinicopathologic study in 152 patients. *J Nephrol* **16**, 126–32.

31. Kasitanon, N., Petri, M., Haas, M., Magder, L.S., and Fine, D.M. (2008) Mycophenolate mofetil as the primary treatment of membranous lupus nephritis with and without concurrent proliferative disease: a retrospective study of 29 cases. *Lupus* **17**, 40–5.

32. Mok, C.C., Wong, R.W., and Lau, C.S. (1999) Lupus nephritis in Southern Chinese patients: clinicopathologic findings and long-term outcome. *Am J Kidney Dis* **34**, 315–23.

33. Sun, H.O., Hu, W.X., Xie, H.L., Zhang, H.T., Chen, H.P., Zeng, C.H., *et al.* (2008) Long-term outcome of Chinese patients with membranous lupus nephropathy. *Lupus* **17**, 56–61.

34. Appel, G.B., Silva, F.G., Pirani, C.L., Meltzer, J.I., and Estes, D. (1978) Renal involvement in systemic lupus erythematosus (SLE): a study of 56 patients emphasizing histologic classification. *Medicine (Baltimore)* **57**, 371–410.

35. Gonzalez-Dettoni, H., and Tron, F. (1984) Membranous glomerulopathy in systemic lupus erythematosus. *Adv Nephrol* **14**, 347–364.

36. Pasquali, S., Banfi, G., Zucchelli, A., Moroni, G., Ponticelli, C., and Zucchelli, P. (1993) Lupus membranous nephropathy: long-term outcome. *Clin Nephrol* **39**, 175–82.

37. Chan, T.M., Li, F.K., Hao, W.K., Chan, K.W., Lui, S.L., Tang, S., Lai, K.N. (1999) Treatment of membranous lupus nephritis with nephrotic syndrome by sequential immunosuppression. *Lupus* **8**, 545–51.

38. Moroni, G., Maccario, M., Banfi, G., Quaglini, S., and Ponticelli, C. (1998) Treatment of membranous lupus nephritis. *Am J Kidney Dis* **31**, 681–6.

39. Pollak, V.E., Pirani, C.L., and Schwartz, F.D. (1964) The natural history of the renal manifestations of systemic lupus erythematosus. *J Lab Clin Med* **63**, 537–50.

40. Tateno, S., Kobayashi, Y., Shigematsu, H., and Hiki, Y. (1983) Study of lupus nephritis: its classification and the significance of subendothelial deposits. *Q J Med* **52**, 311–31.

41. Mok, C.C. (2009) Membranous nephropathy in systemic lupus erythematosus: a therapeutic enigma. *Nat Rev Nephrol* **5**, 212–20.

42. Banfi, G., Mazzucco, G., di Barbiano, B.G., Bestetti, B.M., Stratta, P., Confalonieri, R., *et al.* (1985) Morphological parameters in lupus nephritis: their relevance for classification and relationship with clinical and histological findings and outcome. *Q J Med* **55**, 153–68.

43. Adu, D., Williams, D.G., Taube, D., Vilches, A.R., Turner, D.R., Cameron, J.S., Ogg, C.S. (1983) Late onset systemic lupus erythematosus and lupus-like disease in patients with apparent idiopathic glomerulonephritis. *Q J Med* **52**, 471–87.

44. Kallen, R.J., Lee, S.K., Aronson, A.J., and Spargo, B.H. (1977) Idiopathic membranous glomerulopathy preceding the emergence of systemic lupus erythematosus in two children. *J Pediatr* **90**, 72–6.

45. Shearn, M.A., Hopper, J., Jr., and Biava, C.G. (1980) Membranous lupus nephropathy initially seen as idiopathic membranous nephropathy. Possible diagnostic value of tubular reticular structures. *Arch Intern Med* **140**, 1521–3.

46. Jennette, J.C., Iskandar, S.S., and Dalldorf, F.G. (1983) Pathologic differentiation between lupus and nonlupus membranous glomerulopathy. *Kidney Int* **24**, 377–85.

47 Gruppo Italiano per lo Studio della Nefrite Lupica (GISNEL) (1992) Lupus nephritis: prognostic factors and probability of maintaining life-supporting renal function 10 years after the diagnosis. *Am J Kidney Dis* 19, 473–9.

48. Appel, G.B., Cohen, D.J., Pirani, C.L., Meltzer, J.I., and Estes, D. (1987) Long-term follow-up of patients with lupus nephritis. A study based on the classification of the World Health Organization. *Am J Med* **83**, 877–85.

49. Austin, H.A., III, Klippel, J.H., Balow, J.E., le Riche, N.G., Steinberg, A.D., Plotz, P.H., Decker, J.L. (1986) Therapy of lupus nephritis. Controlled trial of prednisone and cytotoxic drugs. *N Engl J Med* **314**, 614–19.

50. Bakir, A.A., Levy, P.S., and Dunea, G. (1994) The prognosis of lupus nephritis in African-Americans: a retrospective analysis. *Am J Kidney Dis* **24**, 159–71.

51. Bono, L., Cameron, J.S., and Hicks, J.A. (1999) The very long-term prognosis and complications of lupus nephritis and its treatment. *QJM* **92**, 211–18.

52. Huong, D.L., Papo, T., Beaufils, H., Wechsler, B., Bletry, O., Baumelou, A, *et al.* (1999) Renal involvement in systemic lupus erythematosus. A study of 180 patients from a single center. *Medicine (Baltimore)* **78**, 148–66.

53. Leaker, B., Fairley, K.F., Dowling, J., and Kincaid-Smith, P. (1987) Lupus nephritis: clinical and pathological correlation. *Q J Med* **62**, 163–79.

54. Mercadal, L., Montcel, S.T., Nochy, D., Queffeulou, G., Piette, J.C., Isnard-Bagnis, C., and Martinez, F. (2002) Factors affecting outcome and prognosis in membranous lupus nephropathy. *Nephrol Dial Transplant* **17**, 1771–8.

55. Wang, F., Looi, L.M. (1984) Systemic lupus erythematosus with membranous lupus nephropathy in Malaysian patients. *Q J Med* **53**, 209–26.

56. Mok, C.C., Ying, K.Y., Lau, C.S., Yim, C.W., Ng, W.L., Wong, W.S., and Au, T.C. (2004) Treatment of pure membranous lupus nephropathy with prednisone and azathioprine: an open-label trial. *Am J Kidney Dis* **43**, 269–76.

57. Cattran, D.C., Pei, Y., Greenwood, C.M., Ponticelli, C., Passerini, P., and Honkanen, E. (1997) Validation of a predictive model of idiopathic membranous nephropathy: its clinical and research implications. *Kidney Int* **51**, 901–7.

58. Pei, Y., Cattran, D., and Greenwood, C. (1992) Predicting chronic renal insufficiency in idiopathic membranous glomerulonephritis. *Kidney Int* **42**, 960–6.

59. Austin, H.A., III, Illei, G.G., Braun, M.J., and Balow, J.E. (2009) Randomized, controlled trial of prednisone, cyclophosphamide, and cyclosporine in lupus membranous nephropathy. *J Am Soc Nephrol* **20**, 901–11.

60. Troyanov, S., Wall, C.A., Miller, J.A., Scholey, J.W., Cattran, D.C. (2004) Idiopathic membranous nephropathy: definition and relevance of a partial remission. *Kidney Int* **66**, 1199–205.

61. Barr, R.G., Seliger, S., Appel, G.B., Zuniga, R., D'Agati, V., Salmon, J., Radhakrishnan, J. (2003) Prognosis in proliferative lupus nephritis: the role of socio-economic status and race/ethnicity. *Nephrol Dial Transplant* **18**, 2039–46.

62. Alarcon, G.S., McGwin, G., Jr., Bartolucci, A.A., Roseman, J., Lisse, J., Fessler, B.J., *et al.* (2001) Systemic lupus erythematosus in three ethnic groups. IX. Differences in damage accrual. *Arthritis Rheum* **44**, 2797–806.

63. Alarcon, G.S., McGwin. G., Jr., Petri, M., Reveille, J.D., Ramsey-Goldman, R., Kimberly, R.P. (2002) Baseline characteristics of a multiethnic lupus cohort: PROFILE. *Lupus* **11**, 95–101.

64. Austin, H.A., III, Boumpas, D.T., Vaughan, E.M., Balow, J.E. (1994) Predicting renal outcomes in severe lupus nephritis: contributions of clinical and histologic data. *Kidney Int* **45**, 544–50.

65. Austin, H.A., III, Boumpas, D.T., Vaughan, E.M., and Balow, J.E. (1995) High-risk features of lupus nephritis: importance of race and clinical and histological factors in 166 patients. *Nephrol Dial Transplant* **10**, 1620–8.

66. Contreras, G., Lenz, O., Pardo, V., Borja, E., Cely, C., Iqbal, K., *et al.* (2006) Outcomes in African Americans and Hispanics with lupus nephritis. *Kidney Int* **69**, 1846–51.

67. Dooley, M.A., Hogan, S., Jennette, C., and Falk, R. (1997) Cyclophosphamide therapy for lupus nephritis: poor renal survival in black Americans. Glomerular Disease Collaborative Network. *Kidney Int* **51**, 1188–95.

68. Korbet, S.M., Schwartz, M.M., Evans, J., and Lewis, E.J. (2007) Severe lupus nephritis: racial differences in presentation and outcome. *J Am Soc Nephrol* **18**, 244–54.

69. Ward, M.M. (1999) Premature morbidity from cardiovascular and cerebrovascular diseases in women with systemic lupus erythematosus. *Arthritis Rheum* **42**, 338–46.

70. Petri, M., Spence, D., Bone, L.R., and Hochberg, M.C. (1992) Coronary artery disease risk factors in the Johns Hopkins Lupus Cohort: prevalence, recognition by patients, and preventive practices. *Medicine (Baltimore)* **71**, 291–302.

71. Esdaile, J.M., Abrahamowicz, M., Grodzicky, T., Li, Y., Panaritis, C., du, B.R., *et al.* (2001) Traditional Framingham risk factors fail to fully account for accelerated atherosclerosis in systemic lupus erythematosus. *Arthritis Rheum* **44**, 2331–7.

72. Rahman, P., Urowitz, M.B., Gladman, D.D., Bruce, I.N., Genest, J., Jr. (1999) Contribution of traditional risk factors to coronary artery disease in patients with systemic lupus erythematosus. *J Rheumatol* **26**, 2363–8.

73. Ordonez, J.D., Hiatt, R.A., Killebrew, E.J., and Fireman, B.H. (1993) The increased risk of coronary heart disease associated with nephrotic syndrome. *Kidney Int* **44**, 638–42.

74. Neumann, K., Wallace, D.J., Azen, C., Nessim, S., Fichman, M., Metzger, A.L., and Klinenberg, J.R. (1995) Lupus in the 1980s: III. Influence of clinical variables, biopsy, and

treatment on the outcome in 150 patients with lupus nephritis seen at a single center. *Semin Arthritis Rheum* **25**, 47–55.

75. Radhakrishnan, J., Appel, A.S., Valeri, A., and Appel, G.B. (1993) The nephrotic syndrome, lipids, and risk factors for cardiovascular disease. *Am J Kidney Dis* **22**, 135–42.

76. Sahadevan, M., and Kasiske, B.L. (2002) Hyperlipidemia in kidney disease: causes and consequences. *Curr Opin Nephrol Hypertens* **11**, 323–9.

77. Jafar, T.H., Schmid, C.H., Landa, M., Giatras, I., Toto, R., Remuzzi, G., *et al.* (2001) Angiotensin-converting enzyme inhibitors and progression of nondiabetic renal disease. A meta-analysis of patient-level data. *Ann Intern Med* **135**, 73–87.

78. Gupta, A., Khaira, A., Singh, B., Bhowmik, D.M., and Tiwari, S.C. (2009) Aliskiren as an antiproteinuric add-on therapy in primary membranous nephropathy. *Clin Exp Nephrol* **13**, 402–3.

79. Radhakrishnan, J., Szabolcs, M., D'Agati, V., Nicolaides, M., Wharton, R., and Appel, G.B. (1993) Lupus membranous nephropathy: course and prognosis in 50 patients [Abstract]. *J Am Soc Nephrol* **4**, 284.

80. Bellomo, R., and Atkins, R.C. (1993) Membranous nephropathy and thromboembolism: is prophylactic anticoagulation warranted? *Nephron* **63**, 249–54.

81. Sarasin, F.P., and Schifferli, J.A. (1994) Prophylactic oral anticoagulation in nephrotic patients with idiopathic membranous nephropathy. *Kidney Int* **45**, 578–85.

82. Cattran, D. (2005) Management of membranous nephropathy: when and what for treatment. *J Am Soc Nephrol* **16**, 1188–94.

83. Donadio, J.V., Jr., Burgess, J.H., and Holley, K.E. (1977) Membranous lupus nephropathy: a clinicopathologic study. *Medicine (Baltimore)* **56**, 527–36.

84. Mok, C.C., Ying, K.Y., Yim, C.W., Ng, W.L., and Wong, W.S. (2009) Very long-term outcome of pure lupus membranous nephropathy treated with glucocorticoid and azathioprine. *Lupus* **18**, 1091–5.

85. Wang, A.Y., Li, P.K., Lai, F.M., Chow, K.M., Szeto, C.C., Leung, C.B., and Lui, SF. (2001) Severe bone marrow failure associated with the use of alternating steroid with chlorambucil in lupus membranous nephropathy in Chinese. *Lupus* **10**, 295–8.

86. Lewis, E.J., Hunsicker, L.G., Lan, S.P., Rohde, R.D., and Lachin, J.M. (1992) A controlled trial of plasmapheresis therapy in severe lupus nephritis. The Lupus Nephritis Collaborative Study Group. *N Engl J Med* **326**, 1373–9.

87. Ambalavanan, S., Fauvel, J.P., Sibley, R.K., and Myers, B.D. (1996) Mechanism of the antiproteinuric effect of cyclosporine in membranous nephropathy. *J Am Soc Nephrol* **7**, 290–8.

88. Faul, C., Donnelly, M., Merscher-Gomez, S., Chang, Y.H., Franz, S., Delfgaauw, J., *et al.* (2008) The actin cytoskeleton of kidney podocytes is a direct target of the antiproteinuric effect of cyclosporine A. *Nat Med* **14**, 931–8.

89. Schreiber, S.L., and Crabtree, G.R. (1992) The mechanism of action of cyclosporin A and FK506. *Immunol Today* **13**, 136–42.

90. Hallegua, D., Wallace, D.J., Metzger, A.L., Rinaldi, R.Z., and Klinenberg, J.R. (2000) Cyclosporine for lupus membranous nephritis: experience with ten patients and review of the literature. *Lupus* **9**, 241–51.

91. Hu, W., Liu, Z., Shen, S., Li, S., Yao, X., Chen, H., and Li, L. (2003) Cyclosporine A in treatment of membranous lupus nephropathy. *Chin Med J (Engl)* **116**, 1827–30.

92. Maruyama, M., Yamasaki, Y., Sada, K., Sarai, A., Ujike, K., Maeshima, Y., et al. (2006) Good response of membranous lupus nephritis to tacrolimus. *Clin Nephrol* **65**, 276–9.

93. Radhakrishnan, J., Kunis, C.L., D'Agati, V., and Appel, G.B. (1994) Cyclosporine treatment of lupus membranous nephropathy. *Clin Nephrol* **42**, 147–54.

94. Szeto, C.C., Kwan, B.C., Lai, F.M., Tam, L.S., Li, E.K., Chow, K.M., et al. (2008) Tacrolimus for the treatment of systemic lupus erythematosus with pure class V nephritis. *Rheumatology (Oxford)* **47**, 1678–81.

95. Tam, L.-S., Li, E.K., Szeto, C.-C., Wong, S.-M., Leung, C.-B., Lai, F.M., et al. (2001) Treatment of membranous lupus nephritis with prednisone, azathioprine and cyclosporin A. *Lupus* **10**, 827–9.

96. Tse, K.C., Lam, M.F., Tang, S.C., Tang, C.S., and Chan, T.M. (2007) A pilot study on tacrolimus treatment in membranous or quiescent lupus nephritis with proteinuria resistant to angiotensin inhibition or blockade. *Lupus* **16**, 46–51.

97. Waldman, M., and Austin, H.A., III. (2009) Controversies in the treatment of idiopathic membranous nephropathy. *Nat Rev Nephrol* **5**, 469–79.

98. Cattran, D.C., Alexopoulos, E., Heering, P., Hoyer, P.F., Johnston, A., Meyrier, A., et al. (2007) Cyclosporin in idiopathic glomerular disease associated with the nephrotic syndrome: workshop recommendations. *Kidney Int* **72**, 1429–47.

99. Garjau, M., Segarra, A., Ramos, N., Quiroz, A., Carreras, J., Gomez, M.R., et al. (2008) Efficacy of combined therapy with rituximab and tacrolimus in the induction of stable remission of proteinuria in patients with primary membranous glomerulonephritis [Abstract]. *J Am Soc Nephrol* **19**, 561.

100. Borba, E.F., Guedes, L.K., Christmann, R.B., Figueiredo, C.P., Goncalves, C.R., and Bonfa, E. (2006) Mycophenolate mofetil is effective in reducing lupus glomerulonephritis proteinuria. *Rheumatol Int* **26**, 1078–83.

101. Kapitsinou, P.P., Boletis, J.N., Skopouli, F.N., Boki, K.A., and Moutsopoulos, H.M. (2004) Lupus nephritis: treatment with mycophenolate mofetil. *Rheumatology (Oxford)* **43**, 377–380.

102. Karim, M.Y., Pisoni, C.N., Ferro, L., Tungekar, M.F., Abbs, I.C., D'Cruz, D.P., et al. (2005) Reduction of proteinuria with mycophenolate mofetil in predominantly membranous lupus nephropathy. *Rheumatology (Oxford)* **44**, 1317–21.

103. Radhakrishnan, J., Ginzler, E., and Appel, G. (2005) Mycophenolate mofetil (MMF) vs. intravenous cyclophosphamide (IVCY) for severe lupus nephritis (LN): subgroup analysis of patients (pts) with membranous nephropathy (SLE-V) [Abstract]. *J Am Soc Nephrol* **16**, 8.

104. Spetie, D.N., Tang, Y., Rovin, B.H., Nadasdy, T., Nadasdy, G., Pesavento, T.E., and Hebert, L.A. (2004) Mycophenolate therapy of SLE membranous nephropathy. *Kidney Int* **66**, 2411–15.

105. Appel, G.B., Contreras, G., Dooley, M.A., Ginzler, E.M., Isenberg, D., Jayne, D., et al. (2009) Mycophenolate mofetil versus cyclophosphamide for induction treatment of lupus nephritis. *J Am Soc Nephrol* **20**, 1103–12.

106. Ginzler, E.M., Dooley, M.A., Aranow, C., Kim, M.Y., Buyon, J., Merrill, J.T., et al. (2005) Mycophenolate mofetil or intravenous cyclophosphamide for lupus nephritis. *N Engl J Med* **353**, 2219–28.

107. Radhakrishnan, J., Moutzouris, D.A., Ginzler, E.M., Solomons, N., Siempos, I.I., and Appel, G.B. (2010) Mycophenolate mofetil and intravenous cyclophosphamide are similar as induction therapy for class V lupus nephritis. *Kidney Int* **77**, 152–60.

108. Bomback, A.S., Derebail, V.K., McGregor, J.G., Kshirsagar, A.V., Falk, R.J., and Nachman, P.H. (2009) Rituximab therapy for membranous nephropathy: a systematic review. *Clin J Am Soc Nephrol* **4**, 734–44.

109. Furie, R., Looney, R.J., Rovin, B., Latinis, K.M., Appel, G., Sanchez-Guerrero, J., et al. (2009) Efficacy and safety of rituximab in subjects with active proliferative lupus

nephritis (LN): Results from the randomized double blind phase III Lunar study. [Abstract]. *Arthritis Rheum* **60**, S249.

110. Fra, G.P., Avanzi, G.C., and Bartoli, E. (2003) Remission of refractory lupus nephritis with a protocol including rituximab. *Lupus* **12**, 783–87.

111. Jacobson, S.H., van, V.R., and Gunnarsson, I. (2006) Rituximab-induced long-term remission of membranous lupus nephritis. *Nephrol Dial Transplant* **21**, 1742–3.

112. Melander, C., Sallee, M., Trolliet, P., Candon, S., Belenfant, X., Daugas, E., *et al.* (2009) Rituximab in severe lupus nephritis: early B-cell depletion affects long-term renal outcome. *Clin J Am Soc Nephrol* **4**, 579–87.

113. Finck, B.K., Linsley, P.S., and Wofsy, D. (1994) Treatment of murine lupus with CTLA4Ig. *Science* **265**, 1225–7.

114. Appel, G., Nachman, P., Hogan, S., Radhakrishnan, J., Old, C., Hebert, L., *et al.* (2002) Eculizumab (C5 complement inhibitor) in the treatment of idiopathic membranous nephropathy (IMN): preliminary baseline and pharmacokinetic (PK)/pharmacodynamic (PD) data [Abstract]. *J Am Soc Nephrol* **13**, 668.

115. Gross, J.A., Johnston, J., Mudri, S., Enselman, R., Dillon, S.R., Madden, K., *et al.* (2000) TACI and BCMA are receptors for a TNF homologue implicated in B-cell autoimmune disease. *Nature* **404**, 995–9.

116. Navarra, S., Guzman, R., Gallacher, A., Levy, R.A., Li, E.K., Thomas, M., *et al.*, and BLIS-52 Study Group. (2009) Belimumab, a BLyS-specific inhibitor, reduced disease activity, flares and prednisone use in patients with active SLE: Efficacy and safety results from the phase 3 BLISS-52 Study. [Abstract]. *Arthritis Rheum* **60**, 3859.

117. Yao, Y., Richman, L., Higgs, B.W., Morehouse, C.A., de los, R.M., Brohawn, P., *et al.* (2009) Neutralization of interferon-alpha/beta-inducible genes and downstream effect in a phase I trial of an anti-interferon-alpha monoclonal antibody in systemic lupus erythematosus. *Arthritis Rheum* **60**, 1785–96.

118. Aringer, M., Graninger, W.B., Steiner, G., and Smolen, J.S. (2004) Safety and efficacy of tumor necrosis factor alpha blockade in systemic lupus erythematosus: an open-label study. *Arthritis Rheum* **50**, 3161–9.

119. Balow, J.E., and Austin, H.A., III. (2003) Therapy of membranous nephropathy in systemic lupus erythematosus. *Semin Nephrol* **23**, 386–91.

Chapter 8

Lupus podocytopathy

Edmund J. Lewis

Introduction

The term lupus podocytopathy has been formulated in order to describe the renal lesion in a group of patients with systemic lupus erythematosus (SLE) who present with a marked degree of proteinuria, often causing the characteristic clinical changes of the nephrotic syndrome with massive amounts of albuminuria, hypoalbuminemia, and edema. Unlike the classic patient with membranous glomerulonephritis or severe inflammatory lupus nephritis, who may present in this manner, these patients have biopsy findings revealing either no glomerular immune deposits or sparse deposits, which are confined to the glomerular mesangium (Figure 8.1). The characteristic pathological glomerular abnormality observed among these patients is ultrastructural and resides in the visceral glomerular epithelial cells, and is characterized as glomerular epithelial foot process fusion (Figure 8.2). The glomerular lesions are identical to those described in idiopathic minimal change glomerulopathy (MCG) (Figure 8.3), the most common cause of the nephrotic syndrome in children. In some cases there may be glomerular scars, in which case the histological diagnosis fits with the diagnosis of focal and segmental glomerulosclerosis (FSGS) (Figure 8.4). Although usually a primary lesion, MCG can also rarely occur in patients with Hodgkin's disease,[1] has also been associated with lithium administration, and can occur in occasional cases of patients receiving nonsteroidal anti-inflammatory agents (NSAIA).[2–4] Children with MCG almost always respond promptly to the use of high-dose prednisone or prednisolone therapy. Adults with MCG also tend to respond to high-dose steroid therapy, but often do so less rapidly than children.

The pathogenesis of scars in FSGS is variable and complex. As is the case with MCG, FSGS has also only recently been associated with SLE.[5,6] A diverse number of inherited and acquired abnormalities of the structural proteins associated with the glomerular epithelial cell have been associated with FSGS. There is evidence that a circulating factor is responsible for the proteinuria that occurs in idiopathic FSGS.[7–11] Some of this evidence implies the possibility that the factor that may promote proteinuria could be a T cell cytokine. As indicated by the histopathological term, FSGS is characterized by glomerular scars, which affect a portion of the glomerular tuft of some glomeruli (Figure 8.4). Often, when seen in SLE, very few glomeruli may be scarred. These patients are less likely to be prednisone-responsive than those with MCG, and other immunosuppressive agents have generally been required in order to induce a partial or complete remission of the proteinuria.

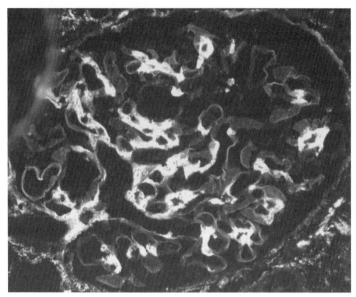

Fig. 8.1 Fluorescence microscopy for immunoglobulin (Ig)G in a renal glomerulus in a patient who has the nephrotic syndrome due to lupus podocytopathy. There are no IgG deposits in the peripheral capillary loops and all deposits are confined to the glomerular mesangium. Magnification, 40× (see Plate 15).

Clinical association of active systemic disease of lupus with the onset of nephrotic syndrome

The finding of MCG or FSGS as the glomerular lesion in SLE patients with proteinuria and the nephrotic syndrome has raised the question of whether these patients, coincidentally, could have two uncommon but distinct diseases. However, the frequency of patients with podocytopathy lesions and their temporal relationship to the onset of acute systemic activity of SLE would appear to make it unlikely that their coincidence in a given patient is unrelated. Hertig *et al.* reported 11 patients with podocytopathy, four of whom had MCG and seven FSGS.[12] Several of the FSGS patients had ≤10% of glomeruli scarred. They recognized that six patients (two MCG, four FSGS) had the simultaneous onset of systemic manifestations of SLE and the nephrotic syndrome. In six cases polyarthralgia was present; however, other lupus manifestations including pleurisy, pericarditis, malar rash, necrotizing skin lesions, seizures, and fever were also noted.[13] Kraft *et al.* described eight patients, six of whom had systemic manifestations of lupus associated with the onset of nephrotic syndrome concomitant or within 1 month of the onset of clinical manifestations of renal disease.

We do not have a detailed understanding of all the humoral and cellular events that underlie the pathophysiological spectrum of lesions seen in the glomerular abnormalities associated with SLE. Logically, the attention of physicians with regard to the pathogenetic mechanisms of lupus nephritis has resided in the well-defined spectrum

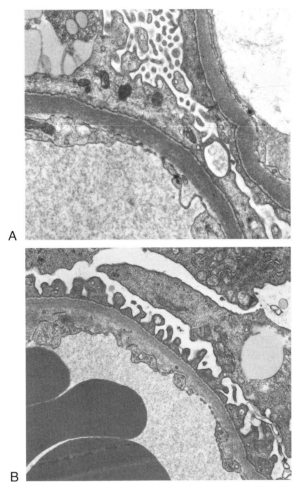

Fig. 8.2 (A) Electron microscopic photograph of a glomerular capillary in which the visceral epithelial cells on the outer side of the glomerular basement membrane demonstrate diffuse foot process effacement, which is the characteristic finding seen in lupus podocytopathy. (B) Ultrastructure of a glomerular capillary loop revealing normal visceral epithelial cell foot processes (pedicels). Magnification, A and B, 12,000×.

of glomerular lesions that appear to be associated with immune deposits. Only recently has it become acknowledged that renal biopsy findings in patients with lupus who have the nephrotic syndrome may reveal few or no histological changes on light microscopy. When limited histological changes are present, they are confined to the glomerular mesangium (Figure 8.5). The histological abnormality of lupus podocytopathy has not appeared in previous World Health Organization (WHO) classifications of lupus nephritis, or in the current International Society of Nephrology/Renal Pathology Society (ISN/RPS) classification.[14–16]

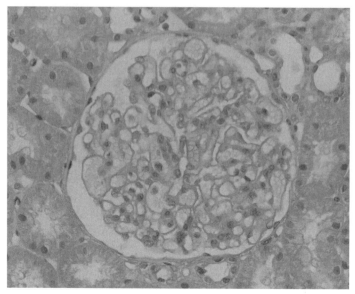

Fig. 8.3 Lupus podocytopathy with minimal change lesion by light microscopy. There are no morphological abnormalities noted. Hematoxylin and eosin, magnification 66× (see Plate 16).

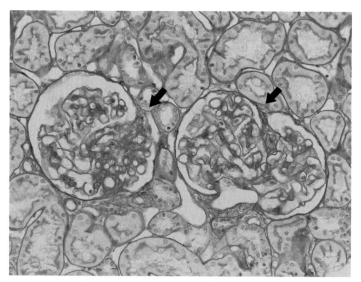

Fig. 8.4 Lupus podocytopathy with focal segmental glomerular sclerosis by light microscopy. There are small segmental glomerular scars with adhesions (arrows) that do not involve the glomerular hilum, in two glomeruli. In some cases this can be accompanied by increased numbers of visceral epithelial cells in the area of the scar and increased mesangial cellularity. Neither of these abnormalities is noted in this example. Periodic acid Schiff stain, magnification 50× (see Plate 17).

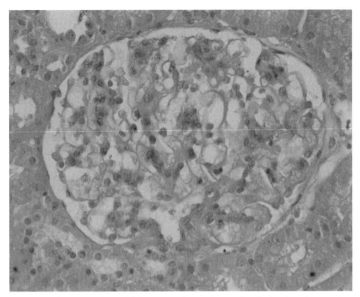

Fig. 8.5 Lupus podocytopathy with increased numbers of cells in the glomerular mesangium. Increased connective tissue components in the mesangium can accompany this abnormality. Otherwise the glomerular histological structure is normal. In lupus, this structural abnormality is usually associated with some mesangial immune deposits, which contain IgG, but may also contain other immunoglobulins and complement components. Hematoxylin and eosin, magnification 66× (see Plate 18).

Nephrotic syndrome and acute renal failure

It is of importance to note that patients with podocytopathy tend to have a dramatic clinical appearance of their renal disease (Table 8.1). As noted, they usually have the nephrotic syndrome with an acute onset, which is often associated with the acute onset of other systemic manifestations of lupus, either as the initial clinical onset of lupus or as a recrudescence of the disease. The amount of proteinuria can be massive and may be associated with acute renal failure in addition to the nephrotic syndrome. Hertig *et al.* reported that two of their 11 patients also had acute renal failure.[12] Kraft *et al.* reported that four of their eight patients had acute renal failure (Table 8.1).[13] Three of these latter patients required hemodialytic therapy. Decreased glomerular filtration rate is a common finding in patients with idiopathic MCG or FSGS; however, acute renal failure, although seen less often, can be a complication in the idiopathic setting of severe acute nephrotic syndrome. The concurrence of the nephrotic syndrome and acute renal failure obliges the clinician to undertake a differential diagnosis to determine whether the patient has diffuse crescentic glomerulonephritis. Several explanations for the concurrence of acute nephrotic syndrome due to podocytopathy and acute renal failure have been offered including (a) sudden plasma volume depletion due to acute hypoalbuminemia, (b) nephrotoxic injury associated with the formation of oxygen-derived free radicals associated with plasma protein reabsorption by proximal tubular cells, and (c) an acute increase in intrarenal pressure

Table 8.1 Clinical features of lupus podocytopathy with nephrotic syndrome

	N	Age mean yrs	Gender F/M	Proteinuria mean g/24 hour	Serum albumin mean g/dl	Serum creatinine mean mg/dl	Serum creatinine mean ≥1.5 mg/dl
Hertig et al.[12]	11	27	10/1	9.2	1.48	2.5	5
Dube et al.[20]	7	33	6/1	9.6	1.81	1.8	4
Kraft et al.[13]	8	32	7/1	7.2	2.10	3.8	6
Han et al.[33]	5	29	4/1	8.4	2.93	0.9	1

associated with edema of the kidney.[17] In the latter case it has been implied that the increase in intrarenal pressure due to edema and increased renal volume of the kidney, which is restricted in size by the renal capsule, could decrease the capillary filtration pressure, thus preventing the movement of fluid across the glomerular capillary wall into Bowman's space.[18,19]

Minimal change glomerulopathy: a manifestation of lupus

Although generally overlooked, a number of authors have, over the past two decades, called attention to the association of minimal change glomerulopathy and the nephrotic syndrome in one or more of their patients who had active SLE.[12,13,20–28] Often, the patient was treated with high-dose prednisone therapy and had a prompt remission of the nephrotic syndrome. Certainly, these clinical experiences suggested that the presence of SLE and MCG in these patients was not a coincidence. Makino reported such a patient in 1995 and raised the intriguing possibility that the spectrum of immunological injury occurring as a consequence of SLE, might be expanded to include damage related to sensitized T cells, which could be releasing a cytokine that might be responsible for increased glomerular permeability due to podocyte injury.[24] The hypothesis that T cells are somehow involved in the generation of podocyte pathology and proteinuria in idiopathic MCG was proposed over 30 years ago.[29]

The reports of Dube et al.[20] and Hertig et al.[12] strengthened the position that the concurrence of MCG and FSGS with the nephrotic syndrome and SLE was indeed not coincidence. Dube et al. reported the clinical and pathological findings in seven patients with MCG, all of whom presented with the nephrotic syndrome. In every case there was diffuse foot process effacement in the absence of significant peripheral capillary wall immune deposits.[20] Five of these patients displayed some electron-dense deposits, which were limited to the mesangium and were so sparse that it was believed that they could not possibly explain the clinical abnormality (Figure 8.6). In all cases the nephrotic syndrome remitted with treatment with high-dose corticosteroids. Importantly, several of the patients in this study had used a NSAIA; these drugs are capable of causing MCG with the nephrotic syndrome.[2–4] However, in most cases the temporal relationship between NSAIA administration and the occurrence of proteinuria did not support this explanation of clinical course of these patients. As would also be further described in subsequent publications, the nephrotic syndrome was

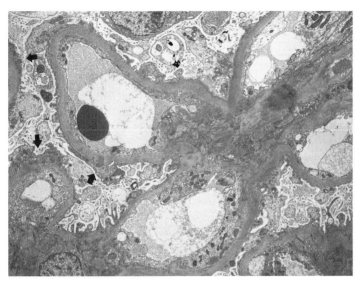

Fig. 8.6 Electron microscopic photograph of several glomerular capillary loops revealing a few scattered electron-dense immune aggregates on the epithelial cell side of the glomerular basement membrane (arrows). The prominent abnormality noted here is the generalized visceral epithelial cell foot process effacement. This biopsy was taken from a patient with active SLE and the nephrotic syndrome. Uranyl acetate and lead citrate, magnification 3000×.

profound among these patients with an average 24-hour urine protein excretion of 9.6 g/day and an average serum albumin of 1.8 g/dl (range 0.6–2.4 g/dl) (Table 8.1).

Mesangial lupus nephritis

In retrospect, it would appear that the relationship between lupus podocytopathy and the nephrotic syndrome has not only been long recognized, but some cases may have been misinterpreted in the literature. Reports have noted the presence of immune deposits in the glomerular mesangium in biopsies of patients who had the nephrotic syndrome, some of whom have responded to steroid therapy.[30] These observations have, therefore, focused attention upon mesangial deposits, implying that WHO Class II (ISN/RPS Class I or II) lesions could rarely cause severe proteinuria while overlooking the relevance of glomerular epithelial cell changes (Figures 8.2 and 8.3). In fact, the majority of patients with mesangial lupus glomerulonephritis manifest no proteinuria at all, and when they do the proteinuria is rarely greater than 1 g/day. It is clear that the nephrotic syndrome would be an extremely rare phenomenon in WHO Class II (ISN/RPS Class I patients). Dube *et al.* noted immunoglobulin (Ig)G and other immunoproteins in five of six of their cases in which immunofluorescence was available. In addition, electron-dense deposits were seen in six of seven of their cases, and the diagnosis of mild or moderate mesangial proliferative lupus nephritis was reported in five of the seven cases, which would place these patients in category II of the 1982 and 1995 WHO classifications and category 1 of the 2002 ISN/RPS classification (Figure 8.5).[20] Kraft *et al.* reported significant mesangial proliferation in seven of their eight cases and positive immunofluorescence for IgG in six cases, with electron-dense deposits in five cases (Figure 8.1). Hertig *et al.* reported mesangial IgG, IgM, C3, and C1q in three cases.[3] The recognition of the extensive visceral epithelial cell changes and the limited mesangial changes that characterize podocytopathy in patients with active systemic lupus leads one to suspect that reports of "mesangial lupus" with extensive proteinuria[30] actually better fit the concept of epithelial cell damage and podocytopathy as the primary pathogenic lesion.

SLE and podocytopathy: not a coincidence

In addition to their own experience, Hertig *et al.* reviewed the existing literature and concluded that the temporal relationship between the appearance of systemic features of SLE and the onset of nephrotic syndrome was almost always concurrent, and that in only one patient reported in the literature were the two syndromes apparently independent.[12] On the basis of the prevalence of two relatively unusual diagnoses, the idiopathic nephrotic syndrome and SLE among adults in France, they proposed that the prevalence of SLE associated with MCG or FSGS, i.e. lupus podocytopathy, could be estimated to be 0.4–1 case per 10,000 people.[12,31,32] It was concluded that this relationship is far more common in the clinic than would be expected if SLE and idiopathic MCG or FSGS were occurring in individual patients by chance alone, and, therefore supports the proposal that Makino *et al.* had initially implied, that MCG was not a coincidence but rather a manifestation of SLE.[24]

Hence, epidemiological and clinical data support the notion that nephrotic-range proteinuria does occur in patients with SLE in the absence of notable immunohistopathological changes and inflammation abnormalities on light microscopy when epithelial cell foot process fusion is the single morphological feature associated with this clinical phenomenon, which appears to be a manifestation of SLE.

With the recognition of the epithelial cell lesion one might propose that lupus podocytopathy is even more common than current literature suggests. Certainly, it has been accepted that more than a single immunopathogenetic manifestation of lupus may be present in the glomeruli of patients with lupus nephritis. For example, membranous lupus nephritis is frequently associated with subendothelial immune deposits in the peripheral capillary loops, and, therefore, is classified as a complex lesion involving membranous and proliferative components. Other examples abound including the concurrence of immune deposit-associated glomerular disease and a lesion analogous to pauci-immune vasculitic glomerulopathy. Thus, it is possible that podocytopathy may accompany minor glomerular lesions other than the mesangial abnormalities previously described. Han *et al.* studied a subset of patients with nephrotic syndrome and SLE who had mesangial lupus nephritis (WHO Class II, ISN/RPS Class I or II) and also had extremely rare subepithelial capillary wall electron-dense deposits (Figure 8.6).[33] These patients did not have enough subepithelial immune aggregate deposition to classify the biopsy as membranous lupus nephritis (WHO-V, ISN/RPS-V); however, neither could the case be made that they had MCG because of the presence of some rare electron-dense subepithelial deposits. The primary distinguishing pathological feature in these nephrotic patients was the presence of diffuse visceral epithelial cell foot process fusion and the clinical features of the nephrotic syndrome were similar to those previously reported. Thus, the intriguing possibility is raised that a spectrum of immunological injury causing the nephrotic syndrome that is the consequence of SLE is not related to apparent minimal and presumed insignificant subepithelial immune deposits, but rather the result of glomerular visceral epithelial cell damage analogous to that seen in idiopathic nephrotic syndrome due to MCG.

Glomerular epithelial cell damage and the nephrotic syndrome

For decades, aberrant T cell function has been held to be responsible for glomerular epithelial cell injury in the idiopathic minimal change glomerulopathy. It deserves emphasis that MCG is a structural lesion. Certainly, there could be significant patho-genetic differences between the mechanism that ultimately causes the glomerular epithelial cell injury pattern in idiopathic MCG of children and that noted in SLE, Hodgkin's disease, lithium intoxication, or NSAIA-associated nephrotic syndrome. Nonetheless, in the absence of glomerular immune deposits, the involvement of a T cell activation mechanism that could result in elaboration of a cytokine causing epithelial cell dysfunction is an attractive hypothesis. This hypothesis was first attrib-uted to Shalhoub, who proposed that MCG represented a renal manifestation of sys-temic immunological abnormality, which involved activated T cell dysregulation.[29] His reasons included: (a) children with MCG could have a measles-induced remis-sion, measles virus being a known inhibitor of T cell mediated immunity; (b) MCG occurred in the occasional patient with Hodgkin's disease, a disease later to be demon-strated as being associated with abnormal T cell regulation; (c) the absence of immune reactants in the glomerulus; and (d) the therapeutic effectiveness of corticosteroid and cyclophosphamide therapy in MCG. A number of specific alterations in the immune system in MCG have been identified since Shalhoub's hypothesis. In fact, although the underlying basis of MCG is elusive, there is growing evidence that activated T cells may elaborate factors that could be responsible for abnormal urine protein excretion. Abnormal T cell cytokine expression has been described in minimal change glomeru-lopathy.[34] Sahali *et al.* suggested abnormal T cell activation on the basis of overexpres-sion of several DNA transcripts from patients with MCG.[35,36] Studies of children with MCG have demonstrated a proinflammatory profile involving Th2 predominance on the basis of increased number of CD4+ and CD69+ activation markers.[37–41] The CXC chemokine, GRO-γ has been suggested to be responsible for these observed T cell activation abnormalities.[42] In addition, a "circulating factor," presumed to be a cytokine of T cell origin has been implicated in the lesions of FSGS.[7–11] These findings raise the question of whether activated T cells could similarly be implicated in the pathogenesis of the podocyte lesion and proteinuria here described. Certainly, T cell dysfunction is present in both SLE and MCG.[43,44] Although abnormalities of helper T and suppressor T cell ratios have been described in SLE and in severe lupus nephritis, one must admit that MCG is a relatively unusual consequence of SLE, and that any T cell functional abnormality must be quite specific. Nevertheless, it is intriguing to consider that an unknown activated T cell clone does exist in some patients, which produces a glomerular capillary permeability factor that might explain lupus podocytopathy.

Clinical recommendations

The nephrotic syndrome is commonly associated with the severe proliferative segmental and diffuse glomerulopathies of SLE, as well as with membranous lupus nephritis. In the case of an abrupt onset of the nephrotic syndrome with the onset of active systemic lupus, lupus podocytopathy should be considered and a renal biopsy is required. Most patients with lupus podocytopathy respond to high-dose corticosteroid therapy. The response ranges from the classic response seen in idiopathic MCG, with a sudden decrease and normalization of proteinuria, to a more modest decrease in proteinuria sometimes referred to as an "incomplete remission." Nevertheless, prednisone alone appears to be appropriate therapy without the addition of other immunosuppressant or anti-inflammatory drugs. The occurrence of acute oliguric renal failure associated with the acute onset of profound nephrotic syndrome should suggest to the clinician that lupus podocytopathy is in the differential diagnosis. In the absence of hematuria and red blood cell casts, the possibility that lupus podocytopathy explains the clinical problem should be strongly considered. This is of particular importance given the fact that the immunosuppressive therapy of severe acute inflammatory lupus nephritis or rapidly progressive glomerulonephritis contrasts with the high-dose steroid regimen recommended in lupus podocytopathy. Acute renal failure, which may require dialytic therapy, can be expected to resolve with resolution of the nephrotic syndrome.

References

1. Moorthy, A.V., Zimmerman, S.W., and Burkholder, P.M. (1976) Nephrotic syndrome in Hodgkin's disease: Evidence for pathogenesis alternative to immune complex disposition. *Am J Med* **61**, 471–7.

2. Feinfield, D.A., Olesnicky, L., Pirani, C.L., and Appel, C.B. (1984) Nephrotic syndrome associated with use of the nonsteroidal anti-inflammatory drugs. *Nephron* **37**, 174–9.

3. Abraham, P.A., and Keane, W.F. (1984) Glomerular and interstitial disease induced by non-steroidal anti-inflammatory drugs. *Am J Nephrol* **4**, 1–6.

4. Warren, G.V., Korbet, S.M., Schwartz, M.M., and Lewis, E.J. (1989) Minimal change glomerulopathy associated with non-steroidal antiinflammatory drugs. *Am J Kidney Dis* **13**, 127–30.

5. Papo, T., Faucher, C., Huong, D., Beaufils, H., Piette, and J., Godeau, P. (1994) Idiopathic focal segmental glomerulosclerosis in a patient with systemic lupus erythematosus An unusual combination. *Am J Kidney Dis* **24**, 880–1.

6. Hickman, P.L., Nolph, K.D., Jacobs, R., Luger, A.M., and Walker, S.E. (1994) Idiopathic focal segmental glomerulosclerosis in a patient with systemic lupus erythematosus: An unusual combination. *Am J Kidney Dis* **23**, 582–6.

7. Savin, V.J. (1993) Mechanisms of proteinuria in noninflammatory glomerular disease. *Am J Kidney Dis* **27**, 347–62.

8. Koyama, A., Fujisaki, M. Kobayashi, M., Igarasm, M., and Narita, M. (1991) A glomerular permeability factor produced by human T Cell hybridomas. *Kidney Int* **40**, 453–60.

9. Yoshizawa, N., Kusumi, Y., Matsumoto, K., Oshima, S., Takeuchi, A., Kawamura, O., *et al.* (1989) Studies of a glomerular permeability factor in patients with minimal change nephrotic syndrome. *Nephron* **51**, 370–6.

10. Trachtman, H., Greenbaum, L.A., McCarthy, E.T., Sharma, M., Gauthier, B.G., Frank, R., *et al.* (2004) Prevalence and prognostic value in pediatric patients with idiopathic nephrotic syndrome. *Am J Kidney Dis* **44**, 604–10.

11. McCarthy, E.T., Sharma, M., Sharma, R., Falk, R.J., and Jennette, J.C. (2004) Sera from patients with collapsing focal segmental glomerulosclerosis increase albumin permeability of isolated glomeruli. *J Lab Clin Med* **143**, 225–9.

12. Hertig, A., Droz, D., Lesavre, P., Grünfield, J., and Rieu, P. (2002) SLE and idiopathic nephrotic syndrome: Coincidence or not? *Am J Kidney Dis* **40**, 1179–84.

13. Kraft, S., Korbet, S.M., and Lewis, E.J. (2005) Glomerular podocytopathy in patients with systemic lupus erythematosus. *J Am Nephrol* **16**, 175–9.

14. Churg, J., Bernstein, J., and Glassock, R. (1995) *Renal Disease*, pp. 151–79. Ikagu-Shoin, Tokyo, Japan.

15. Tan, E.M., Cohen, A.S., Fires, J.F., Masi, A.T., McShane, D.J., Rothfield, N.F., *et al.* (1982) The 1982 revised criteria for the classification of systemic lupus erythematosus. *Arthritis Rheum* **25**, 1271–5.

16 International Society of Nephrology and Renal Pathology Society Working Group on the Classification of Lupus Nephritis. (2004) The classification of Glomerulonephritis in systemic lupus erythematosus revisited. *J Am Soc Nephrol* **15**, 241–50.

17. Erkan, E., Garcia, C.D., Patterson, L.T., Mishra, J., Mitsnefes, M.M., Kaskel, F.J., Devarajan, P. (2005) Induction of renal tubular cell apoptosis in focal segmental glomerulosclerosis: Roles of proteinuria and Fas-dependent pathways. *J Am Soc Nephrol* **16**, 398–407.

18. Lowenstein, J., Schacht, R.G., and Baldwin, D.S. (1981) Renal failure in minimal change nephrotic syndrome. *Am J Med* **70**, 227–33.

19. Bernard, D.B., Alexander, E.A., Couser, W.G., and Levinsky, N.G. (1978) Renal sodium retention during volume expansion in experimental nephrotic syndrome. *Kidney Int* **14**, 478–85.

20. Dube, G.K., Markowitz, G.S., Radhakrishnan, J., Appel, G.B., and D'Agati, V.D. (2002) Minimal change disease in systemic lupus erythematosus. *Clin Nephrol* **57**, 120–6.

21. Abuelo, J., Esparza, A., and Garella, S. (1984) Steroid-dependent nephrotic syndrome in lupus nephritis. Response to chlorambucil. *Arch Intern Med* **144**, 2411–12.

22. Matsumura, N., Dohi, K., Shiiki, H., Morita, H., Yamada, H., Fujimoto, J., *et al.* (1989) Three cases presenting with systemic lupus erythematosus and minimal-change nephrotic syndrome. *Nippon Jinzo Gakkai Shi* **31**, 991–9.

23. Okai, T., Soejima, A., Suzuki, M., Yomogida, S., Nakabayashi, K., Kitamoto, K., and Nagasawa, T. (1992) A case report of lupus nephritis associated with minimal-change nephrotic syndrome – comparison of various histological types of 67 cases with lupus nephritis. *Nippon Jinzo Gakkai Shi* **34**, 835–40.

24. Makino, H., Haramoto, T., Shikata, K., Ogura, T., and Ota, Z. (1995) Minimal-change nephrotic syndrome associated with systemic lupus erythematosus. *Am J Nephrol* **15**, 439–41.

25. Horita, Y., Nazneen, A., Cheng, M., Razzaque, M.S., Namie, S., Tadokoro, M., *et al.* (1997) A case of systemic lupus erythematosus associated with minimal-change nephrotic syndrome. *Nippon Jinzo Gakkai Shi* **39**, 759–64.

26. Nishihara, G., Nakamoto, M., Yasunaga, C., Takeda, K., Matsuo, K., Urabe, M., *et al.* (1997) Systemic lupus erythematosus in a patient with remitting minimal change nephrotic syndrome. *Clin Nephrol* **48**, 327–30.

27. Perakis, C., Arvanitis, A., Sotsiou, F., and Emmanouel, D.S. (1998) Nephrotic syndrome caused by minimal-change disease in a patient with focal proliferative SLE nephritis (WHO III) in remission. *Nephrol Dial Transplant* **13**, 467–70.

28. Hunley, T.E., Yared, A., Fogo, A., and MacDonnell, R.C. (1998) Nephrotic syndrome in an adolescent: The cry of the wolf. *Am J Kidney Dis* **31**, 155–60.

29. Shaloub, R.J. (1974) Pathogenesis of lipoid nephrosis: A disorder of T-cell function. *Lancet* **ii**, 556–60.

30. Stankeviciute, N., Jao, W., Bakir, A., and Lash, J.P. (1997) Mesangial lupus nephritis with associated nephrotic syndrome. *J Am Soc Nephrol* **8**, 1199–204.

31. Simon, P., Ramee, M., Ang, K., and Cam, G. (1988) Epidemiology of glomerular diseases in a region in France. Changes as a function of periods and the age of patients. *Presse Med* **17**, 2175–8.

32. Abdulmassih, Z., Makdassi, R., Bove, N., *et al.* (1990) Epidemiology of primary glomerulonephritis in Picardie. *Ann Med Interne* **141**, 129–33.

33. Han, T.S., Schwartz, M.M., and Lewis, E.J. (2006) Association of glomerular podocytopathy and nephrotic proteinuria in mesangial lupus nephritis. *Lupus* **15**, 71–5.

34. Cunard, R., and Kelly, C.J. (2002) T Cells and minimal change disease. *J Am Soc Nephrol* **13**, 1409–11.

35. Sahali, D., Pawlak, A., Valanciute, A., *et al.* (2002) A novel approach to investigation of the pathogenesis of active minimal-change nephrotic syndrome using subtracted cDNA library screening. *J Am Soc Nephrol* **13**, 1238–47.

36. Sahali, D., Pawlak, A., Gouvello, S.I., *et al.* (2001) Transcriptional and post-transcriptional alterations of m IκBα in active minimal-change nephrotic syndrome. *J Am Soc Nephrol* **12**, 1648–58.

37. Fiser, R.T., Arnold, W.C., Charlton, R.K., Steel, R.W., Childress, S.H., and Shgirkey, B. (1991) T-lymphocyte subsets in nephrotic syndrome. *Kidney Int* **40**, 913–16.

38. Ozaki, T. (1989) Two-color analysis of lymphocyte subpopulations in membranous nephropathy and minimal change nephrotic syndrome. *Jpn J Nephrol* **31**, 797–806.

39. Koyama, A., Fujisaki, M., Kobayashi, M., Igarashi, M., and Narita, M. (1991) A glomerular permeability factor produced by human T cell hybridomas. *Kidney Int* **40**, 453–60.

40. Yap, H.K., Cheung, W., Murugasu, B., Sim, S.K., Seah, C.C., and Jordan, S.C. (1999) Th1 and Th2 cytokine mRNA profiles in childhood nephrotic syndrome: Evidence for increase IL-13 mRNA expression in relapse. *J Am Soc Nephrol* **10**, 529–37.

41. Van Den Berg, J.G., Aten, J., Annink, C., Ravesloot, J.H., Weber, E., and Weening, J.J. (2002) Interleukin-4 and -13 promote basolateral secretion of H (+) and cathepsin L by glomerular epithelial cells. *Am J Physiol Renal Physiol* **282**, F26–F33.

42. Adrogue, H.E., Borillo, J., Torres, I., Kale, A., Zhou, C., Feig, D., *et al.* (2007) Coincident activation of Th2 T cells with the onset of the disease and differential expression of GRO-γ in peripheral blood leukocytes in minimal change disease. *Am J Nephrol* **27**, 253–61.

43. Morimoto, C., Steinberg, A.D., Letvin, N.L., Hagan, M., Takeuchi, T., Dsaley, J., *et al.* (1987) A defect of immunoregulatory T cell subsets in systemic lupus erythematosus patients demonstrated with anti-2H4 antibody. *J Clin Invest* **79**, 762–8.

44. Smolen, J.S., Chused, T.M., Leiserson, W.M., Reeves, J.P., Alling, D., Steinberg, and A.D. (1982) Heterogeneity of immunoregulatory T-cell subsets in systemic lupus erythematosus: Correlation with clinical features. *Am J Med* **72**, 783–90.

Chapter 9

Renal vascular involvement in SLE

Ben Sprangers and Gerald B. Appel

Introduction

Vascular lesions are an integral part of the spectrum of systemic lupus erythematosus (SLE) and lead to a variety of clinical symptoms depending on the site and severity of organ involvement, the size and nature of the vessels involved, the temporal nature (acute or chronic) of the lesions, and various host factors. A number of different histopathological lesions of the renal vasculature may be involved in SLE and each lesion may have a unique pathogenesis.[1-3]

Renal vasculopathy is an all-inclusive term for the vascular lesions seen in SLE.[1] It is far preferable to the indiscriminate use of the term "lupus vasculitis," which properly refers only to a rare subset of inflammatory vascular lesions. Indeed, in the past virtually all arterial lesions in SLE patients, whether renal or in the vessels of the extremities, mesentery, cerebral or coronary circulations, were attributed to "lupus vasculitis."[4-15] In more recent studies, most such lesions have been appropriately ascribed to one of the other more common forms of lupus vascular involvement.[16,17]

In patients with SLE, renal vascular lesions include: vascular immune complex deposition, noninflammatory necrotizing lupus vasculopathy, true inflammatory vasculitis, and a group of thrombotic vasculopathies including renal vein thrombosis, a thrombotic thrombocytopenic purpura (TTP)-like picture, and vasculopathy associated with antiphospholipid (APL) antibodies (Table 9.1).[1,3,17-22] In many cases these vascular lesions are accompanied by proliferative glomerulonephritis, although thrombotic vasculopathy may develop in all classes of lupus nephritis, and sometimes even in the absence of other forms of renal parenchymal disease.

While most histopathological classifications and prognostic studies of the renal lesions of lupus nephritis have focused on the pattern of glomerular involvement and less frequently on tubulointerstitial involvement, only recently has attention been paid to the renal vascular involvement (Table 9.2).[23-26] As these lesions have been shown to influence both the prognosis and potential treatment of the patients, they deserve the recent emphasis placed upon them. This chapter will review the clinical features, histopathology, proposed pathogenesis, and treatment of the various vasculopathies in SLE.

Immune complex deposits

Immune complex deposition in the walls of small renal arteries, without other associated vascular abnormalities, is a common finding in SLE patients (Table 9.3).[1-3,22,27,28]

Table 9.1 Renal vascular involvement in systemic lupus erythematosus

Uncomplicated vascular immune deposits
Noninflammatory necrotizing vasculopathy
Inflammatory vasculitis
Renal vein thrombosis
Thrombotic thrombocytopenic purpura
Isolated glomerular microthromboses
Antiphospholipid syndrome
Glomerular thrombotic microangiopathy
Renal vein thrombosis
Renal arterial occlusion

In a review of the renal biopsies of 153 lupus patients from Columbia University Medical Center, 39% had evidence of uncomplicated vascular immune deposits. Like virtually all other vascular lesions, most occur in young females, similar to the age and sex distribution of the general SLE population. These lesions appear to be more common in patients with focal and diffuse proliferative lupus nephritis (International Society of Nephrology/Renal Pathology Society (ISN/RPS) classes III and IV), but may be found in association with any glomerular lesion. In our experience, they appear to be more frequent in patients with greater serological activity (higher levels of anti-DNA antibody titers and lower serum complement values), akin to the more frequent occurrence of both glomerular and tubulointerstitial immune deposits in these patients.

The vessels of patients with uncomplicated vascular immune complex deposition typically appear normal on light microscopy (Figure 9.1).[1,3] There is no evidence for necrosis, inflammatory infiltration, or thrombosis. On immunofluorescence microscopy, the deposits may contain immunoglobulin (Ig)G, IgA, or IgM and complement components (Figure 9.2). Electron microscopy reveals the presence of discrete, often granular electron-dense deposits most commonly beneath the vascular endothelium or within the basement membranes around the medial myocytes. Occasionally, a fingerprint or tactoid substructure is noted in the deposit. As the immune deposits may be focal in nature, and the light microscopy picture appears normal, these deposits may easily be overlooked. Although the pathogenesis of the deposits is unknown, it

Table 9.2 Pathology of renal vascular lesions in systemic lupus erythematosus

	Arteries	Arterioles	Veins	Necrosis	Inflammation
Vascular immune deposits	++	+	+	0	0
Necrotizing vasculopathy	+	++	0	+	0
Vasculitis	++	+	0	++	++
Thrombotic microangiopathies	+	++	0	+	0

Modified from[1], p. 1506.

Table 9.3 Incidence (%) of renal vascular lesions in systemic lupus erythematosus

	Immune deposits	Necrotizing vasculopathy	Vasculitis	Microthrombopathy
Lit.*	Common	5–10	0.3–2.8	Variable
Banfi†	?	9.5	2.8	8.4
CUMC‡	39	6.5	1.3	9.2

* Composite from literature.
† Italian Collaborative Study.2
‡ Data from Renal Pathology Division, Columbia University Medical Center.

is likely that these form through deposition of circulating immune complexes as they are frequently found in association with the proliferative SLE lesions thought to be associated with this mechanism of immunological damage.

The presence of uncomplicated vascular immune complex deposits does not appear to influence the course of SLE patients.[1,24,25] When found in patients with more benign glomerular pathology, e.g. mesangial lesions (ISN/RPS Class II), there are no associated clinical features and the course remains benign. No special treatment is needed for these renal findings beyond that which is dictated by the glomerular and tubulointerstitial disease itself.

Noninflammatory necrotizing vasculopathy

A noninflammatory necrotizing vasculopathy has been found not infrequently in biopsies of patients with SLE and does adversely affect the course of the patient (Table 9.3).

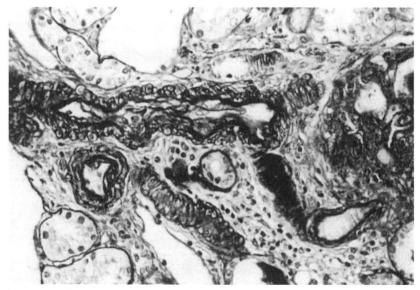

Fig. 9.1 Vascular immune deposits causing mild thickening of the subendothelial basement membrane but no inflammation or necrosis. Periodic acid Schiff (PAS) 320×.

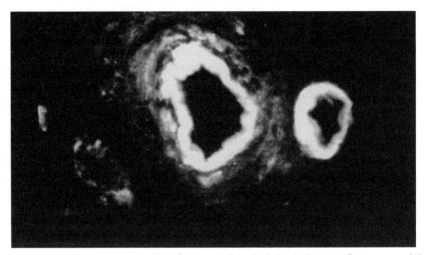

Fig. 9.2 Vascular immune deposits of immunoglobulin (Ig)G by immunofluorescence (IF) in the walls of small arteries. IF 400×.

In a large histopathological review of the renal vascular lesions found in SLE patients, Grishman and Venkataseshan found evidence of vascular damage in 30% of the autopsy specimens in the pre-steroid era, 33% of the autopsies from the post-steroid era, and over 8% of renal biopsies.[3] In most cases this was the noninflammatory necrotizing vasculopathy type. The data from this series must obviously be interpreted in the light of the fact that data came from autopsies on SLE patients who may have had more severe disease resulting in their death, and that biopsies provide less tissue for histopathological analysis than autopsy specimens. Necrotizing and other vasculitic lesions were described in another large series of renal vascular lesions in SLE patients. There were noninflammatory necrotizing vasculopathy in seven of 100 autopsy cases.[29] Baldwin *et al.*[23] found that nine out of 88 SLE patients had necrotizing fibrinoid vasculopathy; and in the Italian Collaborative Study of 285 biopsied lupus patients, noninflammatory necrotizing vasculopathy was found in almost 10% of the biopsies.[2] In our own review of 153 lupus biopsies, we found 7% to have this lesion.[1] With the exception of one study that suggested a higher incidence of vascular lesions in males, all other studies—including the Italian Collaborative Study and our own—have found noninflammatory necrotizing vasculopathy to be most common in young females, akin to the general lupus nephritis population.

The course of the patients with noninflammatory necrotizing vasculopathy appears to be influenced by the vascular lesion. In Baldwin's series, eight out of nine patients had associated severe glomerular lesions, rapid onset of hypertension, and rapid progression to renal failure in a matter of weeks to months.[23] This is true, despite the fact that the serum creatinine level was below 2 mg/dl at onset in most of these patients. Of five patients, in a small series of patients with this lesion, Bhathena *et al.* found a range of serum creatinine levels (0.8 mg/dl to 1.7 mg/dl) and degrees of proteinuria (<1 g/day to >10 g/day), but hypertension was present in 80% of the patients.[19] Most of these patients had associated diffuse proliferative disease, and their course did not differ from other patients without vasculopathy with similar glomerular pathology. In another series of 17 patients with "lupus angiitis," all had diffuse proliferative lupus nephritis (WHO Class IV) and hematuria, decreased glomerular filtration rate, nephrotic range proteinuria, active serology, and a progressive course of renal failure, which were all more common than in patients without vascular lesions.[21] Likewise, an association with diffuse proliferative lupus nephritis, hypertension, and a progressive course to renal failure were more common in the biopsied patients with vascular lesions noted by Grishman and Venkataseshan.[3] The Italian Collaborative Study confirmed that patients with "lupus vasculopathy" have a significantly elevated creatinine level at biopsy versus patients without renal vascular lesions (156 μmol/l versus 108 μmol/l) and greater incidence of hypertension (60% versus 30%), but not a greater degree of proteinuria.[2] These patients with noninflammatory necrotizing vasculopathy were more likely to have severe proliferative glomerular lesions and more active biopsies when graded on a histopathological "activity index" scoring system. In our series, 10 out of 153 biopsies showed the presence of noninflammatory necrotizing vasculopathy.[1] Once again, there was a predominance of patients with associated severe proliferative lesions. In our experience, hypertension and renal dysfunction have also been common with this form of vascular damage.

Noninflammatory necrotizing vasculopathy is characterized by necrotizing changes of the vessel walls, usually pre-glomerular arterioles and less commonly of the interlobular arterioles (Figure 9.3).[19–21,23,24,29] On light microscopy, there is often "smudgy" eosinophilic material (which may stain positive for fibrin derivatives) along the intima of the vessel, extending into the lumen and frequently back into the media of the vessel.

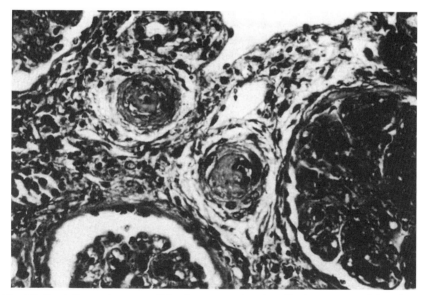

Fig. 9.3 Noninflammatory necrotizing lupus vasculopathy affecting two arterioles. The lumen is occluded by smudgy eosinophilic material but there is no inflammatory infiltrate of the vessel. Hematoxylin and eosin stain (H&E) 320×.

The elastic membrane of the interlobular arteries may be disrupted, but there is no inflammatory infiltrate. Immunofluorescence microscopy reveals the presence of most immunoglobulins and complement components, as well as fibrin-related antigens in the vessel wall.[3,19,23] On electron microscopy, there are massive confluent interluminal and mural granular electron-dense deposits, sometimes along with tactoids of fibrillar protein suggestive of fibrin components. Although the pathogenesis of this lesion is unknown, as most such lesions are associated with diffuse proliferative nephritis, and immune deposits are commonly present, it is likely that immune complex deposition is involved in the pathogenesis of the lesion.[3,19–21,23] As hypertension may be absent in some patients, it makes it unlikely that this is a primary cause of the lesion. However, the frequent occurrence of hypertension in most series argues for a role of elevated blood pressure in the exacerbation of these lesions.[3,23] Initial endothelial damage caused by circulating immune complexes may initiate the renal vascular process followed by associated thrombotic and hypertensive changes.[3,20,21]

In the Italian Collaborative Study of 285 biopsies from lupus patients, the probability of renal survival at 5 years was significantly reduced by the presence of noninflammatory necrotizing vasculopathy (69% versus 90% for patients without renal vascular lesions).[2] However, as most cases of noninflammatory necrotizing vasculopathy occur in patients with diffuse proliferative glomerular lesions, it is possible that the presence of more severe glomerular disease accounts for the worse prognosis of these patients. Nevertheless, the finding of this vascular involvement would still be a marker for a poorer prognosis, and it is just as likely that severe vascular involvement makes a major contribution to the deterioration of renal function and renal survival in this population. Therapy directed at the severe associated proliferative glomerular lesions in most patients should be adequate to counteract the role of the deposition of circulating immune complexes.[1] In most patients this will be intensive corticosteroid and/or cytotoxic therapy (e.g. cyclophosphamide) or mycophenolate mofetil.[30–32] Control of hypertension would be most important to reduce this element of vascular damage; however, there are insufficient data on whether any specific form of antihypertensive therapy (e.g. blockade of the renin–angiotensin system) outweighs another. Although there is some evidence for a contributing pathogenetic role of coagulation in these vascular lesions, there is no evidence that anticoagulants or antiplatelet agents are beneficial here. In conclusion, in noninflammatory necrotizing vasculopathy, the primary goal should be directed at preventing the damage induced by the immune complex deposition, and towards antihypertensive therapy.

Inflammatory vasculitis

Despite the frequent use of the term "lupus vasculitis," true inflammatory renal vasculitis resembling the vasculitis lesions of microscopic polyangiitis is a rare lesion in SLE patients (Table 9.3).[1,2,33] In several series of biopsies and autopsies—accounting for a total histopathological analysis of the kidneys of over 600 SLE patients—the incidence ranged from 0.3 to 2.8% of cases.[2,3,19,23] Indeed, a polling of numerous renal pathologists dealing with SLE nephritis confirms that this lesion is only rarely encountered. The renal vasculitis may occur as an isolated finding or be part of a more systemic disease.

Patients with inflammatory renal vasculitis may have only minimal glomerular involvement with mesangial lesions or diffuse proliferative glomerulonephritis. Hence, their clinical picture will be variable. In the Italian Collaborative series, of the eight patients with true vasculitis, three had associated focal proliferative lesions (WHO Class III), and five had diffuse proliferative glomerular lesions (WHO Class IV). These patients had a higher serum creatinine level than patients without vascular lesions (273 versus 108 µmol/l) and a higher incidence of hypertension (63 versus 30%).[2,33]

The histological lesions found in true vasculitis are identical to those found in micro-scopic polyarteritis.[3,23,24,29,33] Small- and medium-sized arteries are involved (usually the intralobular arteries), with a prominent inflammatory-cell infiltration of the vessel wall by polymorphonuclear cells, mononuclear cells, plasma cells, and lymphocytes (Figure 9.4). The inflammatory response is accompanied by fibrinoid necrosis of the intima and media, and the vessel involvement may be circumferential or eccentric. In some cases, rupture of the elastic lamellae has been noted. On immunofluorescence there is evidence for fibrin-related antigens and a variable deposition of immunoglob-ulins and complement components. Electron microscopy of similar vasculitis lesions in non-SLE patients has not revealed evidence of immune deposits.[34,35]

As the histopathology of this lesion so closely resembles that of polyarteritis, the pathogenesis may be similar. The fact that there is no evidence of immune deposition, and that this vascular lesion may occur in association with any glomerular pathology ranging from mesangial through diffuse proliferative glomerulonephritis, implicates a pathogenesis different from simply immune complex-mediated damage. Neither the

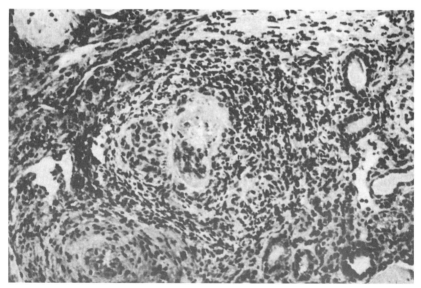

Fig. 9.4 The necrotizing arteritis in a patient with systemic lupus erythematosus. Note the concentric inflammation of the vessel wall and focal fibrinoid necrosis of the intima. Hematoxylin and eosin stain (H&E) 100×.

exact incidence of positive tests for antineutrophil cytoplasmic antibodies (ANCA), nor their role have been fully defined in this rare SLE population.[36] The pathogenesis of the renal vasculitis in SLE and its relationship to ANCA-positive disease and anti-endothelial antibodies remain unclear.[33]

Although the Italian Collaborative Study could not document a poorer 5-year renal survival for patients with true vasculitis versus those without renal vascular lesions (80% versus 90%), this may be due to the small numbers of patients available for study with true inflammatory vasculitis.[2] It is likely that these lesions would have the same effect on prognosis that they do in non-SLE disease states, such as microscopic polyarteritis or ANCA-positive rapidly progressive glomerulonephritis with vascular involvement. Cytotoxic agents have been very successful in the treatment of such patients with polyarteritis, Wegener's granulomatosis, and ANCA-positive rapidly progressive glomerulonephritis.[35,37,38] At the current time, regardless of the associated glomerular pathology, these agents have been recommended as the treatment of choice for true inflammatory vasculitis in SLE patients. It should be emphasized that this is based on a best-guess strategy rather than documented evidence of efficacy, safety, or improved survival in the SLE population.[33]

Thrombotic vascular lesions

Renal vein thrombosis

Renal vein thrombosis (RVT) has been reported in over 50 patients with SLE.[39–54] It has occurred in both sexes and in all age groups, although, as with SLE in general, there is a high incidence in young females. Most cases of documented RVT have occurred in one of two groups of patients with SLE: those with APL antibodies and those with the nephrotic syndrome.[40,49] The former group will be discussed in a separate section. The association of SLE, the nephrotic syndrome, and RVT was first emphasized in 1976.[40] It was apparent that in these patients the RVT was secondary to the associated nephrotic syndrome and was not a cause of the nephrotic syndrome.[40,55,56] Akin to the idiopathic nephrotic syndrome, the vast majority of nephrotic SLE patients suffering RVT have a membranous pattern of nephropathy (International Society of Nephrology (ISN) Class V) as their underlying histopathological lesion. The exact incidence of RVT in nephrotic SLE patients remains uncertain.[43,46,47,55,57] Several studies have reported on the incidence of RVT in patients with lupus membranous nephropathy: an incidence of 2.0–22.7% was found.[58–62] In part, this depends on the technique for diagnosis and whether branches of the renal veins were studied as well as the main renal veins.

In most SLE patients the venous thrombosis is clinically silent, although some patients have increased proteinuria and/or transient worsening of renal function with a rise in their serum creatinine level.[40] Other patients present with symptoms of shortness of breath, dyspnea, and tachypnea associated with pulmonary emboli from the renal vein thromboses.[40,45] Infrequently, patients with more acute and complete thrombosis have developed flank pain, costovertebral angle tenderness, and even gross hematuria.[40,41,45,47]

The radiological signs of RVT vary according to the speed of onset and degree of occlusion of the renal vein. In cases of rapid onset and complete occlusion, the affected kidney becomes enlarged and reaches maximum dimensions within 1 week. Subsequently, however, there is a gradual reduction in the renal size over the following few weeks, and later, renal atrophy. Selective renal venography shows a persistent filling defect in the affected renal veins.[63,64] Renal venography is, however, not widely used as it is invasive, and is associated with complications, e.g. pulmonary embolism (due to clot dislodgement), contrast-induced acute renal failure, and higher radiation exposure.[65] In the past, intravenous urography was frequently used to diagnose RVT. In the acute phase of RVT, absence of visualization of the collecting system (due to poor excretion by the affected kidney), ipsilateral renal enlargement, and pelvicalyceal irregularities were found in almost 80% patients. In more chronic RVT, ureteric notching (due to the development of varicosities) and presence of collateral venous drainage around the kidney were seen.[66–69] Computed tomography (CT) scanning with contrast is currently the imaging of choice for diagnosing RVT as it is relatively noninvasive and has a high diagnostic accuracy. Computed tomography abnormalities, including thrombus in the renal veins and/or inferior vena cava; venous collaterals; enlargement of the affected kidney; delayed, diminished, or absent opacification of the collecting system; a persistent nephrogram attributable to poor venous washout; prolonged corticomedullary differentiation; thickening of the perinephric fascia; and pericapsular whiskering have been described in RVT complicating nephrotic syndrome.[70–73] One study is available prospectively evaluating the role of CT in diagnosis of RVT in patients with nephrotic syndrome:[73] 17 patients underwent both renal venography and CT, including 12 patients who had RVT diagnosed by CT. The estimated sensitivity and specificity of CT with contrast were 92.3% and 100% respectively. One patient had an intrarenal vein thrombosis diagnosed by venography that was missed by CT. Other studies have evaluated the value of magnetic resonance venography imaging (MRI) with or without contrast enhancement in the identification of RVT.[74–76] In a retrospective review of 41 patients who underwent MRI assessment for possible RVT, five patients underwent both renal venography and MRI. Magnetic resonance venography imaging correctly identified three patients who had RVT on venography. Magnetic resonance venography imaging interpretation, however, led to one false-positive and one false-negative result. Magnetic resonance venography imaging is noninvasive, avoids radiation and use of nephrotoxic intravenous iodinated contrast agents. Disadvantages include higher cost, need for anesthesia in children and claustrophobic adults, association of MRI-contrast agents and nephrogenic systemic fibrosis. The comparative safety and efficacy of MR venography versus CT venography using newer techniques is unknown. Ultrasound shows an enlarged kidney and hyperechogenic kidney in approximately 90% of the patients in the early phase of acute RVT.[77] One study has prospectively evaluated Doppler ultrasonography in the diagnosis of RVT in 11 patients with nephrotic syndrome who had also undergone renal venography.[78] The sensitivity of ultrasound was 85% and the specificity 56%, making it useful for screening. However, Doppler ultrasonography has poor yield in detecting segmental venous thrombosis. In renal transplant patients, Doppler ultrasound is being utilized widely to detect RVT in renal transplant patients with a high degree of sensitivity.[79] Abnormalities in renal scintigraphy have been described in RVT using a variety of agents.[80–84] These studies have been primarily limited to case reports but have described decreased blood flow to the affected kidney, an enlarged kidney with decreased uptake, and nonvisualization of the collecting system. Digital subtraction venography has also been suggested as a safer alternative to selective renal venography, but has not been adequately studied to date.[85] The renal histopathology of SLE with RVT typically reveals evidence of underlying membranous lupus nephropathy (ISN Class V), although occasional patients have had mesangial or proliferative lesions.[29,40,48,49] In patients with a biopsy shortly after the venous thrombosis, there is often interstitial edema, tubular degenerative changes, and margination of polymorphonuclear leukocytes in the glomeruli and interstitial capillaries.[40] Infrequently, thrombi may be observed in glomerular capillaries or small renal venules.[41] With a more chronic history of RVT, interstitial fibrosis and tubular atrophy become more prominent on renal biopsies.[39,40,48,53] The pathogenesis of RVT in SLE patients with nephrotic syndrome is thought to be similar to that in non-SLE patients, and to be related to the hypercoagulable state induced by the heavy albuminuria.[86] Several risk factors for the development of thromboembolic or RVT in SLE patients have been identified, e.g. presence of lupus anticoagulant, elevated cholesterol, smoking, disease activity, shorter disease duration, higher mean glucocorticoid dose, and genetic factors (factor V Leiden and prothrombin mutation).[87–91] A prospective trial identified elevated D-dimer level (>2.0 µg/ml) as an accurate predictor of thromboembolic events in SLE patients. In combination with measurements of APL antibodies and lupus anticoagulant, sensitivity and specificity of 100% and 78%, respectively, for the prediction of a thromboembolic event, were obtained.[92]

In our review of 60 patients with membranous lupus, the presence of RVT did not influence the 10-year renal survival of the patients.[58] Patients should be treated with anticoagulants, first with heparin and then with warfarin, irrespective of whether RVT is acute or chronic, unilateral or bilateral, for a minimum period of 6 months.[40] Recanalization of the renal veins occurs and the risk of pulmonary emboli is abolished with adequate anticoagulation. Only rarely have streptokinase or surgical techniques been used to treat the RVT.[41,49] In some patients, the risk of recurrent thrombotic events can be abrogated by obtaining remission of the nephrotic syndrome with immunosuppression, or at least a major reduction in proteinuria with nonspecific proteinuria-reducing medications such as angiotensin converting enzyme inhibitors, angiotensin II receptor antagonists, or cyclosporine. Some clinicians feel that patients with recurrence of persistent RVT, or nephrotic patients who remain severely hypoalbuminemic deserve life-long anticoagulation.[93]

Thrombotic microangiopathies

Patients with SLE may develop renal vascular damage from a thrombotic microangiopathy as part of a TTP-like syndrome, in association with APL antibodies, or as an isolated feature in association with their immune complex glomerulonephritis.[94–96] Each is associated with distinct clinical features, pathogenesis, and potential therapy.

Classic TTP is characterized by the presence of thrombocytopenia, fever, microangiopathic hemolytic anemia, and the combination of neurological and renal involvement by the thrombotic process.[97] Great progress has been made in the unraveling of the pathophysiology of TTP in recent years. It was demonstrated that most patients affected by

TTP have a deficiency of the plasma metalloprotease ADAMTS-13 (A Disintegrin-like And Metalloprotease with ThromboSpondin type 1 motif).[98,99] Deficiency of ADAMTS-13 is associated with the appearance of ultralarge thrombogenic multimers of von Willebrand factor (VWF) triggering intravascular formation of aggregates and occlusive thrombi in terminal arterioles causing the ischemic symptoms typical of TTP. The main causes of ADAMTS-13 deficiency are mutations in the gene encoding the protein, or, more frequently, the development of IgG autoantibodies that inactivate protease activity.

Reduced ADAMTS-13 activity has been found in SLE patients without signs of TTP.[100–102] In these patients, no mutations or autoantibodies to ADAMTS-13 were demonstrated,[101] and the deficiency of ADAMTS-13 was not as profound as in patients with TTP.[100] The deficiency in SLE patients most likely results from increased consumption of ADAMTS-13 due to increased release of VWF into the circulation as a result of SLE-associated endothelial damage.

Thrombotic thombocytopenic purpura and SLE have long been associated. Reportedly, in 0.5–4% of patients, SLE complicates TTP.[103,104] Furthermore, in autopsy studies, pathological findings suggestive of TTP were noted in 28% of cases of SLE.[105] In SLE patients with clinical TTP, levels of ADAMTS-13 are very low or undetectable and Güngör et al. reported the presence of an inhibitor in the plasma of one patient.[106] Of note, Coppo et al. found a high prevalence of antinuclear antibodies, anti-double-stranded DNA antibodies, and anticardiolipin antibodies in patients with idiopathic TTP and severe deficiency of ADAMTS-13, suggesting an association between idiopathic TTP and an autoimmune predilection.[107]

Thrombotic thombocytopenic purpura complicating SLE tends to present more diverse clinical pictures and to be more resistant to treatment in comparison with idiopathic TTP.[103,108,109] The onset of TTP precedes, concurs, or follows the onset of SLE in 12%, 21%, and 67% of cases respectively.[110] Of clinical significance, a fatal outcome occurs in 30% of those patients, even while SLE is in a stable condition. Both presence and absence of antiphospholipid antibodies have been reported.[110–113]

Patients with TTP and SLE may present with clinical manifestations of either syndrome first, or both concurrently, and the SLE may be clinically and serologically active or inactive.[22,114–120] The manifestations of the TTP syndrome include all those found in classical TTP, with microthrombotic occlusion of small vessels in different organ systems.[97] These findings include fever, malaise, neurological signs and symptoms (headache, confusion, disorientation, seizures, paralyses, and coma), petechiae and purpuric skin lesions, abdominal pain, and gastrointestinal bleeding. Thrombocytopenia, often less than 20,000/mm^3, is frequent, as is the presence of schistocytes and other evidence of microangiopathic hemolytic anemia. The renal manifestations of TTP in SLE patients are quite varied and have included varying degrees of proteinuria, reduced renal function with elevated serum creatinine levels, acute renal failure leading to requirement for dialytic support, and hypertension.[114–118,120] In one large series, the mean serum creatinine level in SLE patients with TTP-like lesions was 286 µmol/l versus 108 µmol/l for patients without vascular lesions, and hypertension was significantly more frequent (91% versus 30%).[2] The patients in this series with TTP did, however, more frequently have severe associated proliferative lupus lesions with more activity and chronicity on their renal biopsies as well.

These associated findings may, in part, explain the worse renal function and higher incidence of hypertension.

The histopathological changes of TTP in SLE patients have only infrequently been described.[1,2,22,116–118] Involvement of the interlobular arteries and arterioles is characterized by intimal proliferation with mucoid edema and narrowing of vascular lumens (Figure 9.5).[1,2] At times, focal arteriolar thrombi may be present with necrosis of the vessel walls but no inflammatory infiltrate. Glomeruli often have ischemic changes with thickening and wrinkling of the glomerular capillary walls. Glomerular microthrombi are typically present (Figure 9.6). In some cases, thrombi in small arterioles and glomeruli have stained positive for fibrin-related products by both the phosphotungstic acid–hematoxylin (PTAH) stain and the picro-Mallory (Lendrum) stain (Figure 9.7).[116] The glomeruli have shown a spectrum of involvement ranging from mesangial lesions (ISN/RPS Class II) to diffuse proliferative lesions (ISN/RPS Class IV) with endothelial immune complex deposits. On electron microscopy, in addition to

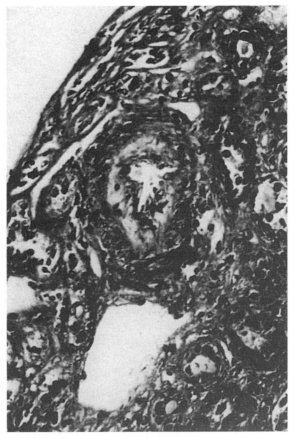

Fig. 9.5 Intimal mucoid edema of an interlobular artery in thrombotic thombocytopenic purpura-like syndrome in systemic lupus erythematosus. Phosphotungstic acid–hematoxylin (PTAH) 320×.

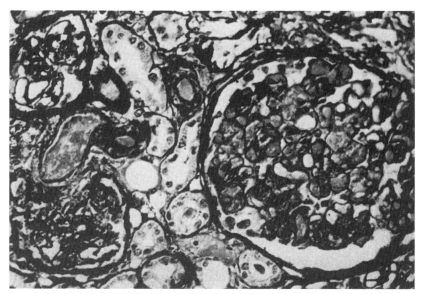

Fig. 9.6 Multiple glomerular capillary and arteriolar occlusion by thrombi in the biopsy of a systemic lupus erythematosus patient with thrombotic thombocytopenic purpura-like syndrome. Jones'–Methenamine–silver 320×.

immune complex type deposits, there is often widening of the subendothelial space by electron-lucent flocculent and fibrillar material, a characteristic finding for the thrombotic microangiopathies.[22,116]

The 5-year survival for SLE patients with TTP-like renal lesions is worse than that of biopsied SLE patients without renal vascular lesions (80% versus 90%).[2] In the past, akin to idiopathic TTP, SLE patients with TTP were treated with corticosteroids, antiplatelet agents, heparin, and, at times, splenectomy, which was associated with a high morbidity and mortality rate. Some patients, however, appeared to benefit from the therapy.[120] More recently, the use of plasma-exchange and plasma-infusion

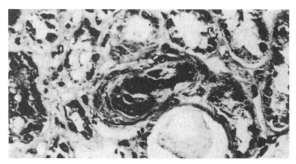

Fig. 9.7 An arteriole involved by thrombosis in thrombotic thombocytopenic purpura-like syndrome, showing positive staining for fibrin. Phosphotungstic acid–hematoxylin (PTAH) 320×.

therapy has been successful in idiopathic TTP and in isolated cases of TTP in SLE patients.[97,116,117,121,122] However, there is no controlled trial documenting the benefit of such therapy in SLE patients, and neither the exact amount nor nature of the plasma product to be infused have been defined. For those patients with associated severe proliferative glomerular lesions, corticosteroids and/or cytotoxic therapy are indicated. Rituximab, a chimeric anti-CD20 monoclonal antibody, has been used with some success in both TTP and SLE;[123–127] however, no controlled trials in SLE patients with TTP are available at this time.

Antiphospholipid antibody syndrome

A variety of APL antibodies, including anticardiolipin antibodies and the lupus anticoagulant, have been noted in both SLE patients and in patients without autoimmune disorders.[128–131] The presence of APL antibodies has been associated with glomerular disease, large vessel renal involvement, as well as coagulation problems in dialysis and renal transplant patients.[49,132–136] The presence of APL antibodies has also been associated with increased risk for chronic renal insufficiency.[137] Antiphospholipid antibodies have been found in 25–45% of SLE patients, although most of these patients never experience the clinical features of the APL syndrome (APS).[134,138,139] In an analysis of 29 published series comprising over 1000 SLE patients, 34% were found to be positive for the lupus anticoagulant and 44% for anticardiolipin antibodies.[139]

The clinical features of the APS, whether in SLE patients or as part of a primary disorder, relate to thrombotic events and consequent ischemia. Systemic features include superficial and deep venous thromboses; arterial thromboses; fetal miscarriages (due to placental thrombosis); pulmonary hypertension; cerebral infarcts with transient ischemic attacks, strokes, memory impairment, and other neurological manifestations; and livedo reticularis.[128–131,138] Patients may also experience fever, malaise, and constitutional symptoms, all of which may be confused with active systemic lupus. In SLE the clinical features correlate well with the presence of high titers of IgG antiphospholipid antibodies as well as thrombocytopenia, the presence of false-positive venereal disease research laboratory test (VDRL) for syphillis (fluorescent treponemal antibody (FTA)-negative), and a prolonged activated partial thromboplastin time (APTT).[131,140,141] Neither the titer of anti-DNA antibody nor the serum complement levels correlate well with the APL antibody levels. In SLE, high titers of IgG anticardiolipin antibody do correlate well with the risk of thromboses.[140]

Recently the term antiphospholipid nephropathy (APSN) was introduced to denote renal thrombotic microangiopathy (in the absence of immune complex-mediated glomerular lesions) showing fresh organizing thrombi, cellular, mucoid or fibrous intimal hyperplasia, occlusion of small arteries/arterioles, and glomerular thrombi, and on electron microscopy evidence of glomerular endothelial injury.[142,143] Histologically, APSN is a vaso-occlusive process associating, side-by-side, acute thromboses (thrombotic microangiopathy) and chronic vascular lesions with arterial fibrous intimal hyperplasia, arteriosclerosis, and organized thromboses, with or without recanalization (Figure 9.8). These progress to fibrous occlusion of the involved vessels and lead to the development of zones of subcapsular ischemic cortical atrophy

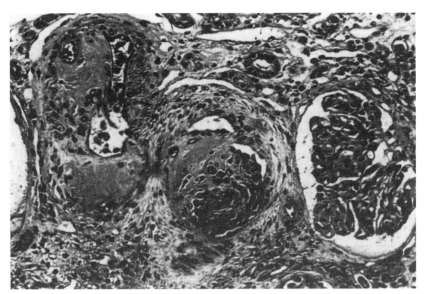

Fig. 9.8 An interlobular artery of a patient with systemic lupus erythematosus and high titers of immunoglobulin (Ig)G anticardiolipin antibody showing organizing recanalized thrombus. Hematoxylin and eosin stain (H&E) 250×.

in the regions served by these vessels.[132,133,144] In 1999, a group of French investigators described for the first time the presence of APS nephropathy in patients with primary APS.[145] In 2002, the prevalence of APSN in SLE patients was reported to be 32% of patients.[143,146] Antiphospholipid nephropathy was found to be associated with APL antibodies and APS (in particular arterial thrombosis and fetal loss),[143,147] although this has not been confirmed in all populations studied.[146] Daugas *et al.* found APSN in 63% of SLE patients with APS, 22% of SLE patients without APS but with antiphospholipid antibodies, and 15% of SLE patients without APS and without antiphospholipid antibodies.[143] Although in one study there was an association of APSN with proliferative lupus glomerulonephritis (WHO Class IV), other studies report that APSN was associated with all forms of lupus glomerulonephritis.[143,147] The presence of APSN was associated with increased risk for hypertension, and, in those patients without APS, increased risk for the subsequent development of APS. With major renal arterial involvement there may be evidence of renal infarction.[148] Renal vein thrombosis may be silent or present with sudden flank pain and a decrease in renal function.[49] As far as renal outcome is concerned, although all studies found an association between APSN and increased creatinine and increased interstitial fibrosis,[143,146,147] only some have found an association between APSN and increased frequency of end stage renal disease (ERSD).[146]

Studies of patients with ESRD have shown a high prevalence of APL antibodies in patients on hemodialysis (10–30%).[141,149–151] Studies of patients with renal insufficiency and patients on peritoneal dialysis have shown much lower incidence of

APL antibodies. In a review from our medical center of 230 hemodialyzed patients, titers of IgG anticardiolipin antibodies were elevated in 26% of patients, as opposed to elevated titers of IgM antibodies in only 4%, and elevated titers of both antibody subtypes in 3%.[152] The vast majority of such patients have not had SLE as the cause of their renal failure, and the relationship of these antibodies to those found in lupus patients with preserved renal function is unknown. The presence of APL antibodies may also damage the renal allograft.[153] In one study, four out of eight SLE patients with APL antibodies who received renal transplants had evidence of related problems with venous thromboses, pulmonary emboli, or persistent thrombocytopenia, as opposed to no patients in a control group of SLE patients without ACL antibodies transplanted in the same time period. Treatment with anticoagulants proved successful in preventing recurrent thromboses and graft loss.[153]

The optimal treatment of patients with APL antibodies and/or APS remains to be defined.[136,154–160] Many SLE patients with APL antibodies do not experience thrombotic events. Vigorous anticoagulation therapy would put this large population at risk for bleeding complications, with questionable benefits. On the other hand, patients with evidence of glomerular microthrombopathy or active coagulation must be treated to avoid life-threatening vascular damage. Several studies have addressed the relationship between the APL antibody class and titer, and the risk of thrombotic events. Lupus anticoagulant and continuous, higher titers of IgG APL antibody have been related to a greater incidence of thrombotic events (transient positive anticardiolipin antibodies in the absence of lupus anticoagulant were not associated with an increased risk for thromboembolic events).[140,161–164] In patients without evidence of the APS, and no thrombotic events and risk factors (e.g. lupus anticoagulant), some clinicians recommend daily aspirin therapy.[165,166] In patients with the full APS, either primary or secondary to SLE, high-dose anticoagulation has proven to be more effective than either no therapy, aspirin, or low-dose anticoagulation in preventing recurrent thromboses.[155] A retrospective analysis of the course of 147 patients with the APS and documented prior thromboses (62 had primary disease, 66 had SLE, and 19 a lupus-like syndrome) recorded 186 recurrent thrombotic events in 69% of the patients.[154] The median time between the initial thrombosis and the first recurrence was 12 months, but with a huge range (0.5–144 months). Treatment with warfarin to produce an international normalized ratio (INR) >3 was significantly more effective than treatment with low-dose (INR <3) warfarin, or treatment with aspirin alone (rates of recurrence per patient-year: 0.0013, 0.23, and 0.18 respectively).[154] The highest rate of thrombosis (1.3 per patient-year) occurred in patients in the 6 months after discontinuing anticoagulation with warfarin. Bleeding complications occurred in 29 of the 147 patients, but were severe in only seven patients.[154] In general, immunosuppressive agents have not been very successful in treating this syndrome. Thus, in SLE patients, the anti-DNA antibody titer and the serum complement may normalize in response to corticosteroid or other immunosuppressive medication without a significant change in a high titer of IgG APL antibody. In rare patients who cannot tolerate anticoagulation due to recent bleeding, who have thromboembolic events despite adequate anticoagulation, or who are pregnant and have the APS, plasmapheresis with corticosteroids, other immunosuppressives, and rituximab have been used with anecdotal success.[156–159]

Conclusions

Renal vascular lesions in patients with SLE range from those of minor clinical relevance to those associated with marked renal impairment and a major increase in morbidity in patients. They may complicate any pattern of glomerular lesion ranging from mesangial involvement to severe proliferative disease. The thrombotic microangiopathies may cause major glomerular and large vessel involvement in SLE patients, and require intervention with anticoagulation and other modalities not usually included in the immunosuppressive treatment of these patients. Although overlooked in many recent histological studies of chronicity and activity on lupus renal biopsies, there is little doubt that vascular lesions can greatly influence the course and treatment of patients with SLE.

References

1. Appel, G.B., Pirani, C.L., and D'Agati, V. (1994) Renal vascular complications of systemic lupus erythematosus. *J Am Soc Nephrol* **4**, 1499–515.

2. Banfi, G., Bertani, T., Boeri, V., Faraggiana, T., Mazzucco, G., Monga, G. *et al.* (1991) Renal vascular lesions as a marker of poor prognosis in patients with lupus nephritis. Gruppo Italiano per lo Studio della Nefrite Lupica (GISNEL). *Am J Kidney Dis* **18**, 240–8.

3. Grishman, E. and Venkataseshan, V.S. (1988) Vascular lesions in lupus nephritis. *Mod Pathol* **1**, 235–41.

4. Asherson, R.A., Derksen, R.H., Harris, E.N., Bingley, P.J., Hoffbrand, B.I., Gharavi, A.E. *et al.* (1986) Large vessel occlusion and gangrene in systemic lupus erythematosus and "lupus-like" disease. A report of six cases. *J Rheumatol* **13**, 740–7.

5. Adelman, D.C., Saltiel, E., and Klinenberg, J.R. (1986) The neuropsychiatric manifestations of systemic lupus erythematosus: an overview. *Semin Arthritis Rheum* **15**, 185–99.

6. Newbold, K.M., Allum, W.H., Downing, R., Symmons, D.P., and Oates, G.D. (1987) Vasculitis of the gall bladder in rheumatoid arthritis and systemic lupus erythematosus. *Clin Rheumatol* **6**, 287–9.

7. Sanders, E.A. and Hogenhuis, L.A. (1986) Cerebral vasculitis as presenting symptom of systemic lupus erythematosus. *Acta Neurol Scand* **74**, 75–7.

8. Kaufman, J.L., Bancilla, E., and Slade, J. (1986) Lupus vasculitis with tibial artery thrombosis and gangrene. *Arthritis Rheum* **29**, 1291–2.

9. Hochberg, M.C., Boyd, R.E., Ahearn, J.M., Arnett, F.C., Bias, W.B., Provost, T.T. *et al.* (1985) Systemic lupus erythematosus: a review of clinico-laboratory features and immunogenetic markers in 150 patients with emphasis on demographic subsets. *Medicine (Baltimore)* **64**, 285–95.

10. Alarcon, S.D., and Osmundson, P.J. (1965) Peripheral vascular syndromes associated with systemic lupus erythematosus. *Ann Intern Med* **62**, 907–19.

11. McCluskey, R.T., and Fienberg, R. (1983) Vasculitis in primary vasculitides, granulomatoses, and connective tissue diseases. *Hum Pathol* **14**, 305–15.

12. Steinman, C.R. (1979) Circulating DNA in systemic lupus erythematosus. Association with central nervous system involvement and systemic vasculitis. *Am J Med* **67**, 429–35.

13. Dubois, E.L., and Arterberry, J.D. (1962) Gangrene as a manifestation of systemic lupus erythematosus. *JAMA* **181**, 366–74.

14. Mintz, G., and Fraga, A. (1965) Arteritis in systemic lupus erythematosus. *Arch Intern Med* **116**, 55–66.

15. Cupps, T. R., and Fauci, A. S. (1981) Hypersensitivity vasculitis. In: *The vasculitides* (L.H. Smith, ed.), pp. 70–1. W.B. Saunders, Philadelphia.

16. Balow, J.E. (1985) Renal vasculitis. *Kidney Int* **27**, 954–64.

17. Schwartz, M. M. Lupus vasculitis. (1992) In: *Systemic Lupus Erythematosus: Renal Vasculitis. Contributions in Nephrology* (A. Sessa, M. Meroni, and G. Battini, eds), pp. 35–46. Karger, Basel.

18. Schwartz, M.M. (1985) The role of renal biopsy in the management of lupus nephritis. *Semin Nephrol* **5**, 255–63.

19. Bhathena, D.B., Sobel, B.J., and Migdal, S.D. (1981) Noninflammatory renal microangiopathy of systemic lupus erythematosus ('lupus vasculitis'). *Am J Nephrol* **1**, 144–59.

20. Grishman, E., Gerber, M.A., and Churg, J. (1982) Patterns of renal injury in systemic lupus erythematosus: light and immunofluorescence microscopic observations. *Am J Kidney Dis* **2**, 135–41.

21. Bhuyan, U.N., Malaviya, A.N., Dash, S.C., and Malhotra, K.K. (1983) Prognostic significance of renal angiitis in systemic lupus erythematosus (SLE). *Clin Nephrol* **20**, 109–13.

22. Magil, A.B., McFadden, D., and Rae, A. (1986) Lupus glomerulonephritis with thrombotic microangiopathy. *Hum Pathol* **17**, 192–4.

23. Baldwin, D.S., Gluck, M.C., Lowenstein, J., and Gallo, G.R. (1977) Lupus nephritis. Clinical course as related to morphologic forms and their transitions. *Am J Med* **62**, 12–30.

24. Appel, G.B., Silva, F.G., Pirani, C.L., Meltzer, J.I., and Estes, D. (1978) Renal involvement in systemic lupus erythematosus (SLE): a study of 56 patients emphasizing histologic classification. *Medicine (Baltimore)* **57**, 371–410.

25. Appel, G.B., Cohen, D.J., Pirani, C.L., Meltzer, J.I., and Estes, D. (1987) Long-term follow-up of patients with lupus nephritis. A study based on the classification of the World Health Organization. *Am J Med* **83**, 877–85.

26. Park, M.H., D'Agati, V., Appel, G.B., and Pirani, C.L. (1986) Tubulointerstitial disease in lupus nephritis: relationship to immune deposits, interstitial inflammation, glomerular changes, renal function, and prognosis. *Nephron* **44**, 309–19.

27. Brentjens, J.R. and Andres, G. (1985) Immunopathogenesis of renal vasculitis. *Semin Nephrol* **5**, 3–14.

28. Pirani, C.L. and Olesnicky, L. (1982) Role of electron microscopy in the classification of lupus nephritis. *Am J Kidney Dis* **2**, 150–63.

29. Tsumagari, T., Fukumoto, S., Kinjo, M., and Tanaka, K. (1985) Incidence and significance of intrarenal vasculopathies in patients with systemic lupus erythematosus. *Hum Pathol* **16**, 43–9.

30. Houssiau, F.A., Vasconcelos, C., D'Cruz, D., Sebastiani, G.D., de Ramon Garrido, E., Danieli, M.G., *et al* (2010) The 10-year follow-up data of the Euro-Lupus Nephritis trial comparing low-dose and high-dose intravenous cyclophosphamide. *Ann Rheum Dis* **69**, 61–4.

31. Appel, G.B., Contreras, G., Dooley, M.A., Ginzler, E.M., Isenberg, D., Jayne, D. *et al.* (2009) Mycophenolate mofetil versus cyclophosphamide for induction treatment of lupus nephritis. *J Am Soc Nephrol* **20**, 1103–12.

32. Ginzler, E.M., Dooley, M.A., Aranow, C., Kim, M.Y., Buyon, J., Merrill, J.T. *et al.* (2005) Mycophenolate mofetil or intravenous cyclophosphamide for lupus nephritis. *N Engl J Med* **353**, 2219–28.

33. Abdellatif, A.A., Waris, S., Lakhani, A., Kadkoy, H., Truong, L.D. (2010) True vasculitis in lupus nephritis. *Clin Nephrol* **74**(2), 106–12.

34. D'Agati, V., Chander, P., Nash, M., and Mancilla-Jimenez, R. (1986) Idiopathic microscopic polyarteritis nodosa: ultrastructural observations on the renal vascular and glomerular lesions. *Am J Kidney Dis* **7**, 95–110.

35. D'Agati, V, and Appel, G B. (1989) Polyarteritis nodosa, Wegener's granulomatosis, Churg-Strauss syndrome, temporal arteritis, and lymphomatoid granulomatosis. In: *Renal Pathology* (C. Tischer, and B. Brenner, eds), pp. 1087–153. J.B. Lippincott, London, Mexico City, New York, St. Louis, Sao Paulo, Sydney.

36. Kuster, S., Apenberg, S., Andrassy, K., and Ritz, E. (1992) Antineutrophilic cytoplasmic antibodies in systemic lupus erythematosus. In: *Systemic Lupus Erythematosus: Renal Vasculitis. Contributions to Nephrology* (A. Sessa, M. Meroni, and G. Battini, eds), pp. 94–8. Karger, Basel.

37. Hoffman, G.S., Kerr, G.S., Leavitt, R.Y., Hallahan, C.W., Lebovics, R.S., Travis, W.D. *et al.* (1992) Wegener granulomatosis: an analysis of 158 patients. *Ann Intern Med* **116**, 488–98.

38. Falk, R.J., Hogan, S., Carey, T.S., and Jennette, J.C. (1990) Clinical course of anti-neutrophil cytoplasmic autoantibody-associated glomerulonephritis and systemic vasculitis. The Glomerular Disease Collaborative Network. *Ann Intern Med* **113**, 656–63.

39. Hamilton, C.R., Jr. and Tumulty, P.A. (1968) Thrombosis of renal veins and inferior vena cava complicating lupus nephritis. *JAMA* **206**, 2315–17.

40. Appel, G.B., Williams, G.S., Meltzer, J.I., and Pirani, C.L. (1976) Renal vein thrombosis, nephrotic syndrome, and systemic lupus erythematosus: an association in four cases. *Ann Intern Med* **85**, 310–17.

41. Moore, H.L., Katz, R., McIntosh, R., Smith, F., Michael, A.F., and Vernier, R.L. (1972) Unilateral renal vein thrombosis and the nephrotic syndrome. *Pediatrics* **50**, 598–608.

42. Disney, T.F., Sullivan, S.N., Haddad, R.G., Lowe, D., and Goldbach, M.M. (1984) Budd-Chiari syndrome with inferior vena cava obstruction associated with systemic lupus erythematosus. *J Clin Gastroenterol* **6**, 253–6.

43. Bradley, W.G., Jr., Jacobs, R.P., Trew, P.A., Biava, C.G., and Hopper, J., Jr. (1981) Renal vein thrombosis: occurrence in membranous glomerulonephropathy and lupus nephritis. *Radiology* **139**, 571–6.

44. Dubois, E.L. (1974) *Lupus Erythematosus*. University of Southern California Press, Los Angeles.

45. Khan, M.A., Ricanati, E.S., and Park, M.J. (1977) Lupus nephritis and renal vein thrombosis. *Ann Intern Med* **86**, 114.

46. Gilsanz, V., Estrada, V., Malillos, E., and Barrio, E. (1971) Transparietal renal phlebography, in the nephrotic syndrome. Renal vein thrombosis: cause or complication of the nephrotic syndrome. *Angiology* **22**, 431–47.

47. Mintz, G., Acevedo-Vazquez, E., Gutierrez-Espinosa, G., and Avelar-Garnica, F. (1984) Renal vein thrombosis and inferior vena cava thrombosis in systemic lupus erythematosus. Frequency and risk factors. *Arthritis Rheum* **27**, 539–44.

48. Gutierrez, M., V, Usera, G., Alcazar de la Ossa JM, Ruilope, L.M., Ortuno, M.T., and Rodicio, J.L. (1978) Renal vein thrombosis, nephrotic syndrome, and focal lupus glomerulonephritis. *Br Med J* **1**, 24–5.

49. Asherson, R.A., Lanham, J.G., Hull, R.G., Boey, M.L., Gharavi, A.E., and Hughes, G.R. (1984) Renal vein thrombosis in systemic lupus erythematosus: association with the "lupus anticoagulant". *Clin Exp Rheumatol* **2**, 75–9.

50. Gladman, D.D., and Urowitz, M.B. (1980) Venous syndromes and pulmonary embolism in systemic lupus erythematosus. *Ann Rheum Dis* **39**, 340–3.

51. Kanfer, A., Kleinknecht, D., Broyer, M., and Josso, F. (1970) Coagulation studies in 45 cases of nephrotic syndrome without uremia. *Thromb Diath Haemorrh* **24**, 562–71.

52. Peck, B., Hoffman, G.S., and Franck, W.A. (1978) Thrombophlebitis in systemic lupus erythematosus. *JAMA* **240**, 1728–30.

53. Cade, R., Spooner, G., Juncos, L., Fuller, T., Tarrant, D., Raulerson, D. *et al.* (1977) Chronic renal vein thrombosis. *Am J Med* **63**, 387–97.

54. Bridi, G.S. and Frayha, R.A. (1976) Lupus glomerulitis and renal vein thrombosis. *Br Med J* **1**, 750.

55. Llach, F., Koffler, A., Finck, E., and Massry, S.G. (1977) On the incidence of renal vein thrombosis in the nephrotic syndrome. *Arch Intern Med* **137**, 333–6.

56. Llach, F. (1982) Nephrotic syndrome: hypercoagulability, renal vein thrombosis, and other thromboembolic complications. In: *Nephrotic Syndrome* (B.M. Brenner, and J.M. Stein, eds) pp. 121–44. Churchill Livingstone, New York.

57. Gonzalez-Dettoni, H., and Tron, F. (1984) Membranous glomerulopathy in systemic lupus erythematosus. In: *Advances in Nephrology* (J. Hamburger, J. Crosnier, and M.H. Maxwell, eds), pp. 347–64. Yearbook Medical Publishers, Chicago.

58. Radhakrishnan, J., Szaboles, J., D'Agati, V.D., *et al.* (1993) Lupus membranous nephropathy: course and prognosis [abstract]. *J Am Soc Nephrol* **4**, 284.

59. Pasquali, S., Banfi, G., Zucchelli, A., Moroni, G., Ponticelli, C., and Zucchelli, P. (1993) Lupus membranous nephropathy: long-term outcome. *Clin Nephrol* **39**, 175–82.

60. Mercadal, L., Montcel, S.T., Nochy, D., Queffeulou, G., Piette, J.C., Isnard-Bagnis, C. *et al.* (2002) Factors affecting outcome and prognosis in membranous lupus nephropathy. *Nephrol Dial Transplant* **17**, 1771–8.

61. Mok, C.C., Ying, K.Y., Lau, C.S., Yim, C.W., Ng, W.L., Wong, W.S., *et al.* (2004) Treatment of pure membranous lupus nephropathy with prednisone and azathioprine: an open-label trial. *Am J Kidney Dis* **43**, 269–76.

62. Sun, H.O., Hu, W.X., Xie, H.L., Zhang, H.T., Chen, H.P., Zeng, C.H., *et al.* (2008) Long-term outcome of Chinese patients with membranous lupus nephropathy. *Lupus* **17**, 56–61.

63. Trew, P.A., Biava, C.G., Jacobs, R.P., and Hopper, J., Jr. (1978) Renal vein thrombosis in membranous glomerulonephropathy: incidence and association. *Medicine (Baltimore)* **57**, 69–82.

64. Harris, R.C. and Ismail, N. (1994) Extrarenal complications of the nephrotic syndrome. *Am J Kidney Dis* **23**, 477–97.

65. Wagoner, R.D., Stanson, A.W., Holley, K.E., and Winter, C.S. (1983) Renal vein thrombosis in idiopathic membranous glomerulopathy and nephrotic syndrome: incidence and significance. *Kidney Int* **23**, 368–74.

66. Froment, J.C., Zergui, F., and Makhlouf, M.B. (1983) Urographic signs of thrombosis of the inferior vena cava and renal veins. *J Radiol* **64**, 729–32.

67. Llach, F., Papper, S., and Massry, S.G. (1980) The clinical spectrum of renal vein thrombosis: acute and chronic. *Am J Med* **69**, 819–27.

68. Chugh, K.S., Malik, N., Uberoi, H.S., Gupta, V.K., Aggarwal, M.L., Singhal, P.C. *et al.* (1981) Renal vein thrombosis in nephrotic syndrome–a prospective study and review. *Postgrad Med J* **57**, 566–70.

69. Velasquez, F.F., Garcia, P.N., and Ruiz, M.N. (1988) Idiopathic nephrotic syndrome of the adult with asymptomatic thrombosis of the renal vein. *Am J Nephrol* **8**, 457–62.

70. Gatewood, O.M., Fishman, E.K., Burrow, C.R., Walker, W.G., Goldman, S.M., and Siegelman, S.S. (1986) Renal vein thrombosis in patients with nephrotic syndrome: CT diagnosis. *Radiology* **159**, 117–22.

71. Ogunbiyi, O.A. (1995) Renal vein thrombosis in patients with nephrotic syndrome: CT diagnosis. *Afr J Med Med Sci* **24**, 33–40.

72. Glazer, G.M., Francis, I.R., Gross, B.H., and Amendola, M.A. (1984) Computed tomography of renal vein thrombosis. *J Comput Assist Tomogr* **8**, 288–93.

73. Wei, L.Q., Rong, Z.K., Gui, L., and Shan, R.D. (1991) CT diagnosis of renal vein thrombosis in nephrotic syndrome. *J Comput Assist Tomogr* **15**, 454–7.

74. Kanagasundaram, N.S., Bandyopadhyay, D., Brownjohn, A.M., and Meaney, J.F. (1998) The diagnosis of renal vein thrombosis by magnetic resonance angiography. *Nephrol Dial Transplant* **13**, 200–2.

75. Rahmouni, A., Jazaerli, N., Radier, C., Mathieu, D., Vasile, N., Ben Maadi, A. *et al.* (1994) Evaluation of magnetic resonance imaging for the assessment of renal vein thrombosis in the nephrotic syndrome. *Nephron* **68**, 271–2.

76. Tempany, C.M., Morton, R.A., and Marshall, F.F. (1992) MRI of the renal veins: assessment of nonneoplastic venous thrombosis. *J Comput Assist Tomogr* **16**, 929–34.

77. Ricci, M.A. and Lloyd, D.A. (1990) Renal venous thrombosis in infants and children. *Arch Surg* **125**, 1195–9.

78. Avasthi, P.S., Greene, E.R., Scholler, C., and Fowler, C.R. (1983) Noninvasive diagnosis of renal vein thrombosis by ultrasonic echo-Doppler flowmetry. *Kidney Int* **23**, 882–7.

79. Clark, R.A., and Colley, D.P. (1980) Radiological evaluation of renal vein thrombosis. *Crit Rev Diagn Imaging* **13**, 337–88.

80. Quigley, J.M., Druy, E.M., and Rich, J.I. (1981) Acute renal vein thrombosis with a diagnostic renal scintigram. *AJR Am J Roentgenol* **137**, 1066–8.

81. Sfakianakis, G.N., Zilleruelo, G., Thompson, T., Al Sheikh, W., and Strauss, J. (1985) Tc-99m glucoheptonate scintigraphy in a case of renal vein thrombosis. *Clin Nucl Med* **10**, 75–9.

82. Mettler, F.A., Jr. and Christie, J.H. (1980) The scintigraphic pattern of acute renal vein thrombosis. *Clin Nucl Med* **5**, 468–70.

83. Loges, R.J., Tulchinsky, M., Boal, D.K., Tulli, M.A., and Eggli, D.F. (1994) Tc-99m MAG3 renography in renal vein thrombosis secondary to Finnish-type congenital nephrotic syndrome. *Clin Nucl Med* **19**, 888–91.

84. Nielander, A.J., Bode, W.A., and Heidendal, G.A. (1983) Renography in diagnosis and follow-up of renal vein thrombosis. *Clin Nucl Med* **8**, 56–9.

85. Said, R. and Hamzeh, Y. (1991) Digital subtraction venography in the diagnosis of renal vein thrombosis. *Am J Nephrol* **11**, 305–8.

86. Singhal, R. and Brimble, K.S. (2006) Thromboembolic complications in the nephrotic syndrome: pathophysiology and clinical management. *Thromb Res* **118**, 397–407.

87. Wahl, D.G., Guillemin, F., de Maistre, E., Perret, C., Lecompte, T., and Thibaut, G. (1997) Risk for venous thrombosis related to antiphospholipid antibodies in systemic lupus erythematosus–a meta-analysis. *Lupus* **6**, 467–73.

88. Somers, E., Magder, L.S., and Petri, M. (2002) Antiphospholipid antibodies and incidence of venous thrombosis in a cohort of patients with systemic lupus erythematosus. *J Rheumatol* **29**, 2531–6.

89. Ho, K.T., Ahn, C.W., Alarcon, G.S., Baethge, B.A., Tan, F.K., Roseman, J. *et al.* (2005) Systemic lupus erythematosus in a multiethnic cohort (LUMINA): XXVIII. Factors predictive of thrombotic events. *Rheumatology (Oxford)* **44**, 1303–7.

90. Brouwer, J.L., Bijl, M., Veeger, N.J., Kluin-Nelemans, H.C., and van der, M.J. (2004) The contribution of inherited and acquired thrombophilic defects, alone or combined with antiphospholipid antibodies, to venous and arterial thromboembolism in patients with systemic lupus erythematosus. *Blood* **104**, 143–8.

91. Calvo-Alen, J., Toloza, S.M., Fernandez, M., Bastian, H.M., Fessler, B.J., Roseman, J.M. *et al.* (2005) Systemic lupus erythematosus in a multiethnic US cohort (LUMINA). XXV. Smoking, older age, disease activity, lupus anticoagulant, and glucocorticoid dose as risk factors for the occurrence of venous thrombosis in lupus patients. *Arthritis Rheum* **52**, 2060–8.

92. Wu, H., Birmingham, D.J., Rovin, B., Hackshaw, K.V., Haddad, N., Haden, D. *et al.* (2008) D-dimer level and the risk for thrombosis in systemic lupus erythematosus. *Clin J Am Soc Nephrol* **3**, 1628–36.

93. Glassock, R.J. (2007) Prophylactic anticoagulation in nephrotic syndrome: a clinical conundrum. *J Am Soc Nephrol* **18**, 2221–5.

94. Kant, K.S., Pollak, V.E., Weiss, M.A., Glueck, H.I., Miller, A.N., and Hess, E.V. (1981) Glomerular thrombosis in systemic lupus erythematosus: prevalence and significance. *Medicine (Baltimore)* **60**, 71–86.

95. Dosekun, A.K., Pollak, V.E., Glas-Greenwalt, P., Kant, K.S., Penovich, P., Lebron-Berges, A. *et al.* (1984) Ancrod in systemic lupus erythematosus with thrombosis. Clinical and fibrinolysis effects. *Arch Intern Med* **144**, 37–42.

96. Glueck, H.I., Kant, K.S., Weiss, M.A., Pollak, V.E., Miller, M.A., and Coots, M. (1985) Thrombosis in systemic lupus erythematosus. Relation to the presence of circulating anticoagulants. *Arch Intern Med* **145**, 1389–95.

97. Remuzzi, G. and Ruggenenti, P. (1995) The hemolytic uremic syndrome. *Kidney Int* **48**, 2–19.

98. Furlan, M., Robles, R., Galbusera, M., Remuzzi, G., Kyrle, P.A., Brenner, B. *et al.* (1998) von Willebrand factor-cleaving protease in thrombotic thrombocytopenic purpura and the hemolytic-uremic syndrome. *N Engl J Med* **339**, 1578–84.

99. Tsai, H.M., and Lian, E.C. (1998) Antibodies to von Willebrand factor-cleaving protease in acute thrombotic thrombocytopenic purpura. *N Engl J Med* **339**, 1585–94.

100. Liu, F., Feys, H.B., Dong, N., Zhao, Y., and Ruan, C. (2006) Alteration of ADAMTS13 antigen levels in patients with idiopathic thrombotic thrombocytopenic purpura, idiopathic thrombocytopenic purpura and systemic lupus erythematosus. *Thromb Haemost* **95**, 749–50.

101. Mannucci, P.M., Vanoli, M., Forza, I., Canciani, M.T., and Scorza, R. (2003) Von Willebrand factor cleaving protease (ADAMTS-13) in 123 patients with connective tissue diseases (systemic lupus erythematosus and systemic sclerosis). *Haematologica* **88**, 914–18.

102. Moore, J.C., Hayward, C.P., Warkentin, T.E., and Kelton, J.G. (2001) Decreased von Willebrand factor protease activity associated with thrombocytopenic disorders. *Blood* **98**, 1842–6.

103. Porta, C., Caporali, R., and Montecucco, C. (1999) Thrombotic thrombocytopenic purpura and autoimmunity: a tale of shadows and suspects. *Haematologica* **84**, 260–9.

104. Vasoo, S., Thumboo, J., and Fong, K.Y. (2002) Thrombotic thrombocytopenic purpura in systemic lupus erythematosus: disease activity and the use of cytotoxic drugs. *Lupus* **11**, 443–50.

105. Devinsky, O., Petito, C.K., and Alonso, D.R. (1988) Clinical and neuropathological findings in systemic lupus erythematosus: the role of vasculitis, heart emboli, and thrombotic thrombocytopenic purpura. *Ann Neurol* **23**, 380–4.

106. Güngör, T., Furlan, M., Lammle, B., Kuhn, F., and Seger, R.A. (2001) Acquired deficiency of von Willebrand factor-cleaving protease in a patient suffering from acute systemic lupus erythematosus. *Rheumatology (Oxford)* **40**, 940–2.

107. Coppo, P., Bengoufa, D., Veyradier, A., Wolf, M., Bussel, A., Millot, G.A. *et al.* (2004) Severe ADAMTS13 deficiency in adult idiopathic thrombotic microangiopathies defines a subset of patients characterized by various autoimmune manifestations, lower platelet count, and mild renal involvement. *Medicine (Baltimore)* **83**, 233–44.

108. Porta, C., Bobbio-Pallavicini, E., Centurioni, R., Caporali, R., and Montecucco, C.M. (1993) Thrombotic thrombocytopenic purpura in systemic lupus erythematosus. Italian Cooperative Group for TTP. *J Rheumatol* **20**, 1625–6.

109. Letchumanan, P., Ng, H.J., Lee, L.H., and Thumboo, J. (2009) A comparison of thrombotic thrombocytopenic purpura in an inception cohort of patients with and without systemic lupus erythematosus. *Rheumatology (Oxford)* **48**, 399–403.

110. Musio, F., Bohen, E.M., Yuan, C.M., and Welch, P.G. (1998) Review of thrombotic thrombocytopenic purpura in the setting of systemic lupus erythematosus. *Semin Arthritis Rheum* **28**, 1–19.

111. Caramaschi, P., Riccetti, M.M., Pasini, A.F., Savarin, T., Biasi, D., and Todeschini, G. (1998) Systemic lupus erythematosus and thrombotic thrombocytopenic purpura. Report of three cases and review of the literature. *Lupus* **7**, 37–41.

112. Jorfen, M., Callejas, J.L., Formiga, F., Cervera, R., Font, J., and Ingelmo, M. (1998) Fulminant thrombotic thrombocytopenic purpura in systemic lupus erythematosus. *Scand J Rheumatol* **27**, 76–7.

113. Montecucco, C., Longhi, M., Caporali, R., and De Gennaro, F. (1989) Hematological abnormalities associated with anticardiolipin antibodies. *Haematologica* **74**, 195–204.

114. Siegel, B.M., Friedman, I.A., Kessler, S., and Schwartz, S.O. (1957) Thrombohemolytic thrombocytopenic purpura and lupus erythematosus. *Ann Intern Med* **47**, 1022–9.

115. Ramkissoon, R.A. (1966) Thrombotic thrombocytopenic purpura and systemic lupus erythematosus. *Calif Med* **104**, 212–14.

116. Gelfand, J., Truong, L., Stern, L., Pirani, C.L., and Appel, G.B. (1985) Thrombotic thrombocytopenic purpura syndrome in systemic lupus erythematosus: treatment with plasma infusion. *Am J Kidney Dis* **6**, 154–60.

117. Ruggenenti, P. and Remuzzi, G. (1996) The pathophysiology and management of thrombotic thrombocytopenic purpura. *Eur J Haematol* **56**, 191–207.

118. Cecere, F.A., Yoshinoya, S., and Pope, R.M. (1981) Fatal thrombotic thrombocytopenic purpura in a patient with systemic lupus erythematosus. Relationship to circulating immune complexes. *Arthritis Rheum* **24**, 550–3.

119. Alpert, L.I. (1968) Thrombotic thrombocytopenic purpura and systemic lupus erythematosus. Report of a case with immunofluorescence investigation of vascular lesions. *J Mt Sinai Hosp N Y* **35**, 165–73.

120. Gatenby, P.A., Smith, H., Kirwan, P., and Lauer, C.S. (1981) Systemic lupus erythematosus and thrombotic thrombocytopenic purpura. A case report and review of relationship. *J Rheumatol* **8**, 504–8.

121. Rock, G.A., Shumak, K.H., Buskard, N.A., Blanchette, V.S., Kelton, J.G., Nair, R.C. *et al.* (1991) Comparison of plasma exchange with plasma infusion in the treatment of thrombotic thrombocytopenic purpura. Canadian Apheresis Study Group. *N Engl J Med* **325**, 393–7.

122. Bell, W.R., Braine, H.G., Ness, P.M., and Kickler, T.S. (1991) Improved survival in thrombotic thrombocytopenic purpura-hemolytic uremic syndrome. Clinical experience in 108 patients. *N Engl J Med* **325**, 398–403.

123. Limal, N., Cacoub, P., Sene, D., Guichard, I., and Piette, J.C. (2008) Rituximab for the treatment of thrombotic thrombocytopenic purpura in systemic lupus erythematosus. *Lupus* **17**, 69–71.

124. Bresin, E., Gastoldi, S., Daina, E., Belotti, D., Pogliani, E., Perseghin, P. *et al.* (2009) Rituximab as pre-emptive treatment in patients with thrombotic thrombocytopenic purpura and evidence of anti-ADAMTS13 autoantibodies. *Thromb Haemost* **101**, 233–8.

125. Smith, K.G., Jones, R.B., Burns, S.M., and Jayne, D.R. (2006) Long-term comparison of rituximab treatment for refractory systemic lupus erythematosus and vasculitis: Remission, relapse, and re-treatment. *Arthritis Rheum* **54**, 2970–82.

126. Walsh, M. and Jayne, D. (2007) Rituximab in the treatment of anti-neutrophil cytoplasm antibody associated vasculitis and systemic lupus erythematosus: past, present and future. *Kidney Int* **72**, 676–82.

127. Melander, C., Sallee, M., Trolliet, P., Candon, S., Belenfant, X., Daugas, E. *et al.* (2009) Rituximab in severe lupus nephritis: early B-cell depletion affects long-term renal outcome. *Clin J Am Soc Nephrol* **4**, 579–87.

128. Anonymous. Anticardiolipin antibodies: a risk factor for venous and arterial thrombosis (Editorial). (1985) *Lancet* **20**, 912–13.

129. Harris, E.N., Asherson, R.A., and Hughes, G.R. (1988) Antiphospholipid antibodies–autoantibodies with a difference. *Annu Rev Med* **39**, 261–71.

130. Eisenberg, G.M. (1992) Antiphospholipid syndrome: the reality and implications. *Hosp Pract (Off Ed)* **27**, 119–31.

131. Hughes, G.R. (1993) The antiphospholipid syndrome: ten years on. *Lancet* **342**, 341–4.

132. Amigo, M.C., Garcia-Torres, R., Robles, M., Bochicchio, T., and Reyes, P.A. (1992) Renal involvement in primary antiphospholipid syndrome. *J Rheumatol* **19**, 1181–5.

133. Kincaid-Smith, P., Fairley, K.F., and Kloss, M. (1988) Lupus anticoagulant associated with renal thrombotic microangiopathy and pregnancy-related renal failure. *Q J Med* **68**, 795–815.

134. Farrugia, E., Torres, V.E., Gastineau, D., Michet, C.J., and Holley, K.E. (1992) Lupus anticoagulant in systemic lupus erythematosus: a clinical and renal pathological study. *Am J Kidney Dis* **20**, 463–71.

135. Frampton, G., Hicks, J., and Cameron, J.S. (1991) Significance of anti-phospholipid antibodies in patients with lupus nephritis. *Kidney Int* **39**, 1225–31.

136. Nicholls, K. and Kincaid-Smith, P. (1995) Antiphospholipid syndrome and renal thrombotic microangiopathy. *J Nephrol* **8**, 123–5.

137. Moroni, G., Ventura, D., Riva, P., Panzeri, P., Quaglini, S., Banfi, G. *et al.* (2004) Antiphospholipid antibodies are associated with an increased risk for chronic renal insufficiency in patients with lupus nephritis. *Am J Kidney Dis* **43**, 28–36.

138. Asherson, R.A. and Harris, E.N. (1986) Anticardiolipin antibodies–clinical associations. *Postgrad Med J* **62**, 1081–7.

139. Love, P.E. and Santoro, S.A. (1990) Antiphospholipid antibodies: anticardiolipin and the lupus anticoagulant in systemic lupus erythematosus (SLE) and in non-SLE disorders. Prevalence and clinical significance. *Ann Intern Med* **112**, 682–98.

140. Escalante, A., Brey, R.L., Mitchell, B.D., Jr., and Dreiner, U. (1995) Accuracy of anticardiolipin antibodies in identifying a history of thrombosis among patients with systemic lupus erythematosus. *Am J Med* **98**, 559–65.

141. Sitter, T., Spannagl, M., and Schiffl, H. (1992) Anticardiolipin antibodies and lupus anticoagulant in patients treated with different methods of renal replacement therapy in comparison to patients with systemic lupus erythematosus. *Ann Hematol* **65**, 79–82.

142. Hughson, M.D., Nadasdy, T., McCarty, G.A., Sholer, C., Min, K.W., and Silva, F. (1992) Renal thrombotic microangiopathy in patients with systemic lupus erythematosus and the antiphospholipid syndrome. *Am J Kidney Dis* **20**, 150–8.

143. Daugas, E., Nochy, D., Huong, D.L., Duhaut, P., Beaufils, H., Caudwell, V. *et al.* (2002) Antiphospholipid syndrome nephropathy in systemic lupus erythematosus. *J Am Soc Nephrol* **13**, 42–52.

144. D'Agati, V., Kunis, C., Williams, G., and Appel, G.B. (1990) Anti-cardiolipin antibody and renal disease: a report three cases. *J Am Soc Nephrol* **1**, 777–84.

145. Nochy, D., Daugas, E., Droz, D., Beaufils, H., Grunfeld, J.P., Piette, J.C. *et al.* (1999) The intrarenal vascular lesions associated with primary antiphospholipid syndrome. *J Am Soc Nephrol* **10**, 507–18.

146. Cheunsuchon, B., Rungkaew, P., Chawanasuntorapoj, R., Pattaragarn, A., and Parichatikanond, P. (2007) Prevalence and clinicopathologic findings of antiphospholipid syndrome nephropathy in Thai systemic lupus erythematosus patients who underwent renal biopsies. *Nephrology (Carlton)* **12**, 474–80.

147. Tektonidou, M.G., Sotsiou, F., Nakopoulou, L., Vlachoyiannopoulos, P.G., and Moutsopoulos, H.M. (2004) Antiphospholipid syndrome nephropathy in patients with systemic lupus erythematosus and antiphospholipid antibodies: prevalence, clinical associations, and long-term outcome. *Arthritis Rheum* **50**, 2569–79.

148. Drew, P., Asherson, R.A., Zuk, R.J., Goodwin, F.J., and Hughes, G.R. (1987) Aortic occlusion in systemic lupus erythematosus associated with antiphospholipid antibodies. *Ann Rheum Dis* **46**, 612–16.

149. Garcia-Martin, F., De Arriba, G., Carrascosa, T., Moldenhauer, F., Martin-Escobar, E., Val, J. *et al.* (1991) Anticardiolipin antibodies and lupus anticoagulant in end-stage renal disease. *Nephrol Dial Transplant* **6**, 543–7.

150. Prakash, R., Miller, C.C., III, and Suki, W.N. (1995) Anticardiolipin antibody in patients on maintenance hemodialysis and its association with recurrent arteriovenous graft thrombosis. *Am J Kidney Dis* **26**, 347–52.

151. Brunet, P., Aillaud, M.F., San Marco, M., Philip-Joet, C., Dussol, B., Bernard, D. *et al.* (1995) Antiphospholipids in hemodialysis patients: relationship between lupus anticoagulant and thrombosis. *Kidney Int* **48**, 794–800.

152. Valeri, A., Joseph, R., and Radhakrishnan, J. (1999) A large prospective survey of anti-cardiolipin antibodies in chronic hemodialysis patients. *Clin Nephrol* **51**, 116–121.

153. Radhakrishnan, J., Williams, G.S., Appel, G.B., and Cohen, D.J. (1994) Renal transplantation in anticardiolipin antibody-positive lupus erythematosus patients. *Am J Kidney Dis* **23**, 286–9.

154. Khamashta, M.A., Cuadrado, M.J., Mujic, F., Taub, N.A., Hunt, B.J., and Hughes, G.R. (1995) The management of thrombosis in the antiphospholipid-antibody syndrome. *N Engl J Med* **332**, 993–7.

155. Lockshin, M.D. (1995) Answers to the antiphospholipid-antibody syndrome? *N Engl J Med* **332**, 1025–7.

156. Kobayashi, S., Tamura, N., Tsuda, H., Mokuno, C., Hashimoto, H., and Hirose, S. (1992) Immunoadsorbent plasmapheresis for a patient with antiphospholipid syndrome during pregnancy. *Ann Rheum Dis* **51**, 399–401.

157. Silver, R.K., MacGregor, S.N., Sholl, J.S., Hobart, J.M., Neerhof, M.G., and Ragin, A. (1993) Comparative trial of prednisone plus aspirin versus aspirin alone in the treatment of anticardiolipin antibody-positive obstetric patients. *Am J Obstet Gynecol* **169**, 1411–17.

158. Carreras, L.D., Perez, G.N., Vega, H.R., and Casavilla, F. (1988) Lupus anticoagulant and recurrent fetal loss: successful treatment with gammaglobulin. *Lancet* **2**, 393–4.

159. Cowchock, F.S., Reece, E.A., Balaban, D., Branch, D.W., and Plouffe, L. (1992) Repeated fetal losses associated with antiphospholipid antibodies: a collaborative randomized trial comparing prednisone with low-dose heparin treatment. *Am J Obstet Gynecol* **166**, 1318–23.

160. Lim, W., Crowther, M.A., and Eikelboom, J.W. (2006) Management of antiphospholipid antibody syndrome: a systematic review. *JAMA* **295**, 1050–7.

161. Tarr, T., Lakos, G., Bhattoa, H.P., Shoenfeld, Y., Szegedi, G., and Kiss, E. (2007) Analysis of risk factors for the development of thrombotic complications in antiphospholipid antibody positive lupus patients. *Lupus* **16**, 39–45.

162. Martinez-Berriotxoa, A., Ruiz-Irastorza, G., Egurbide, M.V., Garmendia, M., Gabriel, E.J., Villar, I. *et al.* (2007) Transiently positive anticardiolipin antibodies and risk of thrombosis in patients with systemic lupus erythematosus. *Lupus* **16**, 810–16.

163. Galli, M., Luciani, D., Bertolini, G., and Barbui, T. (2003) Lupus anticoagulants are stronger risk factors for thrombosis than anticardiolipin antibodies in the antiphospholipid syndrome: a systematic review of the literature. *Blood* **101**, 1827–32.

164. Male, C., Foulon, D., Hoogendoorn, H., Vegh, P., Silverman, E., David, M. *et al.* (2005) Predictive value of persistent versus transient antiphospholipid antibody subtypes for the risk of thrombotic events in pediatric patients with systemic lupus erythematosus. *Blood* **106**, 4152–8.

165. Wahl, D.G., Bounameaux, H., de Moerloose, P., and Sarasin, F.P. (2000) Prophylactic antithrombotic therapy for patients with systemic lupus erythematosus with or without antiphospholipid antibodies: do the benefits outweigh the risks? A decision analysis. *Arch Intern Med* **160**, 2042–8.

166. Hereng, T., Lambert, M., Hachulla, E., Samor, M., Dubucquoi, S., Caron, C. *et al.* (2008) Influence of aspirin on the clinical outcomes of 103 anti-phospholipid antibodies-positive patients. *Lupus* **17**, 11–15.

Chapter 10

Mycophenolate mofetil as treatment in lupus nephritis

Daniel Tak Mao Chan

Introduction

Mycophenolic acid (MPA) is a highly selective, potent, and noncompetitive inhibitor of inosine monophosphate dehydrogenase (IMPDH), the rate-limiting enzyme in the synthesis of guanosine nucleotides through the *de novo* pathway.[1] The guanosine nucleotides are precursors for DNA and RNA synthesis, and the *de novo* synthesis pathway is crucial to B and T lymphocytes that are involved in a proliferative response to antigenic stimuli. The type II isoform of IMPDH, which is expressed in activated lymphocytes, is five times more susceptible to the inhibitory action of MPA compared to the type I isoform, which is expressed in most cell types. In addition, MPA also induces apoptosis in activated T lymphocytes, suppresses glycosylation and expression of adhesion molecules, and depletes tetrahydrobiopterin, a cofactor for inducible nitric oxide synthase. These actions of MPA are the basis of its antiproliferative effect on lymphocytes, its inhibitory effect on inflammatory cell recruitment into inflamed tissues, and the reduction of oxidative damage mediated by peroxynitrite.[2]

Mycophenolate mofetil (MMF) is a 2-morpholinoethyl ester prodrug, which is rapidly hydrolyzed, mostly in the upper gastrointestinal tract, to produce MPA and hydroxyethyl morpholine, an inactive metabolite that is rapidly metabolized and excreted in urine. Over 95% of MPA is bound to serum albumin. The level of pharmacologically active free MPA increases when there is renal dysfunction. Mycophenolic acid is metabolized primarily by uridine diphosphate glucuronyltransferase, mostly in the liver with a minor contribution by the jejunum, to form the inactive 7-hydroxy-beta-glucuronide.[3] Although some of the glucuronide conjugate is excreted by the kidneys, it is also transported into bile and catalyzed back to MPA by glucuronidase that is shed from the intestinal flora. The MPA thus formed is then recycled into the bloodstream, thereby forming an enterohepatic circulation.[4] The result is a sharp first peak of blood MPA level at about 1 hour, followed by secondary peaks 4–8 hours after an oral dose. Also, the resultant accumulation of MPA in the gastrointestinal tract contributes to its gastrointestinal adverse effects.

Mycophenolate mofetil is often used in prophylactic immunosuppressive regimens after kidney transplantation, following reports on three randomized controlled trials in the early 1990s that showed that MMF was more effective than placebo and azathioprine in reducing the incidence of acute rejection after kidney transplantation.[5] Subsequent analysis of follow-up data from these pivotal studies also showed that

MMF treatment was associated with improved preservation of long-term renal allo-graft function.[6] As in the management of patients with lupus, the choice of immuno-suppressive treatment in organ transplant recipients entails a delicate balance between efficacy and risk. In this regard, MMF treatment is generally well tolerated in kidney transplant recipients, and the side effects such as gastrointestinal upset, leucopenia, anemia, and predisposition to infections are relatively mild and easy to manage. Based on the extensive favorable experience, MMF has replaced azathioprine in triple immu-nosuppressant treatment regimens for kidney transplantation.

Since the 1970s the combination of corticosteroid and cyclophosphamide (CTX) has been the conventional treatment for severe lupus nephritis. The addition of CTX to corticosteroid resulted in a higher incidence of sustained renal response and better preservation of renal function compared to treatment with corticosteroid alone.[7–9] Data from recent studies have also demonstrated that corticosteroid and intravenous pulse CTX was more effective than pulse methylprednisolone and azathioprine in reducing chronic renal parenchymal damage and preventing disease flares.[10,11] However, despite its efficacy in improving the renal outcome, CTX is associated with many drawbacks. The immediate adverse effects of CTX include leukopenia, alopecia, and predisposition towards infections, whereas hemorrhagic cystitis, transitional cell tumor in the urinary bladder and other malignancies, and gonadal toxicity are long-term concerns. Reducing the dose or limiting the duration of CTX treatment, approaches adopted by different investigators including the Euro-Lupus trial, can at best reduce some of these adverse effects.[12–16] In addition to the serious side effects induced by CTX, data from long-term studies also showed a high incidence of renal failure despite CTX treatment.[9] Furthermore, treatment with intravenous pulse CTX was associated with a fourfold increase in mortality during long-term follow-up.[9] There was thus a pressing need to look for alternative therapeutic agents that can ensure optimal long-term renal, as well as patient, outcomes.

The pharmacological actions of MMF, and its selectivity for lymphocytes, make it an attractive candidate for the treatment of lupus. The avoidance of nonselective suppression of other cell types not relevant to disease pathogenesis should imply a lower propensity to adverse effects, and the generally favorable tolerability of MMF has been confirmed by the data from kidney transplant recipients. Data from animal experiments showed that MMF could prevent and ameliorate disease manifestations, including nephritis, in lupus-prone mice.[17–21] The therapeutic efficacy was associated with suppression of autoantibodies.[17,22,23] Further to the favorable animal data, early anecdotal observations also suggested that MMF might have a role in the treatment of human lupus nephritis.[24–27]

Mycophenolate mofetil as induction treatment for lupus nephritis

Lupus nephritis is characterized by immune-mediated inflammatory damage to the normal renal parenchyma during the acute stage and a tendency to develop disease flares during the remission phase. In view of the natural course of disease, it is useful to divide treatment into an early "induction" phase and a prolonged "maintenance" phase. The objective of induction treatment, which comprises potent immunosuppression given for 4–6 months, is to achieve rapid abatement of the inflammatory activity in order to ensure prompt and maximal preservation of nephron mass. Although various issues, such as the different degrees of irreversible damage between patients at the time of presentation and the different contributors to persistent proteinuria, confound the definition of "response" or "remission," the important impact of initial therapeutic response on long-term renal outcome is well established, as a favorable response to induction therapy implies minimal attrition of the renal reserve.[14,28] In this regard, a recent report from the Collaborative Study Group showed that renal survival at 10 years was 94% in patients who achieved complete remission, compared to 45% in those who achieved partial remission, and 19% in patients who did not achieve remission, and a similar trend was observed with patient survival.[29]

The first prospective controlled study to investigate MMF as a treatment for lupus nephritis was conducted in 42 Chinese patients with diffuse proliferative lupus nephritis.[30] In this study, prednisolone and MMF was compared to prednisolone and oral CTX given for 6 months then substituted with azathioprine. The investigators had previously reported a response rate of over 90% following treatment with the sequential immunosuppressive regimen as used in the control arm.[13] At the end of this study, after 12 months of treatment, the two groups had comparable response rates, with approximately 80% of patients achieving complete remission and about 15% of patients achieving partial remission. The three patients classified as nonresponders included one who had to stop CTX because of leukopenia, one who had to discontinue MMF because of diarrhea, and one patient who died from miliary tuberculosis in the CTX group. Adverse events were less common in the MMF group, and side effects such as leukopenia, alopecia, and amenorrhea were only observed in CTX-treated patients. Significant gastrointestinal upset affected 5% of MMF treated patients. The lower incidence of all infections, and severe infections that required hospitalization, in MMF-treated subjects compared with CTX induction, achieved statistical significance with a bigger sample size in an extended study.[31] The quality-of-life scores reported by patients were more favorable during MMF treatment than those during induction treatment with CTX, and differences in the SF36 physical and social functioning and energy scores and the World Health Organization Quality of Life (WHOQOL) psychological domain scores reached statistical significance.[32] It is reasonable to speculate that the improved quality-of-life experience with MMF treatment was related to its better risk–benefit profile compared with CTX, especially with regard to the reduced incidence of alopecia and infections. The more favorable subjective experience perceived by patients during MMF treatment compared to CTX induction therapy has important implications on compliance. It is pertinent to note that only Chinese patients were included in these studies, and that the maximum MMF dose was 1 g twice daily. As the investigators had observed disease flares following a 50% dose reduction after 6 months, they subsequently modified the tapering regimen for MMF so that the dose of MMF was reduced by 25%, to 750 mg twice daily, after 6 months, and then to 500 mg twice daily after 12 months of treatment.[31]

Subsequent reports, which compared MMF with intravenous CTX as induction therapy in Chinese, Caucasian, African American, Hispanic, and Malay patients, led to two major conclusions.[33–36] First, the combination of corticosteroid and MMF was better tolerated by patients than corticosteroid and intravenous pulse CTX. Second, the efficacy of MMF-based induction treatment was not inferior to that achieved with CTX and corticosteroid, and could be better than CTX-based induction treatment in certain ethnic groups. The high response rate of over 80% in Chinese subjects was confirmed in a recent cohort study that included 213 patients.[37] It is of interest to note the similarly high response rate, at 83%, in a cohort of 24 Caucasian patients who were treated with prednisolone and MMF 1 g twice daily for 1 year.[38] In addition to clinical outcomes, the data from repeat protocol kidney biopsies in a 6-month study on 46 Chinese patients showed that MMF reduced histological activity and vascular changes, which portended a poor prognosis.[33] In the Malaysian study, which included 44 patients of Malay or Chinese origin with Class III or Class IV lupus nephritis, the results showed comparable efficacy between corticosteroid and either MMF or intravenous CTX as induction treatment at 6 months, with approximately 60% of patients attaining remission.[35] Severe infections such as pneumonia or septicemia occurred in three of 25 patients in the CTX group and in three of 19 patients in the MMF group; and herpes zoster occurred in three patients in each group. In contrast to other reports, the incidence of infection did not differ between the two treatments. Whether this might be related to the relatively high starting dose of prednisolone, at 60 mg daily given for 4–6 weeks, remains speculative. In the induction therapy study reported by Ginzler *et al.* from the USA, 140 patients with Class III, IV, or V lupus nephritis were randomized to treatment with corticosteroid and either MMF or intravenous CTX, and the response to treatment was assessed at 6 months.[36] Over 75% of patients in this study were of African or Hispanic origin, and the target MMF dose was 3 g/day, which was tolerated by 63% of patients. In accordance with previous observations, MMF treatment was associated with a lower incidence of severe infections or hospitalization episodes. Upper gastrointestinal symptoms affected about 25% of patients in each group, and diarrhea was more common in MMF-treated patients. The results showed that MMF treatment resulted in a statistically higher response rate compared with intravenous CTX induction. Using intention-to-treat analysis, the rate of complete remission was 22.5% in the MMF group and 5.8% in the CTX group. In patients with proliferative lupus nephritis, the complete remission rate was 26.3% in the MMF group and 5.4% in the CTX group, whereas the rates of combined complete or partial remission were 52.6% and 30.4% respectively. Two issues deserve attention. First, although the difference between the response rates in the two groups achieved statistical significance, these rates seemed considerably lower than those observed in other studies. Second, 15(21%) of the 71 patients assigned to MMF treatment and 24(35%) of the 69 patients assigned to CTX treatment discontinued their assigned therapy because of adverse effects or inadequate response after 12 weeks of treatment. The relatively high discontinuation rates have thus created difficulties in the interpretation of the results and the conclusions from this study.

The latest data on induction treatment came from the induction phase results of the Aspreva Lupus Management Study (ALMS trial), an international industry sponsored multi-center study.[39] In this trial, 370 patients with Class III, IV, and/or V lupus nephritis were randomized to treatment with either corticosteroid and monthly intravenous pulse CTX at 0.5–1.0 g/m^2 or corticosteroid and MMF at a target dose of 1.5 g twice daily. 16.2% of patients had pure Class V nephritis. The maximum starting dose of prednisone was 60 mg daily. After 24 weeks of induction treatment, 56.2% of patients in the MMF group and 53.0% of patients in the CTX group responded, and the difference in response rates was not statistically significant. Response, being the primary study endpoint in this study, was defined as a reduction in urine protein excretion with stabilization or improvement in serum creatinine. Proteinuria had to decrease to the subnephrotic range or by at least 50% compared with baseline in order to qualify for response. Complete remission, defined as proteinuria not more than 0.5 g daily with normalization of serum creatinine and an inactive urinary sediment, was attained by 8.6% of patients in the MMF group and 8.1% of patients in the CTX group. Racial variation appeared to have an impact on the treatment outcome. Patients in this study were recruited from 88 centers in 20 countries in North and South America, Asia, Australia, and Europe. The ethnicity of the subjects was as follows: 33.2% Asians, 39.7% Caucasians, and 35.4% Hispanic. Although the two treatment regimens gave comparable response rates in Asians and White subjects, in patients under the "other races" category 60.4% responded to MMF and 38.5% responded to CTX, and the difference was statistically significant with a P value of 0.033. Post hoc analysis also showed that Hispanic patients were more likely to respond to MMF (60.9%) than CTX (38.8%). Although the CTX group reported 40.6% more adverse events, the rates of infection and gastrointestinal disorders were similar between the two groups. Of patients in the MMF group, 13.0% withdrew because of adverse events, compared with 7.2% in the CTX group, but the difference did not reach statistical significance. Infections occurred in 12.0% of patients in the MMF group and in 10.0% of patients in the CTX group. Nine of 184 patients treated with MMF and five of 180 patients treated with CTX died. Infections accounted for seven deaths in the MMF group and two deaths in the CTX group. Among the nine Asian mortalities, seven were in the MMF group. The overall response rate of over 50% at 6 months in both treatment groups in the ALMS trial is in keeping with previous experience, except for the report by Ginzler *et al.*, in which the combined complete or partial remission rate at 6 months was 30.4% in the CTX group.[36] The similar treatment efficacy in Asians and White patients between MMF and CTX induction is also in accordance with published experience. The relatively low response rates in the non-Asian, non-White and Hispanic subjects treated with CTX are reminiscent of the data reported by Ginzler *et al.*[36] However, the similar rates of adverse events between MMF and CTX treatment appeared contrary to expectations based on previously published data and prevailing clinical experience. Factors that could have contributed to a relatively high adverse event rate in MMF-treated patients in the ALMS trial should be examined. The target MMF dose in the ALMS trial was 1.5 g twice daily irrespective of ethnicity. Data from kidney transplant recipients have shown a higher incidence of adverse reactions, including infective complications, with an MMF dose of 3 g/day compared with 2 g daily, and that increasing the daily dose from 2 g to 3 g did not improve efficacy except in African Americans.[40,41] Based on these observations, a dose of 3 g MMF per day is recommended for African Americans, and 2 g daily dosage is recommended for non-African Americans, to prevent kidney transplant rejection. The median MMF dose attained in Asian patients in the ALMS trial was 2.6 g daily, and the data suggested excessive infection and mortality in Asian patients treated with MMF. In this regard, the data from 277 Chinese patients in previous studies, based on MMF doses that did not exceed 2 g daily, have shown a relatively low incidence of adverse events.[31,33,34,37] There is thus an interplay between ethnicity and MMF dose to achieve an optimal efficacy–risk balance. In addition to the drug dosage issue, it is also prudent to examine whether there might be a center effect in the incidence of adverse events in multi-center studies on complicated diseases such as severe lupus nephritis. In summary, the induction phase data from the ALMS trial confirmed the efficacy of combined corticosteroid and MMF as treatment for severe proliferative lupus nephritis, but the difference in response to MMF- or CTX-based induction treatment could vary according to ethnicity. In addition, the favorable tolerability profile of MMF appeared dose-dependent, and in Asian patients it could diminish when the daily dose of MMF exceeds 2 g.

Mycophenolate mofetil as maintenance treatment for lupus nephritis

The main objective of maintenance immunosuppressive treatment is to prevent relapse. Disease flares are common in lupus nephritis, and cumulative relapse rates of about 40% over 4–10 years of follow-up have been reported in patients who had received corticosteroid and CTX as induction therapy followed by low-dose corticosteroid with or without azathioprine as maintenance immunosuppression.[16,42,43] Assessment of long-term tolerability of treatment and the detection of adverse effects that emerge late are also issues of pertinence in studies of patients in the maintenance phase.

Investigators in the Netherlands have investigated the efficacy of MMF in averting impending relapse.[44] In 10 patients who showed an increase in the level of anti-dsDNA antibodies by 25% or more, the addition of MMF at 2 g/day for 6 months while keeping the dose of corticosteroid unchanged reduced the titer of anti-dsDNA antibodies, and none of the patients had disease flares during the 6 months of follow-up. A recent retrospective study compared the rates of disease flare before and after the addition of MMF in 67 patients.[45] With the respective mean follow-up durations of 14.1 months and 14.8 months, the investigators observed a reduction of flare rate from 8.9 to 5.3 per 10 patient-years after the addition of MMF, and with concomitant reduction of prednisone dose. Notwithstanding the potential drawbacks, such as possible selection bias, small sample size, short follow-up duration, and the wide range of MMF dose that varied from 250 mg to 3 g daily, these data lent support to the immunosuppressive efficacy and the steroid-sparing action of MMF.

In the study reported by Contreras *et al.*, 59 patients with predominantly WHO Class III or IV lupus nephritis from a single center in Miami, USA, were first treated with corticosteroid and intravenous pulse CTX at 0.5–1.0 g/m^2 body surface area once a month for six to seven pulses, before they were randomized to maintenance immunosuppressive treatment with corticosteroid and MMF, azathioprine, or intravenous

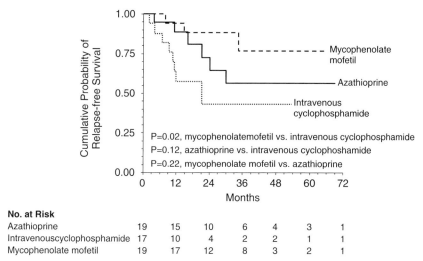

Fig. 10.1 Kaplan–Meier estimates of relapse-free survival in patients with lupus nephritis who were randomized to receive corticosteroid and MMF, azathioprine, or intravenous cyclophosphamide (CTX) given once every 3 months as maintenance immunosuppression after responding to induction therapy consisting of corticosteroid and intravenous pulse CTX. Modified from Figure 3 in[46]. Copyright © Massachusetts Medical Society. All rights reserved.

CTX given once every 3 months.[46] Twenty-nine of the patients were of Hispanic origin, whereas 27 were categorized as Black. Over median follow-up durations of 25–30 months, relapse-free survival was better in the MMF group compared to maintenance with intermittent CTX pulses, but there was no difference between MMF and azathioprine treatment (Figure 10.1). Long-term treatment with MMF or azathioprine was well tolerated, and was associated with lower rates of hospitalization, infection, amenorrhea, and nausea or vomiting compared with the CTX group.

In our extension study we compared 32 patients treated with prednisolone and MMF continuously from the induction phase to the maintenance phase against 30 patients treated with prednisolone and oral CTX for 6 months as induction followed by azathioprine as maintenance immunosuppression, over a median follow-up of 63 months.[31] Similar to our earlier data from the 12-month study, both treatment groups showed high and comparable response rates of approximately 90%. The two treatment groups showed similar relapse-free survival rates and similar hazard ratios for disease flares, with 11 patients in the MMF group and nine patients in the sequential immunosuppression group manifesting disease flares during follow-up. At the latest analysis of updated follow-up data, the two groups continued to show similar rates of disease flare over a mean follow-up of 68.5 months (Figure 10.2). Prolonged treatment with low-dose prednisolone and either MMF or azathioprine was associated with favorable tolerability with minimal side effects.

It is important to note that both the mode of induction immunosuppression and the response to induction therapy have an impact on the subsequent disease course. Although it can be difficult to predict the likelihood of relapse in individual patients,

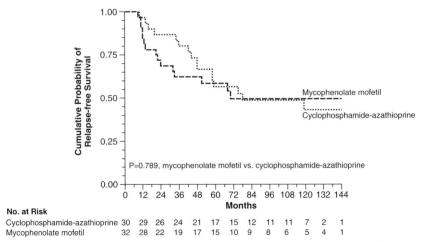

Fig. 10.2 Kaplan–Meier estimates of relapse-free survival in 62 patients with diffuse proliferative lupus nephritis who were randomized to receive corticosteroid and MMF as continuous induction and maintenance immunosuppression or corticosteroid and oral cyclophosphamide (CTX) for 6 months as induction followed by low-dose corticosteroid and azathioprine as maintenance immunosuppression.

lower relapse rates have been observed in patients who achieved complete remission after treatment compared to those who only attained partial remission.[29,42] Cumulative relapse rates of 41% versus 76% over approximately 12 years of follow-up, and median time-to-renal flare of 36 months versus 18 months, have been observed in patients who attained complete remission or partial remission respectively.[42] In addition, an inverse relationship has been noted between time-to-remission and time-to-relapse.[47] In view of the marked heterogeneity between patients in their propensities for flares, and the multiple confounding factors such as prior induction treatment and treatment response, clinical studies aiming to investigate maintenance treatment would require a big sample size and prolonged follow-up.

Impact of mycophenolate mofetil treatment on renal and patient survival

As chronic renal failure is a relatively slow and progressive process following the treatment of acute nephritic flares, a sufficient follow-up duration is required to discern an impact of treatment on renal survival. In this regard, it has been previously reported that in patients with severe lupus nephritis treated with corticosteroid and cytotoxic agents, a follow-up of at least 5 years was required to detect differences in the rates of renal failure associated with different treatments.[8]

In the induction phase study reported by Ginzler *et al.*, death and renal failure were twice as frequent in patients who had received intravenous CTX compared to the MMF group during post-induction follow-up of approximately 37 months, but the difference did not reach statistical significance.[36] The data reported by Contreras *et al.*

showed an excessive risk of death and/or renal failure in patients given intravenous CTX pulses every 3 months as maintenance immunosuppression.[46] The clinical outcomes in this group of patients were extremely poor, with four deaths and three patients developing renal failure over a median treatment duration of 25 months, compared with one death and one renal failure in the MMF group, and one renal failure in the azathioprine group. Although the data clearly demonstrated inferior clinical outcomes with intravenous pulse CTX as maintenance treatment, there was no significant difference in terms of renal or patient survival between MMF and azathioprine maintenance, similar to what had been observed in the prevention of relapses.

Data from our extension study showed that serum creatinine and creatinine clearance remained stable and similar between patients treated with corticosteroid and MMF and those given sequential immunosuppressive treatment with CTX followed by azathioprine, over a median follow-up of 63 months.[31] The incidence of doubling of baseline serum creatinine level was 6% in the MMF group and 10% in the sequential immunosuppression group, with four patients in the latter group reaching the endpoint of death or renal failure, and the difference was not statistically significant. These data demonstrated that in Chinese patients prednisolone and MMF given as continuous induction-then-maintenance immunosuppressive treatment was associated with relatively favorable renal and patient survival rates within the first 5 years of follow-up.

Mycophenolate mofetil and membranous lupus nephritis

Membranous features are present in over 20% of renal biopsies that show lupus nephritis. Pure membranous lupus nephritis usually presents with variable degrees of proteinuria, and it is quite common that the serological parameters are quiescent. These patients usually have a relatively low risk or slow rate of renal function deterioration. The concomitant presence of endocapillary proliferation and/or necrosis indicates more aggressive disease, and thus justifies treatment with potent immunosuppression, as for focal or diffuse proliferative lupus nephritis.[48,49] Diverse approaches have been adopted for the management of pure membranous lupus nephritis, and treatment decisions are often informed by the severity of proteinuria. Inhibition or blockade of the renin–angiotensin pathway and blood pressure control may be the initial treatment in patients with low level proteinuria, normal serum albumin level, and normal renal function, whereas immunosuppressive treatment with corticosteroid, cytotoxic agents, and/or calcineurin inhibitors is justified in nephrotic patients. Corticosteroid combined with cyclophosphamide or azathioprine has been reported to be effective in reducing proteinuria in up to 90% of patients, with over 50% achieving complete remission.[50,51] Calcineurin inhibitors such as cyclosporine or tacrolimus are predictably effective in the reduction of proteinuria, but nephrotoxicity, hypertension, and relapse after discontinuation of treatment are important concerns.[52,53] Although reports from pilot studies suggested that MMF given together with corticosteroid could be a therapeutic option in the treatment of pure membranous lupus nephritis,[54–56] the paucity of data from controlled studies precludes definitive conclusions.

Effects of mycophenolic acid on resident kidney cells

The immunosuppressive actions of MMF account for its efficacy in the prevention of transplant rejection and the treatment of immune-mediated diseases. However, there are accumulating data on the direct effects of MMF on nonlymphoid cells. Mycophenolic acid has been shown to inhibit the proliferation of endothelial cells, smooth muscle cells, fibroblasts, tubular epithelial cells, and mesangial cells *in vitro*.[57–62] Apart from an antiproliferative effect, MPA also decreased mesangial cell activation and matrix synthesis upon stimulation with fetal calf serum or transforming growth factor β1 (TGFβ1).[59] There are also data to show that MMF could reduce renal myofibroblast infiltration, collagen III deposition, and glomerular crescent formation in animal models of glomerulonephritis.[63]

Our group has previously demonstrated that polyclonal anti-DNA antibodies isolated from patients with active lupus nephritis could bind to the surface of human mesangial cells and induce cytokine and extracellular matrix synthesis.[64–66] More recently, we reported that these autoantibodies induced phosphorylation of protein kinase C (PKC) α, βI, and βII, TGFβ1, and fibronectin synthesis in cultured human mesangial cells, and that these effects were abrogated by MPA.[67] Results from experiments in the NZBWF1/J mice with established nephritis showed that the therapeutic effect of MMF was accompanied by decreased phosphorylation of PKCα, βI, and βII, and reduced mesangial fibronectin deposition (Figure 10.3). In addition, MMF treatment was associated with reduced immunoglobulin deposition in the glomerulus, similar to observations in MRL/*lpr* mice by other investigators.[18] These data suggest direct actions of MPA on resident kidney cells, which could contribute to therapeutic benefit in the setting of lupus nephritis.

Other issues related to mycophenolate mofetil treatment

Cost of treatment

The current high cost of MMF could present a significant economic barrier to patients who should benefit from this treatment. An analysis based on mathematical modeling has shown better cost-effectiveness with 6 months of MMF compared to intravenous CTX as induction treatment.[68] However, the conclusions from this analysis might not apply in actual clinical practice, as available data and general experience suggest that the MMF treatment duration of 6 months is probably too short to secure sustained remission. Although it is conceivable that the reduced incidence of adverse events, especially the infective complications, associated with MMF treatment may be able to offset part of its higher medication cost compared with CTX and azathioprine, the financial implications of these treatment regimens have not been examined previously. In this regard, we have compared the costs of immunosuppressive drugs and the treatment costs for complications between patients treated with corticosteroid and MMF and those treated with corticosteroid and oral CTX induction followed by azathioprine maintenance.[69] Our data showed that although the drug cost for MMF was 14-fold higher than that in the CTX and azathioprine regimen, MMF treatment resulted in an 80% reduction in the cost of hospitalization and treatment for infective

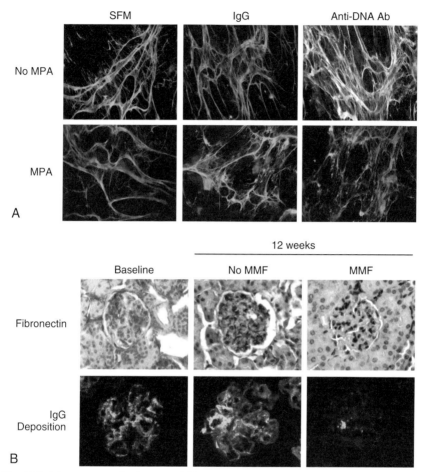

Fig. 10.3 (A) Representative images of fibronectin deposition by cultured human mesangial cells after incubation with serum-free medium (SFM), control immunoglobulin (Ig)G from healthy individuals, or polyclonal anti-dsDNA antibodies isolated from patients with lupus nephritis, in the absence or presence of mycophenolic acid (MPA) (5 μg/ml). Original magnification ×400. (B) Representative images showing fibronectin expression in glomeruli from NZBWF1/J mice after 12 weeks of treatment with vehicle or mycophenolate mofetil (MMF). Original magnification ×200 (upper panels). Immunofluorescence staining showing IgG deposition in the glomeruli after vehicle or MMF treatment (lower panels). Adapted with permission from Figures 5 and 6 in[67].

complications, so that the cost excess associated with MMF treatment in the first 2 years was reduced to 57%.

Crescentic lupus nephritis

Patients with crescentic glomerulonephritis and those who presented with rapidly progressive glomerulonephritis and severe renal failure were often excluded from clinical studies because of research ethics considerations. As a result, the reported experience with MMF treatment may not apply to this group of patients. Recent data from a retrospective study, which included 52 Chinese patients with lupus nephritis and crescent formation in over 50% of glomeruli, showed comparable responses to treatment with corticosteroid and either MMF or CTX.[70] The response rates in both groups were approximately 70% after 12 months of treatment. All the patients received pulse methylprednisolone 500 mg daily for 3 days initially, and CTX was given intravenously at 0.5–0.75/m^2 body surface area once a month, whereas the dose of MMF was 750–1000 mg twice daily. These preliminary data suggest that MMF can be a useful therapeutic option in these patients who present with severe acute renal failure, although they should be monitored closely for the early detection of treatment resistance.

Ethnic variability

The issue of ethnic variability in lupus nephritis, with regard to both disease manifestations and the response to treatment, has been alluded to in the section on induction therapy. Differences in disease presentation and a 23% difference in the proportion of patients achieving remission have been observed between Black and White patient groups in the USA.[71] Genetic and socio-economic factors such as prompt access to healthcare facilities could contribute to the variability in treatment response between different ethnic groups observed with both CTX- and MMF-based therapies. A relatively low incidence of doubling of baseline serum creatinine at 4.4% over 7 years was observed in Chinese patients with diffuse proliferative lupus nephritis who had been treated with prednisolone and oral CTX for 6 months as induction followed by azathioprine during the maintenance phase,[16] in contrast to an incidence of 20% over 3 years in some of the studies in USA, which included a high proportion of African American patients.[42,72] In the Euro-Lupus trial, in which over 80% of patients were Caucasians, the regimen with reduced dosage and duration of intravenous CTX was associated with fewer adverse effects but preserved treatment efficacy.[15,73] The ALMS trial induction phase data showed that Caucasians and Asians had a more favorable response to corticosteroid and MMF treatment when compared with Hispanics and other ethnic groups.[39] A recent single-center study in New York, USA, also reported similar ethnic variation in response to MMF or CTX treatment.[74] It follows then that treatment decisions with regard to the choice and the dose of cytotoxic agents should take into account the differences in the risk–benefit balance across different patient populations.

Pediatric patients with lupus nephritis

Compared with adult patients, there are much less data on MMF treatment in pediatric patients with lupus nephritis. The anecdotal data to date suggest that MMF may have comparable efficacy as CTX when combined with corticosteroid in treating proliferative or membranous lupus nephritis.[75–77] However, there is insufficient information on patients with very severe disease such as crescentic glomerulonephritis.[78] It also remains unknown whether the response rate in children is similar to that in adults.

Therapeutic drug monitoring

The role of MPA therapeutic drug monitoring in routine clinical practice remains an area of uncertainty. The marked pharmacokinetic variability for MMF between individuals, including lupus patients, is well recognized.[79] Various factors can affect circulating drug levels, and these include concomitant corticosteroid dose, renal function, liver function, and serum albumin level.[80,81] Data from patients with lupus nephritis showed that MPA exposure was lower in patients with heavy proteinuria, whereas meta-analysis of pooled data has demonstrated correlations between drug exposure and renal function as well as serum albumin level.[82,83] The practical importance of drug level monitoring depends on its usefulness in predicting efficacy and adverse effects. In kidney transplantation, MPA exposure as measured by the area-under-the-curve correlates with the risk of acute rejection but not with drug-induced adverse effects, which appear better predicted by the free MPA level in the circulation.[80] Although there are preliminary data to suggest that an adequate trough MPA blood level may be important in maintaining remission in patients with vasculitis or systemic lupus erythematosus,[84] it is generally agreed that limited sampling strategies are better than single-point drug level assessments.[79] The data to date suggest that determination of MPA exposure is not routinely required in all lupus patients, but should be considered selectively in nonresponders or frequent relapsers, and those who develop excessive adverse effects during MMF treatment at conventional dosage.

Conclusions

The management of severe lupus nephritis entails considerations of treatment efficacy and the prevention and treatment of disease-related complications and drug-induced toxicities, which can present immediately or emerge during long-term follow-up. The heterogeneity in clinical course and responses to treatment presents additional challenges. Accumulating data over the past decade have substantiated the important role of MMF as first-line treatment of diffuse or focal proliferative lupus nephritis.[85,86] High response rates have been observed in patients treated with corticosteroid and MMF for remission induction, especially in Chinese and Caucasian populations, and the available data from Chinese patients show that the favorable early response is associated with low morbidity, mortality, and rate of renal failure during follow-up. Although the response rates to this induction treatment appeared slightly lower in African Americans and Hispanics, it is in these patients that treatment with MMF has been shown to confer a better efficacy than induction treatment with intravenous CTX. At appropriate dosage, MMF treatment is associated with fewer adverse effects compared to CTX, but careful attention to patient characteristics, including ethnicity, is required to ensure optimization of the efficacy–risk profile during immunosuppressive treatment. Further studies are required to examine the role and optimal dose of MMF in the treatment of crescentic lupus nephritis and membranous lupus nephritis, as well as the impact of MMF treatment in children with lupus nephritis, in comparison with other available therapies. In contrast to the definitive conclusions on MMF as an induction agent, there is considerable uncertainty on the comparative advantage of MMF against azathioprine when given as maintenance immunosuppression. It is intuitive that too rapid tapering or early discontinuation of MMF could precipitate disease flares. The experience to date suggests that the dose of MMF should probably not be reduced by more than 25% after the first 6 months, and that it is advisable to continue treatment for at least 12–18 months, in order to secure a sustained disease response. Effective and safe immunosuppressive treatment plays a critical role in preserving nephron mass and renal reserve. The importance of adjunctive treatments, such as the control of hypertension, the suppression of proteinuria, and the prevention of systemic complications, in ensuring optimal long-term outcomes cannot be overemphasized.

References

1. Allison, A.C., and Eugui, E.M. (1993) Immunosuppressive and other effects of mycophenolic acid and an ester prodrug mycophenolate mofetil. *Immunol Rev* **136**, 5–28.

2. Allison, A.C., and Eugui, E.M. (2000) Mycophenolate mofetil and its mechanisms of action. *Immunopharmacology* **47**, 85–118.

3. Bowalgaha, K., and Miners, J.O. (2001) The glucuronidation of mycophenolic acid by human liver, kidney and jejunum microsomes. *Br J Clin Pharmacol* **52**, 605–9.

4. Shaw, L.M., Figurski, M., Milone, M.C., Trofe, J., and Bloom, R.D. (2007) Therapeutic drug monitoring of mycophenolic acid. *Clin J Am Soc Nephrol* **2**, 1062–72.

5. Halloran, P., Mathew, T., Tomlanovich, S., Groth, C., Hooftman, L., and Barker, C. (1997) Mycophenolate mofetil in renal allograft recipients: a pooled efficacy analysis of three randomized double-blind clinical studies in prevention of rejection. The International Mycophenolate Mofetil Renal Transplant Study Groups. *Transplantation* **63**, 39–47.

6. Meier-Kriesche, H.U., Steffen, B.J., Hochberg, A.M., Gordon, R.D., Liebman, M.N., Morris, J.A., et al. (2003) Mycophenolate mofetil versus azathioprine therapy is associated with a significant protection against long-term renal allograft function deterioration. *Transplantation* **75**, 1341–6.

7. Donadio, J.V. Jr., Holley, K.E., Ferguson, R.H., Ilstrup, D.M. (1978) Treatment of diffuse proliferative lupus nephritis with prednisone and combined prednisone and cyclophosphamide. *N Engl J Med* **299**, 1151–5.

8. Austin, H.A.,III, Klippel, J.H., Balow, J.E., le Riche, N.G., Steinberg, A.D., Plotz, P.H., et al. (1986) Therapy of lupus nephritis. Controlled trial of prednisone and cytotoxic drugs. *N Engl J Med* **314**, 614–9.

9. Illei, G.G., Austin, H.A., Crane, M., Collins, L., Gourley, M.F., Yarboro, C.H., et al. (2001) Combination therapy with pulse cyclophosphamide plus pulse methylprednisolone improves long-term renal outcome without adding toxicity in patients with lupus nephritis. *Ann Intern Med* **135**, 248–57.

10. Grootscholten, C., Ligtenberg, G., Hagen, E.C., van den Wall Bake, A.W., de Glas-Vos, J.W., Bijl, M., et al. (2006) Azathioprine/methylprednisolone versus cyclophosphamide in proliferative lupus nephritis. A randomised controlled trial. *Kidney Int* **70**, 732–42.

11. Grootscholten, C., Bajema, I.M., Florquin, S., Steenbergen, E.J., Peutz-Kootstra, C.J., Goldschmeding, R., et al. (2007) Treatment with cyclophosphamide delays the progression of chronic lesions more effectively than does treatment with azathioprine plus methylprednisolone in patients with proliferative lupus nephritis. *Arthritis Rheum* **56**, 924–37.

12. Feng, P.H., Jayaratnam, F.J., Tock, E.P., and Seah, C.S. (1973) Cyclophosphamide in treatment of systemic lupus erythematosus: 7 years' experience. *Br Med J* **2**, 450–2.

13. Chan, T.M., Li, F.K., Wong, R.W., Wong, K.L., Chan, K.W., and Cheng, I.K. (1995) Sequential therapy for diffuse proliferative and membranous lupus nephritis: cyclophosphamide and prednisolone followed by azathioprine and prednisolone. *Nephron* **71**, 321–7.

14. Korbet, S.M., Lewis, E.J., Schwartz, M.M., Reichlin, M., Evans, J., and Rohde, R.D. (2000) Factors predictive of outcome in severe lupus nephritis. Lupus Nephritis Collaborative Study Group. *Am J Kidney Dis* **35**, 904–4.

15. Houssiau, F.A., Vasconcelos, C., D'Cruz, D., Sebastiani, G.D., Garrido ed Ede, R., Danieli, M.G., *et al.* (2002) Immunosuppressive therapy in lupus nephritis: the Euro-Lupus Nephritis Trial, a randomized trial of low-dose versus high-dose intravenous cyclophosphamide. *Arthritis Rheum* **46**, 2121–31.

16. Chan, T.M., Tse, K.C., Tang, C.S, Lai, K.N., and Li, F.K. (2005) Long-term outcome of patients with diffuse proliferative lupus nephritis treated with prednisolone and oral cyclophosphamide followed by azathioprine. *Lupus* **14**, 265–2.

17. McMurray, R.W., Elbourne, K.B., Lagoo, A., and Lai, S. (1998) Mycophenolate mofetil suppresses autoimmunity and mortality in the female NZBxNZW F1 mouse model of systemic lupus erythematosus. *J Rheumatol* **25**, 2364–70.

18. Van Bruggen, M.C., Walgreen, B., Rijke, T.P., and Berden, J.H. (1998) Attenuation of murine lupus nephritis by mycophenolate mofetil. *J Am Soc Nephrol* **9**, 1407–15.

19. Jonsson, C.A., Svensson, L., and Carlsten, H. (1999) Beneficial effect of the inosine monophosphate dehydrogenase inhibitor mycophenolate mofetil on survival and severity of glomerulonephritis in systemic lupus erythematosus (SLE)-prone MRLlpr/lpr mice. *Clin Exp Immunol* **116**, 534–41.

20. Mehling, A., Grabbe, S., Voskort, M., Schwarz, T., Luger, T.A., and Beissert, S. (2000) Mycophenolate mofetil impairs the maturation and function of murine dendritic cells. *J Immunol* **165**, 2374–81.

21. Zoja, C., Benigni, A., Noris, M., Corna, D., Casiraghi, F., Pagnoncelli, M., *et al.* (2001) Mycophenolate mofetil combined with a cyclooxygenase-2 inhibitor ameliorates murine lupus nephritis. *Kidney Int* **60**, 653–63.

22. Corna, D., Morigi, M., Facchinetti, D., Bertani, T., Zoja, C., and Remuzzi, G. (1997) Mycophenolate mofetil limits renal damage and prolongs life in murine lupus autoimmune disease. *Kidney Int* **51**, 1583–9.

23. Ramos, M.A., Pinera, C., Setien, M.A., Buelta, L., de Cos, M.A., de Francisco, A.L., *et al.* (2003) Modulation of autoantibody production by mycophenolate mofetil: effects on the development of SLE in NZBxNZW F1 mice. *Nephrol Dial Transplant* **18**, 878–83.

24. Glicklich, D., and Acharya, A. (1998) Mycophenolate mofetil therapy for lupus nephritis refractory to intravenous cyclophosphamide. *Am J Kidney Dis* **32**, 318–22.

25. Briggs, W.A., Choi, M.J., and Scheel, P.J., Jr. (1998) Successful mycophenolate mofetil treatment of glomerular disease. *Am J Kidney Dis* **31**, 213–7.

26. Dooley, M.A., Cosio, F.G., Nachman, P.H., Falkenhain, M.E., Hogan, S.L., Falk, R.J., and Hebert, L.A. (1999) Mycophenolate mofetil therapy in lupus nephritis: clinical observations. *J Am Soc Nephrol* **10**, 833–9.

27. Gaubitz, M., Schorat, A., Schotte, H., Kern, P., and Domschke, W. (1999) Mycophenolate mofetil for the treatment of systemic lupus erythematosus: an open pilot trial. *Lupus* **8**, 731–6.

28. Houssiau, F.A., Vasconcelos, C., D'Cruz, D., Sebastiani, G.D., Garrido, E.R., Danieli, M.G., *et al.* (2004) Early response to immunosuppressive therapy predicts good renal outcome in lupus nephritis. *Arthritis Rheum* **50**, 3934–40.

29. Chen, Y.E., Korbet, S.M., Katz, R.S., Schwartz, M.M., Lewis, E.J., for the Collaborative Study Group (2008) Value of a complete or partial remission in severe lupus nephritis. *Clin J Am Soc Nephrol* **3**, 46–53.

30. Chan, T.M., Li, F.K., Tang, C.S., Wong R.W., Fang, G.X., Ji, Y.L., *et al.* (2000) Efficacy of mycophenolate mofetil in patients with diffuse proliferative lupus nephritis. Hong Kong-Guangzhou Nephrology Study Group. *N Engl J Med* **343**, 1156–62.

31. Chan, T.M., Tse, K.C., Tang, C.S., Mok, M.Y., Li, F.K., for the Hong Kong Nephrology Study Group (2005) Long-term study of mycophenolate mofetil as continuous induction and maintenance treatment for diffuse proliferative lupus nephritis. *J Am Soc Nephrol* **16**, 1076–84.

32. Tse, K.C., Tang, C.S, Lio, W.I., Lam, M.F., and Chan, T.M. (2006) Quality of life comparison between corticosteroid-and-mycofenolate mofetil and corticosteroid-and-oral cyclophosphamide in the treatment of severe lupus nephritis. *Lupus* **15**, 371–9.

33. Hu, W., Liu, Z., Chen, H., Tang, Z., Wang, Q., Shen K, *et al.* (2002) Mycophenolate mofetil vs cyclophosphamide therapy for patients with diffuse proliferative lupus nephritis. *Chin Med J (Engl)* **115**, 705–9.

34. Ding, L., Zhao, M., Zou, W., Liu, Y., and Wang, H. (2004) Mycophenolate mofetil combined with prednisone for diffuse proliferative lupus nephritis: a histopathological study. *Lupus* **13**, 113–8.

35. Ong, L.M., Hooi, L.S., Lim, T.O., Goh, B.L., Ahmad, G., Ghazalli, R., *et al.* (2005) Randomized controlled trial of pulse intravenous cyclophosphamide versus mycophenolate mofetil in the induction therapy of proliferative lupus nephritis. *Nephrology* **10**, 504–10.

36. Ginzler, E.M., Dooley, M.A., Aranow, C., Kim, M.Y., Buyon, J., Merrill, J.T., *et al.* (2005) Mycophenolate mofetil or intravenous cyclophosphamide for lupus nephritis. *N Engl J Med* **353**, 2219–28.

37. Lu, F., Tu, Y., Peng, X., Wang, L., Wang, H., Sun, Z, *et al.* (2008) A prospective multicentre study of mycophenolate mofetil combined with prednisolone as induction therapy in 213 patients with active lupus nephritis. *Lupus* **17**, 622–9.

38. Cross, J., Dwomoa, A., Andrews, P., Burns A., Gordon C., Main, J., *et al.* (2005) Mycophenolate mofetil for remission induction in severe lupus nephritis. *Nephron Clin Pract* **100**, c92–100.

39. Appel, G.B., Contreras, G., Dooley, M.A., Ginzler, E.M., Isenberg, D., Jayne, D., *et al.* (2009) Mycophenolate mofetil versus Cyclophosphamide for induction treatment of lupus nephritis. *J Am Soc Nephrol* **20**, 1103–12.

40. Neylan, J.F. (1997) Immunosuppressive therapy in high-risk transplant patients: dose-dependent efficacy of mycophenolate mofetil in African-American renal allograft recipients. U.S. Renal Transplant Mycophenolate Mofetil Study Group. *Transplantation* **64**, 1277–82.

41. Mathew, T.H. (1998) A blinded long-term randomized multicenter study of mycophenolate mofetil in cadaveric renal transplantation: results at three years. Tricontinental Mycophenolate Mofetil Renal Transplant Study Group. *Transplantation* **65**, 956–65.

42. Illei, G.G., Takada, K., Parkin, D., Austin, H.A., Crane, M., Yarboro, C.H., *et al.* (2002) Renal flares are common in patients with severe proliferative lupus nephritis treated with pulse immunosuppressive therapy: long-term followup of a cohort of 145 patients participating in randomized controlled studies. *Arthritis Rheum* **46**, 995–1002.

43. El Hachmi, M., Jadoul, M., Lefebvre, C., Depresseux, G., and Houssiau, F.A. (2003) Relapses of lupus nephritis: incidence, risk factors, serology and impact on outcome. *Lupus* **12**, 692–6.

44. Bijl, M., Horst, G., Bootsma, H., Limburg, P.C., and Kallenberg, C.G.M. (2003) Mycophenolate mofetil prevents a clinical relapse in patients with systemic lupus erythematosus at risk. *Ann Rheum Dis* **62**, 534–9.

45. Nannini, C., Crowson, C., Matteson, E., and Moder, K. (2009) Mycophenolate mofetil is effective in reducing disease flares in systemic lupus erythematosus patients: a retrospective study. *Lupus* **18**, 394–9.

46. Contreras, G., Pardo, V., Leclercq, B., Lenz, O., Tozman, E., O'Nan, P., *et al.* (2004) Sequential therapies for proliferative lupus nephritis. *N Engl J Med* **350**, 971–80.

47. Ioannidis, J.P.A., Boki, K.A., Katsorida, M.E., Drosos, A.A., Skopouli, F.N., Boletis, J.N., *et al.* (2000) Remission relapse and re-remission of proliferative lupus nephritis treated with cyclophosphamide. *Kidney Int* **57**, 258–64.

48. Donadio, J.V. Jr. (1992) Treatment of membranous nephropathy in systemic lupus erythematosus. *Nephrol Dial Transplant* **7** (Suppl 1), 97–104.

49. Sloan, R.P., Schwartz, M.M., Korbet, S.M., Borok, R.Z., and the Lupus Nephritis Collaborative Study Group (1996) Long-term outcome in systemic lupus erythematosus membranous glomerulonephritis. *J Am Soc Nephrol* **7**, 299–305.

50. Chan, T.M., Li, F.K., Hao, W.K., Chan, K.W., Lui, S.L., Tang, S., *et al.* (1999) Treatment of membranous lupus nephritis with nephrotic syndrome by sequential immunosuppression. *Lupus* **8**, 545–51.

51. Mok, C.C., Ying, K.Y., Lau, C.S., Yim, C.W., Ng, W.L., Wong, W.S., *et al.* (2004) Treatment of pure membranous nephropathy with prednisone and azathioprine: an open-label trial. *Am J Kidney Dis* **43**, 269–76.

52. Tam, L.S., Li, E.K., Szeto, C.C., Wong, S.M., Leung, C.B., Lai, F.M., *et al.* (2001) Treatment of membranous lupus nephritis with prednisone, azathioprine, and cyclosporine A. *Lupus* **10**, 827–9.

53. Tse, K.C., Lam, M.F., Tang, S.C., Tang, C.S., and Chan, T.M. (2007) A pilot study on tacrolimus treatment in membranous or quiescent lupus nephritis with proteinuria resistant to angiotensin inhibition or blockade. *Lupus* **16**, 46–51.

54. Spetie, D.N., Tang, Y., Rovin, B.H., Nadasdy, T., Nadasdy, G., Pesavento, T.E., *et al.* (2004) Mycophenolate therapy of SLE membranous nephropathy. *Kidney Int* **66**, 2411–5.

55. Karim, M.Y., Pisoni, C.N., Ferro, L., Tungekar, M.F., Abbs, I.C., D'Cruz, D.P., *et al.* (2005) Reduction of proteinuria with mycophenolate mofetil in predominantly membranous lupus nephropathy. *Rheumatology (Oxford)* **44**, 1317–21.

56. Kasitanon, N., Petri, M., Haas, M., Magder, L.S., and Fine, D.M. (2008) Mycophenolate mofetil as the primary treatment of membranous lupus nephritis with and without concurrent proliferative disease: a retrospective study of 29 cases. *Lupus* **17**, 40–5.

57. Hauser, I.A., Renders, L., Radeke, H.H., Sterzel, R.B., and Goppelt-Struebe, M. (1999) Mycophenolate mofetil inhibits rat and human mesangial cell proliferation by guanosine depletion. *Nephrol Dial Transplant* **14**, 58–63.

58. Baer, P.C., Gauer, S., Hauser, I.A., Scherberich, J.E., and Geiger, H. (2000) Effects of mycophenolic acid on human renal proximal and distal tubular cells in vitro. *Nephrol Dial Transplant* **15**, 184–90.

59. Dubus, I., Vendrely, B., Christophe, I., Labouyrie, J.P., Delmas, Y., Bonnet, J., *et al.* (2002) Mycophenolic acid antagonizes the activation of cultured human mesangial cells. *Kidney Int* **62**, 857–67.

60. Morath, C., and Zeier, M. (2003) Review of the antiproliferative properties of mycophenolate mofetil in non-immune cells. *Int J Clin Pharmacol Ther* **41**, 465–9.

61. Park, J., Ha, H., Seo, J., Kim, M.S., Kim, H.J., Huh, K.H., *et al.* (2004) Mycophenolic acid inhibits platelet-derived growth factor-induced reactive oxygen species and mitogen-activated protein kinase activation in rat vascular smooth muscle cells. *Am J Transplant* **4**, 1982–90.

62. Huang, Y., Liu, Z., Huang, H., Liu, H., and Li, L. (2005) Effects of mycophenolic acid on endothelial cells. *Int Immunopharmacol* **5**, 1029–39.

63. Badid, C., Vincent, M., McGregor, B., Melin, M., Hadj-Aissa, A., Veysseyre, C., *et al.* (2000) Mycophenolate mofetil reduces myofibroblast infiltration and collagen III deposition in rat remnant kidney. *Kidney Int* **58**, 51–61.

64. Chan, T.M., Leung, J.K., Ho, S.K., and Yung, S. (2002) Mesangial cell-binding anti-DNA antibodies in patients with systemic lupus erythematosus. *J Am Soc Nephrol* **13**, 1219–29.

65. Yung, S., Tsang, R.C., Sun, Y., Leung, J.K., and Chan, T.M. (2005) Effect of human anti-DNA antibodies on proximal renal tubular epithelial cell cytokine expression: implications on tubulointerstitial inflammation in lupus nephritis. *J Am Soc Nephrol* **16**, 3281–94.

66. Yung, S., Tsang, R.C., Leung, J.K., and Chan, T.M. (2006) Increased mesangial cell hyaluronan expression in lupus nephritis is mediated by anti-DNA antibody-induced IL-1beta. *Kidney Int* **69**, 272–80.

67. Yung, S., Zhang, Q., Zhang, C.Z., Chan, K.W., Lui, S.L., and Chan, T.M. (2009) Anti-DNA antibody induction of protein kinase C phosphorylation and fibronectin synthesis in human and murine lupus and the effect of mycophenolic acid. *Arthritis Rheum* **60**, 2071–82.

68. Wilson, E.C., Jayne, D.R., Dellow, E., and Fordham, R.J. (2007) The cost-effectiveness of mycophenolate mofetil as firstline therapy in active lupus nephritis. *Rheumatology* **46**, 1096–101.

69. Tse, K.C., Tang, C.S., Lam, M.F., Yap, D.Y., and Chan, T.M. (2009) Cost comparison between mycophenolate mofetil and cyclophosphamide-azathioprine in the treatment of lupus nephritis. *J Rheumatology* **36**, 76–81.

70. Tang, Z., Yang, G., Yu, C., Yu, Y., Wang, J, Hu, W., *et al.* (2008) Effects of mycophenolate mofetil for patients with crescentic lupus nephritis. *Nephrology* **13**, 702–7.

71. Korbet, S.M., Schwartz, M.M., Evans, J., Lewis, E.J., for the Collaborative Study Group. (2007) Severe lupus nephritis: racial differences in presentation and outcome. *J Am Soc Nephrol* **18**, 244–54.

72. Boumpas, D.T., Austin, H.A., III., Vaughn, E.M., Klippel, J.H., Steinberg, A.D., Yarboro, C.H., *et al.* (1992) Controlled trial of pulse methylprednisolone versus two regimens of pulse cyclophosphamide in severe lupus nephritis. *Lancet* **340**, 741–5.

73. Houssiau, F.A., Vasconcelos, C., D'Cruz, D., Sebastiani, GD., de Ramon Garrido, E., Danieli, M.G., *et al.* (2010) The 10-year follow-up data of the Euro-Lupus Nephritis Trial comparing low-dose versus high-dose intravenous cyclophosphamide. *Ann Rheum Dis* **69**, 61–4.

74. Rivera, T.L., Belmont, H.M., Malani, S., Latorre, M., Benton, L., Weisstuch, J., *et al.* (2009) Current therapies for lupus nephritis in an ethnically heterogeneous cohort. *J Rheumatol* **36**, 298–305.

75. Lau, K.K., Jones, D.P., Hastings, M.C., Gaber, L.W., and Ault, B.H. (2006) Short-term outcomes of severe lupus nephritis in a cohort of predominantly African-American children. *Pediatr Nephrol* **21**, 655–62.

76. Lau, K.K., Ault, B.H., Jones, D.P., and Butani, L. (2008) Induction therapy for pediatric focal proliferative lupus nephritis: cyclophosphamide versus mycophenolate mofetil. *J Pediatr Health Care* **22**, 282–8.

77. Cramer, C.H., II, Mills, M., Valentini, R.P., Smoyer, W.E., Haftel, H., and Brophy, P.D. (2007) Clinical presentation and outcome in a cohort of paediatric patients with membranous lupus nephritis. *Nephrol Dial Transplant* **22**, 3495–500.

78. Paredes, A. (2007) Can mycophenolate mofetil substitute cyclophosphamide treatment of pediatric lupus nephritis? *Pediatr Nephrol* **22**, 1077–82.

79. Zahr, N., Amoura, Z., Debord, J., Hulot, J.S., Saint-Marcoux, F., Marquet, P., *et al.* (2008) Pharmacokinetic study of mycophenolate mofetil in patients with systemic lupus erythematosus and design of Bayesian estimator using limited sampling strategies. *Clin Pharmacokinet* **47**, 277–84.

80. Knight, S.R., and Morris, P.J. (2008) Does the evidence support the use of mycophenolate mofetil therapeutic drug monitoring in clinical practice? A systematic review. *Transplantation* **85**, 1675–85.

81. Mino, Y., Naito, T., Matsushita, T., Otsuka, A., Ushiyama, T., Ozono, S., *et al.* (2008) Comparison of pharmacokinetics of mycophenolic acid and its glucuronide between patients with lupus nephritis and with kidney transplantation. *Ther Drug Monit* **30**, 656–61.

82. Joy, M.S., Hilliard, T., Hu, Y., Hogan, S.L., Dooley, M.A., Falk, R.J., *et al.* (2009) Pharmacokinetics of mycophenolic acid in patients with lupus nephritis. *Pharmacotherapy* **29**, 7–16.

83. Van Hest, R.M., Mathot, R.A., Pescovitz, M.D., Gordon, R., Mamelok, R.D., and van Gelder, T. (2006) Explaining variability in mycophenolic acid exposure to optimize mycophenolate mofetil dosing: a population pharmacokinetic meta-analysis of mycophenolic acid in renal transplant recipients. *J Am Soc Nephrol* **17**, 871–80.

84. Neumann, I., Fuhrmann, H., Fang, I.F., Jaeger, A., Bayer, P., and Kovarik, J. (2008) Association between mycophenolic acid 12-h trough levels and clinical endpoints in patients with autoimmune disease on mycophenolate mofetil. *Nephrol Dial Transplant* **23**, 3514–20.

85. Appel, G.B., and Cameron, J.S. (2007) Lupus nephritis. In: *Comprehensive Clinical Nephrology*, *3rd* Edition (J. Feehally, J. Floege, and R.J. Johnson, eds), pp. 291–303. Mosby Elsevier, Philadelphia, USA.

86. Bertsias, G., Ioannidis, J.P., Boletis, J., Bombardieri, S., Cervera, R., Dostal, C., *et al.* (2008) EULAR recommendations for the management of systemic lupus erythematosus. Report of a task force of the EULAR Standing Committee for International Clinical Studies including Therapeutics. *Ann Rheum Dis* **67**, 195–205.

Chapter 11

Lupus nephritis and pregnancy

Kate Bramham, Sarah Germain, and
Catherine Nelson-Piercy

Introduction

Systemic lupus erythematosus (SLE) commonly affects women of childbearing age. Therefore, knowledge of the relationship of the condition with respect to fertility and pregnancy is important for all clinicians involved in management of women with SLE. Pregnancy may affect disease course, and the presence of SLE, diagnosed before, during, and after pregnancy, can influence pregnancy outcome. Women with lupus nephritis have particularly high complication rates in pregnancy. The majority are taking multiple medications, the benefits and risks of which need to be evaluated for the wellbeing of the mother and the fetus.

Numbers affected

Prevalence of SLE in one UK study was 52.0/100,000 in females and 25–45% of patients, depending on racial origin, were less than 40 years old.[1] In another UK study in North West England in 2001, the incidence of lupus nephritis was 0.41 per 100,000/ year with a rate of 0.68 (95% CI 0.40–1.10) in women and 0.09 (95% CI 0.01–0.32) in men, median age 36 in women and 65 in men.[2] Using the assumption of conception at a replacement population birth rate, it is estimated that in a population of 1 million, there will be a birth rate of 5–10 pregnancies/year in women with SLE.[3]

Fertility

Women with SLE generally have normal fertility,[4,5] even if disease is active,[6] but rates of fetal loss are increased, even before the development of clinical manifestations.[4,5,7,8] In the presence of impaired renal function, fertility may be reduced.[9] Women with chronic kidney disease (CKD) develop amenorrhea and anovulation with progressive renal impairment, although it is unclear at exactly what level of renal function this occurs.[9] Renal transplantation rapidly restores fertility and some women with severe renal impairment may be advised to delay conception until after transplantation.[10,11]

Use of cyclophosphamide has previously been associated with ovarian failure.[12] However, it has now been demonstrated that the total dose of cyclophosphamide and age >35 years old are the most important predictors of anovulation.[13,14] The relationship between renal impairment, use of cyclophosphamide, and ovarian failure has not been explored, but in one study two women with serum creatinine >2 mg/dl developed ovarian failure after 2 months of treatment.[12]

Normal renal physiological changes in pregnancy

During pregnancy profound physiological changes occur within the kidney. An increase in glomerular filtration rate (GFR) is detectable within 3–4 weeks of conception. Glomerular filtration rate progressively rises to 50% above nonpregnant levels by the end of the first trimester and is predominantly driven by an 80% increase in renal plasma flow.[15] Glomerular micropuncture studies in rats suggest that this hyperfiltration does not result in increased intraglomerular pressure, as both afferent and efferent arteriolar resistance are reduced in parallel.[16] As a consequence of increased GFR and plasma volume expansion, serum creatinine falls in pregnancy. Modification of diet in renal disease (MDRD) estimation of GFR (eGFR) underestimates creatinine clearance by up to 40% in pregnant women, and therefore should not be used in pregnancy.[17]

Elevated GFR together with changes in glomerular and tubular handling of protein results in an increase in proteinuria, with the upper limit of normal rising to 300 mg/24 hours (30 mg/mmol creatinine). Increased calcium excretion also occurs, which may predispose to calculi in susceptible individuals. Erythropoietin and vitamin D synthesis increase in order to meet elevated requirements.

Dilatation of the renal tract is a normal finding in pregnancy. "Physiological" hydronephrosis occurs in more than half of pregnant women by the middle of the second trimester and renal volume may increase by 30%.[18] Consequent urinary stasis may predispose to the development of urinary tract infection, and therefore screening for asymptomatic bacteriuria is suggested in those at risk as cystitis and pyelonephritis are four times more common in pregnancy than in nonpregnant cases. Furthermore, pyelonephritis has been associated with pre-term labour and low birth weight.[19]

Lupus and pregnancy hormones

There is a 9:1 female to male ratio in those affected by SLE, and it has therefore been proposed that the gender difference is due to sex hormones. Many mechanisms of estrogen action on the immune system have been reported, including upregulation of pathogenic autoreactive B cells[20] and increased production of autoantibodies in murine studies.[21] In the NZB/NZW murine SLE model, removal of estrogen or addition of androgen improves survival,[22] although in the MRL/lpr mouse model, estrogen worsens immune-complex glomerulonephritis but improves T cell-mediated disease manifestations, e.g. peri-articular inflammation.[23] Oral contraceptives and hormone replacement therapy may increase the development of later-onset SLE[24] and one case–control study has suggested that oral contraceptives exacerbate pre-existing lupus nephritis.[25] In contrast, other case–control[26] and cross-sectional[27] studies have not found any association with disease activity and oral contraceptive use. A randomized clinical trial comparing estrogen-containing oral contraceptive with placebo for 1 year in women with inactive SLE did not demonstrate any difference in flare rate,[28] nor did another clinical trial comparing the use of combined oral contraceptives, intrauterine device, or progesterone-only pill,[29] suggesting that estrogen alone is unlikely to be responsible for the female preponderance of SLE.

In men with SLE, higher estrogen levels and lower testosterone levels have been described.[30] Similarly in women, low testosterone is reported as well as reduced dehydroepiandrosterone (DHEA).[31] Replacement of DHEA has been shown to improve outcome in both murine SLE models[32] and randomized controlled trials.[33,34] Recently, it has been suggested that prolactin is also an important mediator of disease in SLE, as high prolactin levels are associated with disease activity.[35] In murine models, hyperprolactinemia exacerbates SLE regardless of estrogen levels,[36] and, in both humans and mice, bromocriptine has been shown to modulate disease activity.[37] Prolactin levels rise throughout pregnancy and peak during lactation, which may contribute to post-partum flare.

Currently it appears that estrogen, prolactin, DHEA, and testosterone may have a role in disease activity in SLE, and it is likely that the complex interaction between these sex hormones contributes to gender differences in prevalence of SLE. Substantial changes occur in sex hormone levels during pregnancy, but how these alterations affect disease activity during pregnancy is currently poorly understood.

Effect of pregnancy on lupus and renal disease

Disease activity during pregnancy

General

Numerous reports with conflicting outcomes have attempted to address the issue of the influence of pregnancy on SLE activity.[38–42] Comparison of these studies is hampered by different definitions of disease activity, diagnosis of renal and extrarenal disease, inclusion of women with active disease at conception or women with disease diagnosed during pregnancy. A study of 73 pregnancies in 53 women with lupus nephritis, compared with 78 nonpregnant controls suggested that pregnancy itself did not influence renal disease activity.[43] Similarly, another study of 51 pregnancies in 38 women with lupus nephritis used as their own controls did not identify an increased incidence of disease flare associated with pregnancy.[44] Renal disease activity appears to be more common post-partum,[43] whereas extrarenal disease flare occurs predominantly in the second and third trimesters.[41,45]

Lupus nephritis flare

Lupus nephritis flare is commonly accompanied by extrarenal disease flare. Studies from 1970 to 1992 have included 276 women who had a diagnosis of lupus nephritis at conception, 133 (48%) had an exacerbation of renal disease during pregnancy, and at least 16% of these women developed nephrotic range proteinuria.[7,46–61] However a more recent multi-center retrospective study[63] reporting renal and pregnancy outcomes of 113 pregnancies in 81 women with lupus nephritis diagnosed before pregnancy between 1984 and 2004 suggests an improvement in rates of renal flare. Fifteen percent of these women had hypertension, 11% had CKD stage 3, and 76% were in remission at conception. Renal flare occurred in only 15% of pregnancies and in another 15% of women up to a year post-partum. Lupus nephritis activity was more common in women with active disease at conception, in partial remission, those with proteinuria >1 g/24 hours or with GFR <60 ml/min/1.73m^2, and those not on treatment. After treatment, complete or partial recovery was achieved in two-thirds of cases.

Another recent small study of women with SLE, which included a group of 11 women with 20 pregnancies with quiescent lupus nephritis, reported a rate of 10% of women developing renal flare.[62] This reduction in rate of renal flare may reflect an improvement in pre-pregnancy counseling, in which more women are advised to delay conception until disease activity is controlled, together with the development of newer immunosuppressive agents used before pregnancy, such as mycophenolate mofetil, which has improved renal outcome for women with lupus nephritis.

Extrarenal disease flare

In a recent study of 113 pregnancies in women with lupus nephritis, 12% of pregnancies were complicated by flare of extrarenal disease without renal involvement.[63] Another study of 53 pregnancies in women with quiescent lupus nephritis only reported one case of extrarenal flare. Disease flare, regardless of the site, in pregnancy is usually no more severe than in the nonpregnant state.[64]

Progression of renal disease

Several retrospective studies and two recent prospective studies have evaluated the risk of progression of renal disease as a result of pregnancy. Women with mild renal impairment can be reassured that there is a less than 3% chance of a permanent deterioration in renal function.[65] In women with creatinine >125 μmol/l, renal function has been reported to deteriorate in 20% of cases during pregnancy and in 23% after 6 weeks to 6 months post-partum. Some of these women recover renal function by 6 months, but 31% have a pregnancy-related persistent decline.[66] Even temporary renal deterioration may have serious consequences, including pre-term iatrogenic delivery. Some women may require temporary hemodialysis to allow the fetus to reach a viable gestation, which may be detrimental not only to the fetus, but also to preservation of maternal renal function.

Imbasciati *et al.* recently published a comprehensive prospective series of 49 women with mean serum creatinine at conception 186±88 μmol/l. They reported that the most important predictors of permanent deterioration of renal disease were pre-pregnancy GFR<40 ml/min/m^2 and level of proteinuria (>1 g/24 hours) and concluded that both factors need to be present for a statistically significant increase in risk of long-term renal damage.[67]

Few studies have specifically studied the effect of pregnancy on long-term renal function in lupus nephritis. Packham *et al.* reported that 19% of 41 pregnancies were complicated by impaired renal function (Cr>110 mmol or an increase in Cr of 50% or more), and in only one case was this irreversible.[55] Four out of 19 women with lupus nephritis, in a study by Imbasciati *et al.*, developed acute renal failure after delivery, two of whom never regained renal function and died.[52] Bobrie *et al.* found that out of 53 pregnancies in women with lupus nephritis, six had severe deterioration in renal function, of whom four progressed rapidly to end stage renal failure.[7]

In a meta-analysis of 17 studies of pregnancies affected by SLE, 10% of women with lupus nephritis developed acute renal failure, in 3% the decline in renal function was permanent, without requiring dialysis, and a further 6% progressed to end stage renal failure or death.[7,46–61] However, a more recent study of lupus nephritis in pregnancy by Imbasciati *et al.*,[63] which included 11% of women with CKD stage 3 found only 2% of women suffered a progressive deterioration in GFR, without requiring dialysis and only 1% needed renal replacement therapy.

Effect of lupus nephritis on pregnancy outcome

Maternal outcome

Pre-eclampsia

Pre-eclampsia is a multi-organ syndrome of placental origin and is characterized by systemic endothelial cell activation. It is more common in SLE patients than in the general population, even in women with matched levels of renal impairment.[53,68] For those with SLE but without renal disease, the incidence of pre-eclampsia is 13–35%.[69] The rate of pre-eclampsia in women with lupus nephritis may be as low 9%,[63] but has been found to occur in up to 35% in women who were diagnosed with lupus nephritis during pregnancy.[70] Higher rates are also described in pregnancies that were unplanned or with active disease at conception.[62,71]

Maternal death

A review of 345 pregnancies in 218 women with lupus nephritis identified a maternal death rate of 3.4%.[59] The majority of deaths were directly attributable to renal disease. The long-term prognosis of lupus nephritis has improved over recent decades due to more effective therapeutic strategies and better patient surveillance.[72] In more recent series only five deaths were reported, all of which were due to maternal sepsis.[44,52,71] Some severe cases of lupus nephritis flare occurring in pregnancy do still result in maternal death,[44,71,73] even in women with quiescent disease at conception.[62]

Fetal outcome

Fetal loss

Successful pregnancy outcome in women with lupus nephritis, excluding terminations, ranges from 65% to 92%.[44,53,59,63,68,71,73,74] Two reports have suggested that active disease at conception is associated with increased fetal loss,[44,62] but this has not been confirmed by another study.[73] Similarly, a significant association between fetal loss and SLE activity during pregnancy has been found in many,[42,44,50,57,71] but not all studies.[7,40,42,75] Inactive lupus nephritis at conception in women with preserved renal function is not associated with higher rates of fetal loss than in women with SLE without lupus nephritis.[62]

Pre-term delivery and small for gestational age (SGA)

Pre-term delivery is a common complication in SLE pregnancies and is further increased in those with renal involvement to a rate of 30–58%.[44,63,76] The pregnancy outcomes of women with lupus nephritis were compared to those in women with SLE but no renal involvement, and, although median gestation was shorter in those women with active disease, it was only statistically significantly shortened in those with active lupus nephritis at conception.[62] In a study of 113 pregnancies in women diagnosed with lupus nephritis before pregnancy, 24% of infants were SGA,[63] although, in another study, rates of SGA were even lower than expected for the normal population, even in women with active lupus nephritis.[62]

Neonatal lupus syndromes

Anti-Ro (SSA) and anti-La (SSB) antibodies are found in approximately a third of women with SLE,[77] and may be asymptomatic. These antibodies can cross the placenta and cause specific fetal complications. Cutaneous neonatal lupus occurs in 5% of women with anti-Ro antibodies.[78] The neonate is affected by a nonscarring photosensitive rash, which usually appears after 2 weeks. It usually resolves by 6 months, which correlates with the disappearance of maternal antibody, and does not require treatment.

Congenital heart block occurs in 2% of babies of women with positive antibodies; however, if a previous child has been affected, the risk increases to 15–20%, and up to 50% if two children have been affected.[79] The usual clinical presentation is fetal bradycardia and/or congestive cardiac failure, and fetal/neonatal mortality may be as high as 30%.[79] Regular assessment, including fetal echocardiography at 18–20 weeks and in the third trimester, is recommended for all women with positive anti-Ro/La antibodies. For affected babies that survive to be born, delivery at a neonatal unit with a pediatric cardiologist is advised as a pacemaker is usually required. Currently, no form of immunosuppressive intervention, including corticosteroids, plasma exchange, or intravenous immunoglobulin, has reliably been shown to reduce the risk of congenital heart block.[79]

Factors influencing pregnancy outcome

Disease activity at conception

Disease activity at conception has been shown by several authors to influence both pregnancy outcome and disease activity.[40,44,50,55,62,63,73,75,80] In a review of pregnancies in women with active lupus at the time of conception, fetal loss was 26%.[63] Flare occurred in 60% of pregnancies in an unselected group,[81] but in planned pregnancies was reduced to 27%.[82] Hypocomplementemia at conception has been identified as a predictor of fetal loss and perinatal death,[40,63,83] although in another study was not associated with worse pregnancy outcome.[59] Quiescent disease at conception was found by one group to be the only predictor of favorable maternal outcomes in women with lupus nephritis.[44]

Level of renal function

Women with CKD have worse pregnancy outcomes than healthy individuals. Even women with normal renal function have an elevated risk of pre-eclampsia, and for those with more severe renal impairment (creatinine >250 µmol/l) successful pregnancy outcome is only reported to occur in 46% of cases, with 57–73% complicated by fetal growth restriction and/or pre-term delivery.[84] In a meta-analysis of pregnancy outcome according to stage of CKD, women with lupus nephritis have worse overall pregnancy outcome than women with the same level of renal function but other causes of CKD.[85] Moroni and Ponticelli described fetal loss in half of all conceptions in women with creatinine >106 µmol/l and 60% fetal loss in pregnancies with creatinine rising above 133 µmol/l during pregnancy.[70] Possible mechanisms underlying this finding have not been explored, but one explanation could be increased systemic inflammation in women with SLE, which has been demonstrated to be a predisposing factor for the development of poor pregnancy outcomes.

Hypertension

Hypertension diagnosed before pregnancy affects up to 25% of pregnancies in women with SLE, and is associated with a risk of superimposed pre-eclampsia, pre-term delivery, fetal growth restriction, and placental abruption.[86–88] Hypertension is even more common in women with lupus nephritis, and occurred in 44% of pregnancies according to Packham et al., was irreversible in 14%, and was more common in pregnancies that predated a diagnosis of SLE.[55] Rates of fetal loss in women with lupus nephritis have been reported to be higher in women with hypertension (29%) compared to those with normal blood pressure.[59]

Treated hypertension was not related to outcome in one study,[59] but this finding may be related to the small number of women included in the study.

Proteinuria

Proteinuria has been associated with worse pregnancy outcome in some series,[50,54,63,71] but not others,[59] although women who developed nephrotic syndrome tended to deliver earlier. A review of pregnancies in women with lupus nephritis found that proteinuria >0.5 g/24 hours was associated with a 57% rate of fetal loss, compared to 9% in women with no proteinuria.[70] Proteinuria may increase due to the physiological changes in pregnancy, but may also be related to the discontinuation of angiotensin converting enzyme inhibitor (ACEI) I. Up to a doubling of proteinuria may be expected as a result of normal physiological response to pregnancy, but more than this would suggest the development of pre-eclampsia or a flare of lupus nephritis.

Histological class

It might be expected that women with more aggressive histological features of lupus nephritis have worse pregnancy outcome. Packham et al. suggested that membranous nephritis was associated with a lower perinatal mortality rate than diffuse proliferative glomerulonephritis,[55] and Oviasu et al. found that pre-term deliveries only occurred in women with Class III, IV, and V lupus nephritis.[59] In addition, half the miscarriages in this study were in women with Class V. Another study identified an increased incidence of hypertension and pre-eclampsia in women with Class III and IV, than Class II and V.[68] However, several small studies have directly addressed this issue, and none has found any direct association between histological class and pregnancy outcome.[59,62,63,68,71,89] As previously described, disease activity at conception, regardless of histological diagnosis, is a more important determinant of pregnancy outcome. Of the small number of cases of lupus nephritis diagnosed *de novo* during pregnancy, classes III and IV appear to develop more severe disease than classes I and II.[44,71]

Antiphospholipid (APL) antibodies

Approximately a third of women with SLE have positive APL antibodies (lupus anticoagulant (LA) or anticardiolipin (ACL) antibodies).[90] Additional features, including arterial or venous thrombosis, recurrent early fetal demise, (more than three miscarriages at <10 weeks' gestation), fetal death at >10 weeks' gestation with normal fetal morphology, or pre-term birth at <34 weeks as a result of pre-eclampsia or placental insufficiency must be present to make a diagnosis of antiphospholipid syndrome (APS).[91] In a prospective study of pregnancies in women with SLE, women with APL antibodies had the highest rate of fetal loss,[42] and complications such as miscarriage, growth restriction, and pre-term delivery have also been reported to occur three times more often when APL antibodies are positive in women with SLE.[92]

Some women with APL antibodies alone have completely unremarkable obstetric histories despite having markedly elevated antibody titers.[93,94] Those at greatest risk appear to be women with previous poor pregnancy outcome.[95-99] Expert opinion suggests that there should be a further subcategorization of APS patients, those with previous recurrent miscarriages or fetal loss, and those with previous thromboembolic events, as there appear to be distinct differences in pregnancy outcome between these two groups, with the former group having fewer complications in pregnancy when on treatment.[100]

Prophylactic low molecular weight heparin (LMWH), together with aspirin 75 mg once daily (od), is given throughout the pregnancy and continued up to 6 weeks postpartum in women with a previous history of thromboembolism or late fetal loss, neonatal death or adverse outcome due to pre-eclampsia, fetal growth restriction, or abruption. Women already taking warfarin should be switched to LMWH twice daily by 6 weeks, or as soon as pregnancy is confirmed. Women with a history of recurrent miscarriage but no other adverse events may be managed with aspirin 75 mg od alone,[101] or aspirin plus LMWH, if they have previously miscarried on aspirin alone. Low molecular weight heparin can be discontinued at 12 weeks' gestation or at 20 weeks if the uterine artery Doppler scan is normal.

Diagnosis during pregnancy

Diagnosis of lupus nephritis during pregnancy is associated with worse outcomes,[4,44,50,52,71] both for the fetus and the mother. Packham *et al.* examined the pregnancy outcome of 41 women and 64 pregnancies from a single center, which included 18 pregnancies during which a diagnosis of lupus nephritis had been made. Pregnancies occurring after the diagnosis of lupus nephritis had been established were complicated by less hypertension, and proteinuria, but there was no difference in the incidence of impaired renal function.[55]

Management

Pre-pregnancy counseling

All women of childbearing age with lupus nephritis should be offered the opportunity for pre-pregnancy counseling. This allows the woman to be informed of the risk of complications during the pregnancy and post-partum to both herself and her baby. Medications can also be reviewed and adjusted if necessary.

During pre-pregnancy counseling a woman needs to be assessed for severity of renal disease, disease activity, and associated antibodies, which may cause further complications (APL and/or anti-Ro/La antibodies). Pulmonary hypertension should be excluded as it is an absolute contraindication to pregnancy due to the high associated maternal mortality. Cardiac status and valvular disease may also need to be investigated. Suggested pre-pregnancy investigations are listed in Table 11.1. Women should have inactive disease for 6 months before attempting to conceive. A period of 3–6 months following changes in medication should be allowed to allow stabilization and dose adjustment on the new drug.

Table 11.1 Pre-pregnancy, baseline, and maternal surveillance investigations

Blood	
Full blood count	
Urea, creatinine, electrolytes	
Uric acid	
Liver function tests	
Antinuclear antibodies	
dsDNA	
C3 and C4	
Anti-Ro and anti-La antibodies (ENA)	
Lupus anticoagulant and anticardiolipin antibodies	
Other	
Urinalysis or protein:creatinine ratio	
Blood pressure	
Pre-pregnancy	**During pregnancy**
Echocardiogram	Assessment of fetal growth
Pulmonary function tests	Fetal heart rate (in those at risk of congenital block)

Antenatal care

During pregnancy women should be regularly reviewed by a multi-disciplinary antenatal team, including obstetricians, midwives, nephrologists, and/or obstetric physicians. Routine investigations at the start and during pregnancy are listed in Table 11.1. All women with lupus nephritis should be advised to take low-dose aspirin unless there are contraindications, as it has been shown to reduce the risk of pre-eclampsia by 17% in high-risk pregnancies[102] and is also associated with improved fetal and neonatal survival in women with lupus nephritis.[63]

Diagnosis of disease flare

Clinicians should remain vigilant for the development of flare of both renal and extrarenal disease in addition to pregnancy complications including pre-eclampsia. Diagnosis of lupus activity may be difficult as many features of pregnancy mimic SLE disease activity (see Table 11.2). There are several indices of lupus activity that have been adapted for use in pregnancy (Lupus Activity Criteria Count (LACC), Systemic Lupus Erythematosus Disease Activity Index (SLEDAI-2K));[103] however, they should be used in centers that routinely report disease activity in this manner, otherwise misdiagnosis may occur. In our experience, one of the most reliable ways of diagnosing disease flare is by asking the woman whether her symptoms are typical of her SLE.

Table 11.2 Common clinical features of pregnancy and systemic lupus erythematosus

Clinical features	SLE	Pregnancy
General	Fatigue and malaise	Fatigue
Hair	Loss	Loss or gain
Skin	Malar rash	Melasma/chloasma
		Facial flushing
Joint pain and swelling	Inflammatory synovitis	Mechanical arthralgia
		Bland knee effusion
Seizure	Neuropsychiatric lupus	Eclampsia
Edema	Lupus nephritis flare	Pre-eclampsia
Anemia	Hemolytic anemia	Hemodilution
	Anemia of chronic disease	Iron deficiency
Thrombocytopenia	Immune thrombocytopenia	Pre-eclampsia
		HELLP syndrome
Deranged LFTs	Lupus hepatitis (usually transaminases)	Pre-eclampsia
		HELLP syndrome
		Obstetric cholestasis
ESR	Elevated	Elevated

ESR, erythrocyte sedimentation rate; HELLP, hemolysis elevated liver enzymes low platelets; LFT, liver function tests; SLE, systemic lupus erythematosus.

Pre-eclampsia and lupus nephritis flare

Distinguishing between pre-eclampsia and active lupus nephritis can be a clinical challenge for both nephrologists and obstetricians, as both conditions are associated with hypertension, proteinuria, thrombocytopenia, and renal impairment. Close monitoring of urine protein is necessary to detect developing pre-eclampsia. Levels of >300 mg/24 hours or a protein:creatinine ratio (p/c) of >30 mg/μmol together with new-onset hypertension (a blood pressure >140/90 mmHg on two separate occasions greater than 6 hours apart) confirms the diagnosis of pre-eclampsia.[104] Diagnosis is more challenging in women with pre-existing hypertension or proteinuria. Other symptoms may include visual disturbance, headache, epigastric pain, and edema. Hypertension should be treated and drugs such as methydopa, nifedipine, hydralazine, labetolol, and doxazocin are safe in pregnancy. A woman with confirmed pre-eclampsia should be monitored for fetal growth restriction.

Table 11.3 shows the features that pre-eclampsia and lupus nephritis have in common, and useful markers to assist discrimination and diagnosis. Biochemical markers such as a rise in uric acid and/or transaminases may help support the diagnosis of pre-eclampsia. The most useful markers of disease activity include the presence of active urinary sediment, active extrarenal disease, and rising lupus serology (anti-dsDNA antibodies). One study suggested that anti-dsDNA antibodies are more useful for distinguishing between pre-eclampsia and active lupus nephritis than low C3 and C4, which are usually elevated in pregnancy, and have been shown to fall in the absence of flare in over 50% of pregnancies complicated by lupus nephritis.[71]

There are few indications for renal biopsy in pregnancy, but if the diagnosis of acute lupus nephritis is suspected at less than 24–28 weeks' gestation a biopsy may be appropriate, as the result is likely to affect management decisions. Despite reports suggesting that renal biopsy is safe in pregnancy,[105] many are reluctant to perform the procedure, as it requires operator experience in taking the biopsy in the upright position.

Table 11.3 Distinguishing features of lupus nephritis and pre-eclampsia

Investigations	Lupus nephritis flare	Pre-eclampsia
Differentiating features		
Urine analysis – blood and or red cell casts	Present	Absent
Anti-DNA antibodies	Raised	Normal
Complement C3 and C4	Low	Normal or raised
Liver function tests	Normal	Normal or raised
Similar features		
Hypertension	Present	Present and rising
Proteinuria	Present	Present
Low platelets	Present	Present
Rising creatinine	Present	Present

If the diagnosis of lupus nephritis is confirmed, steroids are the treatment of choice. For more severe disease, pulsed methyl-prednisolone may be indicated, and, in some cases, adjustment or the introduction of steroid-sparing agents, usually azathioprine, may be necessary. Beyond 28 weeks' gestation when the fetus is viable, delivery may be the most appropriate course if mother or fetus are at risk, in order to allow diagnosis and administration of drugs such as cyclophosphamide and rituximab, which are contraindicated in pregnancy (see Table 11.4). Rituximab has been shown to cross the placenta and inhibit neonatal B lymphocyte development.[106] Some authors have reported miscarriage in the first trimester and fetal demise in the second trimester with the use of cyclophosphamide for the treatment of lupus nephritis;[107] however, others have described successful outcomes for both mother and baby with use in both the first and second trimesters.[108,109] Evidence from studies of women treated with cyclophosphamide for breast cancer and lymphoma in the second and third trimester[110–112] suggest that cyclophosphamide may be less harmful to the fetus than previously considered, therefore it could be used as a last resort in a woman with severe lupus nephritis who is not responding to other treatment. However, in view of its potential tetratogenic effects, it should be avoided in the first trimester. In cases of severe flare, where both mother and baby are at risk, termination of the pregnancy may be discussed in order to allow more aggressive treatment of disease.

Any woman taking >7.5 mg prednisolone daily for more than 2 weeks should have intravenous hydrocortisone to cover the stress of delivery. If delivery is expected within the next 2 weeks and the platelet count is below 50×10^9/l, prednisolone and/or intravenous immunoglobulin is recommended to increase the platelet count, reduce the risk of hemorrhage, and facilitate regional analgesia or anesthesia.

Extrarenal disease flare

Traditional nonsteroidal anti-inflammatory drugs (NSAIDs), e.g. ibuprofen and diclofenac, are usually avoided in pregnancy; paracetamol-based analgesia and corticosteroids are used in preference. However, NSAIDS are generally safe during pregnancy (see Table 11.4) and can occasionally be used to manage some persistent symptoms of extrarenal disease flare (such as pleuritic pain) in pregnancy providing renal function is preserved. They should be avoided after 32 weeks' gestation though, due to risk of premature closure of ductus arteriosus. Misoprostol-containing preparations, e.g. Arthrotec, are contraindicated in pregnancy due to the effects of prostaglandin E on the uterus. Newer NSAIDs, especially COX-2 specific inhibitor, should also be avoided as there are inadequate data regarding safety in pregnancy. Paracetamol and codeine-based analgesia may be used and are preferred for pain relief.

Thromboprophylaxis

All pregnant women become increasingly prothrombotic throughout pregnancy, due to alterations in hemostatic profiles.[113,114] Those with APL antibodies are at particularly high risk, and in one report over half of thromboembolic events in women with APS occurred in association with pregnancy or estrogen-containing contraception.[12] Women with SLE have higher rates of thromboembolism than background and have a further elevated risk in pregnancy, particularly those with a history of thromboembolism.[115]

Table 11.4 Safety of analgesia and immunosuppressants in pregnancy[138,139]

Drug	Transplacental passage	Human teratogenicity	Fetal/neonatal effects	Safe in pregnancy	Safe in breast-feeding
Paracetamol				Yes	Yes
Nonsteroidal anti-inflammatory drugs	Yes	No	Constriction of ductus arteriosus and renal blood flow restriction in late pregnancy	Yes	Yes
Cyclooxygenase II inhibitors	Unknown	Unknown	Unknown	Unknown	Unknown
Prednisolone	Limited	Possible increase in oral clefts	Rare (cataract, adrenal insufficiency, and infection)	Yes	Yes
Hydroxychloroquine	Yes	No	Not at recommended doses	Yes	Yes
Sulfasalazine	Yes	No	Case reports of aplastic anemia and neutropenia at >2g maternal dose	Yes	Yes
Azathioprine	Yes	No	Sporadic congenital abnormalities, transient immune alterations in neonates	Yes	Probably safe
Mycophenolate mofetil	Yes	Three case reports	Not reported	No – stop 3/12 preconception	No
Tacrolimus	Yes	No	Hyperkalemia and renal impairment	Yes	Probably possible
Cyclophosphamide	Yes – animal data	Yes	Chromosomal abnormalities and cytopenia	Yes, late pregnancy for severe disease	No
Cyclosporine	Yes	No	Transient immune alterations	Yes	Probably possible
Intravenous Immunoglobulin	Yes	No	None reported	Yes	Yes
Rituximab	Yes	Not reported	Inhibition of neonatal B lymphocyte development	Limit to severe disease pre fetal viability where no alternative	Probably avoid

Avoid thalidomide, retinoids, and bisphosphonates.

Women with lupus nephritis potentially have the additional complication of proteinuria, which is associated with further procoagulant changes.[116] It is currently recommended that all women with proteinuria >3 g/24 hours or p/c >300 mg/mmol and serum albumin <30 g/l have thromboprophylaxis,[117] which is prescribed according to level of renal impairment. Both LMWH and unfractionated heparin are safe in pregnancy.

Women with renal impairment

Erythropoetin requirements increase during pregnancy, and women with moderate to severe renal impairment may require introduction or increased erythropoesis-stimulating agents. Vitamin D supplementation is recommended, and review by a dietician for calorific, calcium, and phosphate intake may be necessary.

It is recommended for women requiring renal replacement therapy either before or during pregnancy that hemodialysis frequency should be increased to five to seven times per week, aiming for more than 20 hours, in order to improve clearance, and reduce dramatic volume shifts. This regime appears to have been successful in several cases.[118–120]

Medication

See Table 11.4 for safety profiles of medications in pregnancy.

Corticosteroids

Steroids are usually continued in pregnancy as benefits usually outweigh risks.[121] Prednisolone is preferable as it is metabolized by the placenta to relatively inactive 11-ketoforms by 11β-hydroxysteroid dehydrogenase, and only 10% crosses into the fetal circulation at maternal doses of less than 20 mg.[122] Other glucocorticoids, including betamethasone and dexamethasone, are less well metabolized, and therefore larger amounts reach the fetus.[121] Exposure to corticosteroids in the first trimester may slightly increase rates of cleft lip and palate;[123,124] however, this has not been substantiated in all studies.[125,126] There is increased maternal risk of gestational diabetes or infection. Currently, prophylactic steroid treatment is not advised, as it has not been shown to prevent flares.[89]

Other immunosuppression

Cyclosporine[127,128] and tacrolimus[129] are nonteratatogenic; however, there is an increased risk of gestational diabetes and hypertension in women taking tacrolimus[130] and therefore screening with a glucose tolerance test is recommended at 28 weeks or sooner if there are other risk factors. Azathioprine has also been shown to be safe in pregnancy.[121,131,132] Hydroxychloroquine is safe to use throughout pregnancy[121] and should not be discontinued because of pregnancy, especially as this may result in worsening of symptoms. In any case, due to its long half-life, cessation after conception does not prevent exposure of the fetus to the drug.

Mycophenolate mofetil

Mycophenolate mofetil (MMF) is now a first line agent for the treatment of lupus nephritis. An evolving weight of animal data has demonstrated teratogenicity,[133] and, in 2004, the first case of teratogenicity in human pregnancy was described.[134] Since then, 26 cases of early exposure in 18 renal transplant patients have been reported and a clinical syndrome similar to animal studies has been identified, including hypoplastic nails, shortened fifth fingers, diaphragmatic hernia, microtia (ear deformity), micrognathia, cleft lip and palate, and congenital heart defects.[135] This has resulted in a reclassification of MMF status by the US Food and Drug Administration (FDA) to class C. Women are now advised to switch from MMF at least 3 months before conception to an immunosuppressive agent that has a safer profile in pregnancy, e.g. azathioprine, cyclosporine, or tacrolimus. There are some situations where alternatives have been tried without success or with serious side effects and MMF is the only treatment able to achieve disease stability. The woman needs to be counseled carefully about the relative risks to the fetus if she remains on MMF during her pregnancy. It is currently unknown if such defects can be detected by antenatal ultrasonography.

Angiotensin converting enzyme inhibitors (ACEI)/angiotensin receptor blockers(ARB)

Before 2006 ACEI were not advised in the second or third trimester due to an association with fetal complications, including growth restriction, oligohydramnios, hypocalvaria, renal dysplasia, anuria, renal failure, and often fetal death.[136] Cooper *et al.* published a landmark paper in the *New England Journal of Medicine* in 2005, which suggested that ACEI and ARB use in the first trimester is also associated with a 2.7-fold increase in congenital malformations.[137] Abnormalities include cardiovascular, central nervous system, and renal defects.

There are three possible approaches for those women with lupus nephritis taking ACEI/ARBs considering pregnancy. Women with minimal proteinuria taking ACEI/ARB for blood pressure control can be switched to an alternative antihypertensive known to be safe in pregnancy, e.g. nifedipine, amlodipine, labetalol, methyl dopa, or doxazosin. Women with proteinuria controlled by ACEI/ARB with mild renal impairment can be advised to stop taking their medication when they start trying to conceive, with close monitoring of blood pressure. Some women may have heavy proteinuria, which may advance their deterioration in renal function while they are attempting to conceive, particularly older women and those with more severe renal impairment; therefore, having a prolonged period without ACEI/ARB may be ill-advised. It is then recommended that ACEI/ARB are discontinued as soon as the pregnancy is confirmed, as the period of teratogenicity is considered to be from 6 weeks onwards. Women with an irregular menstrual cycle, in whom pregnancy confirmation may be delayed, need to be assessed and advised on an individual basis.

Post-partum

Post-partum monitoring is essential, as many flares of disease and thromboembolic complications occur within 6 months following delivery. All drugs that are recommended during pregnancy are also considered to be safe during breast-feeding, including azothioprine and steroids, although the data supporting cyclosporine and tacrolimus use are still limited. Angiotensin converting enzyme inhibitors may be safely used in women who are breast-feeding (recently, a drug safety article was published saying that ACEIs should be avoided because of neonatal hypotension, but we do not think this is being taken seriously).

Conclusion

Women with lupus nephritis tend to have complicated pregnancies, with increased rates of pre-eclampsia, fetal loss, pre-term delivery, low birth weight infants, and neonatal complications. However, risks are significantly reduced in those with inactive disease at conception, and in the absence of hypertension, renal impairment, and APL antibodies. Renal disease flare does not appear to be increased by pregnancy, but may be difficult to distinguish from pre-eclampsia.

Pre-pregnancy counseling is advised for women to make an informed decision about risks and potential complications associated with pregnancy. Immunosuppression needs to be reviewed, together with other medications such as analgesia and antihypertensives. Careful assessment for complicating factors, including anti-Ro and anti-La antibodies, APL antibodies, and the presence of hypertension, proteinuria, and pulmonary hypertension, is important. Antenatal care should be delivered by a multidisciplinary team with expertise in the care of women with SLE and renal disease. Surveillance for disease flare and pregnancy complications is essential.

References

1. Johnson, A.E., Gordon, C., Palmer, R.G., and Bacon, P.A. (1995) The prevalence and incidence of systemic lupus erythematosus in Birmingham, England. Relationship to ethnicity and country of birth. *Arthritis Rheum* **38**(4), 551–8.
2. Patel, M., Clarke, A.M., Bruce, I.N., and Symmons, D.P. (2006) The prevalence and incidence of biopsy-proven lupus nephritis in the UK: Evidence of an ethnic gradient. *Arthritis Rheum* **54**(9), 2963–9.
3. Venning, M.P.M. (2008) *Renal Disease in Pregnancy* (Daviso, J.M., Nelson-PIercy, C., Kehoe, S., and Baker P. eds), p. 96. RCOG Press.
4. Fraga, A.M.G., and Orozco, H. (1974) Sterility and fertility rates, fetal wastage and maternal morbidity in systemic lupus erythematosus. *J Rheumatol* **1**, 193–8.
5. Grigor, R.R., Shervington, P.C., Hughes, G.R., and Hawkins, D.F. (1977) Outcome of pregnancy in systemic lupus erythematosus. *Proc R Soc Med* **70**(2), 99–100.
6. Ramsey-Goldman, R., Mientus, J.M., Kutzer, J.E., Mulvihill, J.J., and Medsger, T.A., Jr. (1993) Pregnancy outcome in women with systemic lupus erythematosus treated with immunosuppressive drugs. *J Rheumatol* **20**(7), 1152–7.
7. Bobrie, G., Liote, F., Houillier, P., Grunfeld, J.P., and Jungers, P. (1987) Pregnancy in lupus nephritis and related disorders. *Am J Kidney Dis* **9**(4), 339–43.
8. Cameron, J.S., and Hicks, J. (1984) Pregnancy in patients with pre-existing glomerular disease. *Contrib Nephrol* **37**, 149–56.
9. Hou, S. (1999) Pregnancy in chronic renal insufficiency and end-stage renal disease. *Am J Kidney Dis* **33**(2), 235–52.
10. Hou, S. (2003) Pregnancy in renal transplant recipients. *Adv Ren Replace Ther* **10**(1), 40–7.
11. McKay, D.B., and Josephson, M.A. (2006) Pregnancy in recipients of solid organs–effects on mother and child. *N Engl J Med* **354**(12), 1281–93.

12. Warne, G.L., Fairley, K.F., Hobbs, J.B., and Martin, F.I. (1973) Cyclophosphamide-induced ovarian failure. *N Engl J Med* **289**(22), 1159–62.

13. Park, M.C., Park, Y.B., Jung, S.Y., Chung, I.H., Choi, K.H., and Lee, S.K. (2004) Risk of ovarian failure and pregnancy outcome in patients with lupus nephritis treated with intravenous cyclophosphamide pulse therapy. *Lupus* **13**(8), 569–74.

14. Boumpas, D.T., Austin, H.A., III, Vaughan, E.M., Yarboro, C.H., Klippel, J.H., and Balow, J.E. (1993) Risk for sustained amenorrhea in patients with systemic lupus erythematosus receiving intermittent pulse cyclophosphamide therapy. *Ann Intern Med* **119**(5), 366–9.

15. Davison, J.M., and Noble, M.C. (1981) Serial changes in 24 hour creatinine clearance during normal menstrual cycles and the first trimester of pregnancy. *Br J Obstet Gynaecol* **88**(1), 10–7.

16. Baylis, C. (1987) Glomerular filtration and volume regulation in gravid animal models. *Baillieres Clin Obstet Gynaecol* **1**(4), 789–813.

17. Smith, M.C., Moran, P., Ward, M.K., and Davison, J.M. (2008) Assessment of glomerular filtration rate during pregnancy using the MDRD formula. *BJOG* **115**(1), 109–12.

18. Jeyabalan, A., and Lain, K.Y. (2007) Anatomic and functional changes of the upper urinary tract during pregnancy. *Urol Clin North Am* **34**(1), 1–6.

19. Macejko, A.M., and Schaeffer, A.J. (2007) Asymptomatic bacteriuria and symptomatic urinary tract infections during pregnancy. *Urol Clin North Am* **34**(1), 35–42.

20. Grimaldi, C.M., Cleary, J., Dagtas, A.S., Moussai, D., and Diamond, B. (2002) Estrogen alters thresholds for B cell apoptosis and activation. *J Clin Invest* **109**(12), 1625–33.

21. Yurino, H., Ishikawa, S., Sato, T., Akadegawa, K., Ito, T., Ueha, S., *et al.* (2004) Endocrine disruptors (environmental estrogens) enhance autoantibody production by B1 cells. *Toxicol Sci* **81**(1), 139–47.

22. Roubinian, J., Talal, N., Siiteri, P.K., and Sadakian, J.A. (1979) Sex hormone modulation of autoimmunity in NZB/NZW mice. *Arthritis Rheum* **22**(11), 1162–9.

23. Steinberg, A.D., Melez, K.A., Raveche, E.S., Reeves, J.P., Boegel, W.A., Smathers, P.A., *et al.* (1979) Approach to the study of the role of sex hormones in autoimmunity. *Arthritis Rheum* **22**(11), 1170–6.

24. Sanchez-Guerrero, J., Karlson, E.W., Liang, M.H., Hunter, D.J., Speizer, F.E., and Colditz, G.A. (1997) Past use of oral contraceptives and the risk of developing systemic lupus erythematosus. *Arthritis Rheum* **40**(5), 804–8.

25. Jungers, P., Dougados, M., Pelissier, C., Kuttenn, F., Tron, F., Lesavre, P., *et al.* (1982) Influence of oral contraceptive therapy on the activity of systemic lupus erythematosus. *Arthritis Rheum* **25**(6), 618–23.

26. Julkunen, H.A. (1991) Oral contraceptives in systemic lupus erythematosus: side-effects and influence on the activity of SLE. *Scand J Rheumatol* **20**(6), 427–33.

27. Buyon, J.P., Kalunian, K.C., Skovron, M.L., Petri, M., Lahita, R., Merrill, J., *et al.* (1995) Can Women with Systemic Lupus Erythematosus Safely Use Exogenous Estrogens? *J Clin Rheumatol* **1**(4), 205–12.

28. Petri, M., Kim, M.Y., Kalunian, K.C., Grossman, J., Hahn, B.H., Sammaritano, L.R., *et al.* (2005) Combined oral contraceptives in women with systemic lupus erythematosus. *N Engl J Med* **353**(24), 2550–8.

29. Sanchez-Guerrero, J., Uribe, A.G., Jimenez-Santana, L., Mestanza-Peralta, M., Lara-Reyes, P., Seuc, A.H., *et al.* (2005) A trial of contraceptive methods in women with systemic lupus erythematosus. *N Engl J Med* **353**(24), 2539–49.

30. Vennemann, F., and Tholen, S. (1986) [Sex hormones in lupus erythematosus]. *Z Hautkr* **61**(11), 791–9.

31. Dougados, M., Nahoul, K., Benhamou, L., Jungers, P., Laplane, D., and Amor, B. (1984) [Study of plasma androgens in women with autoimmune diseases]. *Rev Rhum Mal Osteoartic* **51**(3), 145–9.

32. Lucas, J.A., Ahmed, S.A., Casey, M.L., and MacDonald, P.C. (1985) Prevention of autoantibody formation and prolonged survival in New Zealand black/New Zealand white F1 mice fed dehydroisoandrosterone. *J Clin Invest* **75**(6), 2091–3.

33. Petri, M.A., Lahita, R.G., Van Vollenhoven, R.F., Merrill, J.T., Schiff, M., Ginzler, E.M., *et al.* (2002) Effects of prasterone on corticosteroid requirements of women with systemic lupus erythematosus: a double-blind, randomized, placebo-controlled trial. *Arthritis Rheum* **46**(7), 1820–9.

34. Petri, M.A., Mease, P.J., Merrill, J.T., Lahita, R.G., Iannini, M.J., Yocum, D.E., *et al.* (2004) Effects of prasterone on disease activity and symptoms in women with active systemic lupus erythematosus. *Arthritis Rheum* **50**(9), 2858–68.

35. Walker, S.E. (1993) Prolactin: an immune-stimulating peptide that regulates other immune-modulating hormones. *Lupus* **2**(2), 67–9.

36. Elbourne, K.B., Keisler, D., and McMurray, R.W. (1998) Differential effects of estrogen and prolactin on autoimmune disease in the NZB/NZW F1 mouse model of systemic lupus erythematosus. *Lupus* **7**(6), 420–7.

37. Walker, S.E. (2001) Modulation of hormones in the treatment of lupus. *Am J Manag Care* **7**(16 Suppl), S486–9.

38. Chakravarty, E.F., Colon, I., Langen, E.S., Nix, D.A., El-Sayed, Y.Y., Genovese, M.C., *et al.* (2005) Factors that predict prematurity and preeclampsia in pregnancies that are complicated by systemic lupus erythematosus. *Am J Obstet Gynecol* **192**(6), 1897–904.

39. Cervera, R., Font, J., Carmona, F., and Balasch, J. (2002) Pregnancy outcome in systemic lupus erythematosus: good news for the new millennium. *Autoimmun Rev* **1**(6), 354–9.

40. Cortes-Hernandez, J., Ordi-Ros, J., Paredes, F., Casellas, M., Castillo, F., and Vilardell-Tarres, M. (2002) Clinical predictors of fetal and maternal outcome in systemic lupus erythematosus: a prospective study of 103 pregnancies. *Rheumatology (Oxford)* **41**(6), 643–50.

41. Ruiz-Irastorza, G., Lima, F., Alves, J., Khamashta, M.A., Simpson, J., Hughes, G.R., *et al.* (1996) Increased rate of lupus flare during pregnancy and the puerperium: a prospective study of 78 pregnancies. *Br J Rheumatol* **35**(2), 133–8.

42. Clowse, M.E., Magder, L.S., Witter, F., and Petri, M. (2005) The impact of increased lupus activity on obstetric outcomes. *Arthritis Rheum* **52**(2), 514–21.

43. Tandon, A., Ibanez, D., Gladman, D.D., and Urowitz, M.B. (2004) The effect of pregnancy on lupus nephritis. *Arthritis Rheum* **50**(12), 3941–6.

44. Moroni, G., Quaglini, S., Banfi, G., Caloni, M., Finazzi, S., Ambroso, G., *et al.* (2002) Pregnancy in lupus nephritis. *Am J Kidney Dis* **40**(4), 713–20.

45. Petri, M. (1997) Hopkins Lupus Pregnancy Center: 1987 to 1996. *Rheum Dis Clin North Am* **23**(1), 1–13.

46. Zulman, J.I., Talal, N., Hoffman, G.S., and Epstein, W.V. (1980) Problems associated with the management of pregnancies in patients with systemic lupus erythematosus. *J Rheumatol* **7**(1), 37–49.

47. Lockshin, M.D., Reinitz, E., Druzin, M.L., Murrman, M., and Estes, D. (1984) Lupus pregnancy. Case-control prospective study demonstrating absence of lupus exacerbation during or after pregnancy. *Am J Med* **77**(5), 893–8.

48. Meehan, R.T., and Dorsey, J.K. (1987) Pregnancy among patients with systemic lupus erythematosus receiving immunosuppressive therapy. *J Rheumatol* **14**(2), 252–8.

49. Petri, M., Howard, D., and Repke, J. (1991) Frequency of lupus flare in pregnancy. The Hopkins Lupus Pregnancy Center experience. *Arthritis Rheum* **34**(12), 1538–45.

50. Hayslett, J.P., and Lynn, R.I. (1980) Effect of pregnancy in patients with lupus nephropathy. *Kidney Int* **18**(2), 207–20.

51. Wong, C.H., Chen, T.L., Lee, C.S., Lin, C.J., and Chen, C.P. (2006) Outcome of pregnancy in patients with systemic lupus erythematosus. *Taiwan J Obstet Gynecol* **45**(2), 120–3.

52. Imbasciati, E., Surian, M., Bottino, S., Cosci, P., Colussi, G., Ambroso, G.C., *et al.* (1984) Lupus nephropathy and pregnancy. A study of 26 pregnancies in patients with systemic lupus erythematosus and nephritis. *Nephron* **36**(1), 46–51.

53. Julkunen, H., Kaaja, R., Palosuo, T., Gronhagen-Riska, C., and Teramo, K. (1993) Pregnancy in lupus nephropathy. *Acta Obstet Gynecol Scand* **72**(4), 258–63.

54. Fine, L.G.B.E.V., Danovitch, G.M., Nissenson, A.R., Conolly, M.F., and Lieb, S.M. (1981) Systemic lupus erthematosus during pregnancy. *Ann Intern Med* **94**, 667–77.

55. Packham, D.K., Lam, S.S., Nicholls, K., Fairley, K.F., and Kincaid-Smith, P.S. (1992) Lupus nephritis and pregnancy. *Q J Med* **83**(300), 315–24.

56. Bear, R. (1976) Pregnancy and lupus nephritis. A detailed report of six cases with a review of the literature. *Obstet Gynecol* **47**(6), 715–8.

57. Mintz, G., Niz, J., Gutierrez, G., Garcia-Alonso, A., and Karchmer, S. (1986) Prospective study of pregnancy in systemic lupus erythematosus. Results of a multidisciplinary approach. *J Rheumatol* **13**(4), 732–9.

58. McGee, C.D., and Makowski, E.L. (1970) Systemic lupus erythematosus in pregnancy. *Am J Obstet Gynecol* **107**(7), 1008–12.

59. Oviasu, E., Hicks, J., and Cameron, J.S. (1991) The outcome of pregnancy in women with lupus nephritis. *Lupus* **1**(1), 19–25.

60. Varner, M.W., Meehan, R.T., Syrop, C.H., Strottmann, M.P., Goplerud, and C.P. (1983) Pregnancy in patients with systemic lupus erythematosus. *Am J Obstet Gynecol* **145**(8), 1025–40.

61. Houser, M.T., Fish, A.J., Tagatz, G.E., Williams, P.P., and Michael, A.F. (1980) Pregnancy and systemic lupus erythematosus. *Am J Obstet Gynecol* **138**(4), 409–13.

62. Wagner, S., Craici, I., Reed, D., Norby, S., Bailey, K., Wiste, H., *et al.* (2009) Maternal and foetal outcomes in pregnant patients with active lupus nephritis. *Lupus* **18**(4), 342–7.

63. Imbasciati, E., Tincani, A., Gregorini, G., Doria, A., Moroni, G., Cabiddu, G., *et al.* (2009) Pregnancy in women with pre-existing lupus nephritis: predictors of fetal and maternal outcome. *Nephrol Dial Transplant* **24**(2), 519–25.

64. Germain, S., and Nelson-Piercy, C. (2006) Lupus nephritis and renal disease in pregnancy. *Lupus* **15**(3), 148–55.

65. Katz, A.I., Davison, J.M., Hayslett, J.P., Singson, E., and Lindheimer, M.D. (1980) Pregnancy in women with kidney disease. *Kidney Int* **18**(2), 192–206.

66. Jones, D.C., and Hayslett, J.P. (1996) Outcome of pregnancy in women with moderate or severe renal insufficiency. *N Engl J Med* **335**(4), 226–32.

67. Imbasciati, E., Gregorini, G., Cabiddu, G., Gammaro, L., Ambroso, G., Del Giudice, A., *et al.* (2007) Pregnancy in CKD stages 3 to 5: fetal and maternal outcomes. *Am J Kidney Dis* **49**(6), 753–62.

68. Carmona, F., Font, J., Moga, I., Lazaro, I., Cervera, R., Pac, V., *et al.* (2005) Class III-IV proliferative lupus nephritis and pregnancy: a study of 42 cases. *Am J Reprod Immunol* **53**(4), 182–8.

69. Clowse, M.E. (2007) Lupus activity in pregnancy. *Rheum Dis Clin North Am* **33**(2), 237–52, v.

70. Moroni, G., and Ponticelli, C. (2005) Pregnancy after lupus nephritis. *Lupus* **14**(1), 89–94.

71. Huong, D.L., Wechsler, B., Vauthier-Brouzes, D., Beaufils, H., Lefebvre, G., and Piette, J.C. (2001) Pregnancy in past or present lupus nephritis: a study of 32 pregnancies from a single centre. *Ann Rheum Dis* **60**(6), 599–604.

72. Abu-Shakra, M., Urowitz, M.B., Gladman, D.D., and Gough, J. (1995) Mortality studies in systemic lupus erythematosus. Results from a single center. II. Predictor variables for mortality. *J Rheumatol* **22**(7), 1265–70.

73. Rahman, F.Z., Rahman, J., Al-Suleiman, S.A., and Rahman, M.S. (2005) Pregnancy outcome in lupus nephropathy. *Arch Gynecol Obstet* **271**(3), 222–6.

74. Soubassi, L., Haidopoulos, D., Sindos, M., Pilalis, A., Chaniotis, D., Diakomanolis, E., *et al.* (2004) Pregnancy outcome in women with pre-existing lupus nephritis. *J Obstet Gynaecol* **24**(6), 630–4.

75. Urowitz, M.B., Gladman, D.D., Farewell, V.T., Stewart, J., and McDonald, J. (1993) Lupus and pregnancy studies. *Arthritis Rheum* **36**(10), 1392–7.

76. Cavallasca, J.A., Laborde, H.A., Ruda-Vega, H., and Nasswetter, G.G. (2008) Maternal and fetal outcomes of 72 pregnancies in Argentine patients with systemic lupus erythematosus (SLE). *Clin Rheumatol* **27**(1), 41–6.

77. Nelson-Piercy C. *Handbook of Obstetric Medicine*. 3rd ed. Informa Healthcare; 2006, pp. 155–6.

78. Cimaz, R., Spence, D.L., Hornberger, L., and Silverman, E.D. (2003) Incidence and spectrum of neonatal lupus erythematosus: a prospective study of infants born to mothers with anti-Ro autoantibodies. *J Pediatr* **142**(6), 678–83.

79. Friedman, D.M., Rupel, A., and Buyon, J.P. (2007) Epidemiology, etiology, detection, and treatment of autoantibody-associated congenital heart block in neonatal lupus. *Curr Rheumatol Rep* **9**(2), 101–8.

80. Jungers, P., Dougados, M., Pelissier, C., Kuttenn, F., Tron, F., Lesavre, P., *et al.* (1982) Lupus nephropathy and pregnancy. Report of 104 cases in 36 patients. *Arch Intern Med* **142**(4), 771–6.

81. Le Thi Huong, D., Weschler, B., Piette, J.-C., Bletry, O., and Godeau, P. (1994) Pregnancy and its outcome in systemic lupus erythematosus. *Q J Med* **87**, 721–9.

82. Le Huong, D., Wechsler, B., Vauthier-Brouzes, D., Seebacher, J., Lefebvre, G., Bletry, O., *et al.* (1997) Outcome of planned pregnancies in systemic lupus erythematosus: a prospective study on 62 pregnancies. *Br J Rheumatol* **36**(7), 772–7.

83. Shibata, S., Sasaki, T., Hirabayashi, Y., Seino, J., Okamura, K., Yoshinaga, K., *et al.* (1992) Risk factors in the pregnancy of patients with systemic lupus erythematosus: association of hypocomplementaemia with poor prognosis. *Ann Rheum Dis* **51**(5), 619–23.

84. Davison, J.M.N.P.C., Kehoe, S., and Baker, P. (eds) (2008) *Renal Disease in Pregnancy*, pp. 25–6. RCOG Press.

85. Stratta, P., Canavese, C., and Quaglia, M. (2006) Pregnancy in patients with kidney disease. *J Nephrol* **19**(2), 135–43.

86. Sibai, B.M., Lindheimer, M., Hauth, J., Caritis, S., VanDorsten, P., Klebanoff, M., *et al.* (1998) Risk factors for preeclampsia, abruptio placentae, and adverse neonatal outcomes among women with chronic hypertension. National Institute of Child Health and Human Development Network of Maternal-Fetal Medicine Units. *N Engl J Med* **339**(10), 667–71.

87. Chappell, L.C., Enye, S., Seed, P., Briley, A.L., Poston, L., and Shennan, A.H. (2008) Adverse perinatal outcomes and risk factors for preeclampsia in women with chronic hypertension: a prospective study. *Hypertension* **51**(4), 1002–9.

88. Chakravarty, E.F., Nelson, L., and Krishnan, E. (2006) Obstetric hospitalizations in the United States for women with systemic lupus erythematosus and rheumatoid arthritis. *Arthritis Rheum* **54**(3), 899–907.

89. Moroni, G., and Ponticelli, C. (2003) The risk of pregnancy in patients with lupus nephritis. *J Nephrol* **16**(2), 161–7.

90. Lim, W., Crowther, M.A., and Eikelboom, J.W. (2006) Management of antiphospholipid antibody syndrome: a systematic review. *JAMA* **295**(9), 1050–7.

91. Miyakis, S., Lockshin, M.D., Atsumi, T., Branch, D.W., Brey, R.L., Cervera, R., *et al.* (2006) International consensus statement on an update of the classification criteria for definite antiphospholipid syndrome (APS). *J Thromb Haemost* **4**(2), 295–306.

92. Nelson Piercy, C., and Rosene-Montella, K. (2008) *Systemic Lupus Erythematosus. Medical Care of the Pregnant Patient* [second edition] (Lee, R.V., Rosene-Montella, K., Barbour, L.A., Garner, P.R., and Keely, E. eds), pp. 513–21. American College Physicians, Philadelphia.

93. Lynch, A., Silver, R., and Emlen, W. (1997) Antiphospholipid antibodies in healthy pregnant women. *Rheum Dis Clin North Am* **23**(1), 55–70.

94. Cowchock, S., and Reece, E.A. (1997) Do low-risk pregnant women with antiphospholipid antibodies need to be treated? Organizing Group of the Antiphospholipid Antibody Treatment Trial. *Am J Obstet Gynecol* **176**(5), 1099–100.

95. Ramsey-Goldman, R., Kutzer, J.E., Kuller, L.H., Guzick, D., Carpenter, A.B., and Medsger, T.A., Jr. (1992) Previous pregnancy outcome is an important determinant of subsequent pregnancy outcome in women with systemic lupus erythematosus. *Am J Reprod Immunol* **28**(3-4), 195–8.

96. Martinez-Rueda, J.O., Arce-Salinas, C.A., Kraus, A., Alcocer-Varela, J., and Alarcon-Segovia, D. (1996) Factors associated with fetal losses in severe systemic lupus erythematosus. *Lupus* **5**(2), 113–9.

97. Out, H.J., Bruinse, H.W., Christiaens, G.C., van Vliet, M., de Groot, P.G., Nieuwenhuis, H.K., *et al.* (1992) A prospective, controlled multicenter study on the obstetric risks of pregnant women with antiphospholipid antibodies. *Am J Obstet Gynecol* **167**(1), 26–32.

98. Lockshin, M.D., Druzin, M.L., and Qamar, T. (1989) Prednisone does not prevent recurrent fetal death in women with antiphospholipid antibody. *Am J Obstet Gynecol* **160**(2), 439–43.

99. Lima, F., Khamashta, M.A., Buchanan, N.M., Kerslake, S., Hunt, B.J., and Hughes, G.R. (1996) A study of sixty pregnancies in patients with the antiphospholipid syndrome. *Clin Exp Rheumatol* **14**(2), 131–6.

100. Branch, D.W., and Khamashta, M.A. (2003) Antiphospholipid syndrome: obstetric diagnosis, management, and controversies. *Obstet Gynecol* **101**(6), 1333–44.

101. Laskin, C.A., Spitzer, K.A., Clark, C.A., Crowther, M.R., Ginsberg, J.S., Hawker, G.A., *et al.* (2009) Low molecular weight heparin and aspirin for recurrent pregnancy loss: results from the randomized, controlled HepASA Trial. *J Rheumatol* **36**(2), 279–87.

102. Duley, L., Henderson-Smart, D.J., Meher, S., and King, J.F. (2007) Antiplatelet agents for preventing pre-eclampsia and its complications. *Cochrane Database Syst Rev* (2), CD004659.

103. Ruiz-Irastorza, G., and Khamashta, M.A. (2004) Evaluation of systemic lupus erythematosus activity during pregnancy. *Lupus* **13**(9), 679–82.

104. Brown, M.A., Lindheimer, M.D., de Swiet, M., Van Assche, A., and Moutquin, J.M. (2001) The classification and diagnosis of the hypertensive disorders of pregnancy: statement from the International Society for the Study of Hypertension in Pregnancy (ISSHP). *Hypertens Pregnancy* **20**(1), IX–XIV.

105. Packham, D., and Fairley, K.F. (1987) Renal biopsy: indications and complications in pregnancy. *Br J Obstet Gynaecol* **94**(10), 935–9.

106. Klink, D.T., van Elburg, R.M., Schreurs, M.W., and van Well, G.T. (2008) Rituximab administration in third trimester of pregnancy suppresses neonatal B-cell development. *Clin Dev Immunol* **271**, 363.

107. Clowse, M.E., Magder, L., and Petri, M. (2005) Cyclophosphamide for lupus during pregnancy. *Lupus* **14**(8), 593–7.

108. Fernandez, M., Andrade, R., and Alarcon, G.S. (2006) Cyclophosphamide use and pregnancy in lupus. *Lupus* **15**(1), 59.

109. Kart Koseoglu, H., Yucel, A.E., Kunefeci, G., Ozdemir, F.N., and Duran, H. (2001) Cyclophosphamide therapy in a serious case of lupus nephritis during pregnancy. *Lupus* **10**(11), 818–20.

110. Berry, D.L., Theriault, R.L., Holmes, F.A., Parisi, V.M., Booser, D.J., Singletary, S.E., *et al.* (1999) Management of breast cancer during pregnancy using a standardized protocol. *J Clin Oncol* **17**(3), 855–61.

111. Gwyn, K.M., and Theriault, R.L. (2000) Breast cancer during pregnancy. *Curr Treat Options Oncol* **1**(3), 239–43.

112. Lishner, M., Zemlickis, D., Sutcliffe, S.B., and Koren, G. (1994) Non-Hodgkin's lymphoma and pregnancy. *Leuk Lymphoma* **14**(5-6), 411–3.

113. Halligan, A., Bonnar, J., Sheppard, B., Darling, M., and Walshe, J. (1994) Haemostatic, fibrinolytic and endothelial variables in normal pregnancies and pre-eclampsia. *Br J Obstet Gynaecol* **101**(6), 488–92.

114. Branch, D.W., and Scott, J.R. (1990) Clinical Implications of Antiphospholipid Antibodies: The Utah Experience. In: *Phospholipid-Binding Antibodies.* Harris EN, Exner T, Hughes GRV *et al.* (eds), pp. 853–84. CRC Press, Boca Raton.

115. Direskeneli, H., Buchanan, N.M., Khamashta, M.A., Keser, G., D'Cruz, D., and Hughes, G.R. (1997) Markers of vascular damage in lupus pregnancy. *Clin Exp Rheumatol* **15**(5), 535–9.

116. Singhal, R., and Brimble, K.S. (2006) Thromboembolic complications in the nephrotic syndrome: pathophysiology and clinical management. *Thromb Res* **118**(3), 397–407.

117. Davison, J.M.N.P.C., Kehoe S., and Baker, P. (eds) (2008) *Renal Disease in Pregnancy*, p. 250. RCOG Press.

118. Bagon, J.A., Vernaeve, H., De Muylder, X., Lafontaine, J.J., Martens, J., and Van Roost, G. (1998) Pregnancy and dialysis. *Am J Kidney Dis* **31**(5), 756–65.

119. Okundaye, I., Abrinko, P., and Hou, S. (1998) Registry of pregnancy in dialysis patients. *Am J Kidney Dis* **31**(5), 766–73.

120. Chan, W.S., Okun, N., and Kjellstrand, C.M. (1998) Pregnancy in chronic dialysis: a review and analysis of the literature. *Int J Artif Organs* **21**(5), 259–68.

121. Ostensen, M., Khamashta, M., Lockshin, M., Parke, A., Brucato, A., Carp, H., *et al.* (2006) Anti-inflammatory and immunosuppressive drugs and reproduction. *Arthritis Res Ther* **8**(3), 209.

122. Benediktsson, R., Calder, A.A., Edwards, C.R., and Seckl, J.R. (1997) Placental 11 beta-hydroxysteroid dehydrogenase: a key regulator of fetal glucocorticoid exposure. *Clin Endocrinol (Oxf)* **46**(2), 161–6.

123. Park-Wyllie, L., Mazzotta, P., Pastuszak, A., Moretti, M.E., Beique, L., Hunnisett, L., *et al.* (2000) Birth defects after maternal exposure to corticosteroids: prospective cohort study and meta-analysis of epidemiological studies. *Teratology* **62**(6), 385–92.

124. Carmichael, S.L., Shaw, G.M., Ma, C., Werler, M.M., Rasmussen, S.A., and Lammer, E.J. (2007) Maternal corticosteroid use and orofacial clefts. *Am J Obstet Gynecol* **197**(6), 585, e1–7; discussion 683–4, e1–7.

125. Kallen, B. (2003) Maternal drug use and infant cleft lip/palate with special reference to corticoids. *Cleft Palate Craniofac J* **40**(6), 624–8.

126. Czeizel, A.E., and Rockenbauer, M. (1997) Population-based case-control study of teratogenic potential of corticosteroids. *Teratology* **56**(5), 335–40.

127. Bar Oz, B., Hackman, R., Einarson, T., and Koren, G. (2001) Pregnancy outcome after cyclosporine therapy during pregnancy: a meta-analysis. *Transplantation* **71**(8), 1051–5.

128. Armenti, V.T., Ahlswede, K.M., Ahlswede, B.A., Jarrell, B.E., Moritz, M.J., and Burke, J.F. (1994) National transplantation Pregnancy Registry–outcomes of 154 pregnancies in cyclosporine-treated female kidney transplant recipients. *Transplantation* **57**(4), 502–6.

129. Kainz, A., Harabacz, I., Cowlrick, I.S., Gadgil, S.D., and Hagiwara, D. (2000) Review of the course and outcome of 100 pregnancies in 84 women treated with tacrolimus. *Transplantation* **70**(12), 1718–21.

130. Armenti, V.T., Radomski, J.S., Moritz, M.J., Gaughan, W.J., Hecker, W.P., Lavelanet, A., *et al.* (2004) Report from the National Transplantation Pregnancy Registry (NTPR): outcomes of pregnancy after transplantation. *Clin Transpl* 103–14.

131. Francella, A., Dyan, A., Bodian, C., Rubin, P., Chapman, M., and Present, D.H. (2003) The safety of 6-mercaptopurine for childbearing patients with inflammatory bowel disease: a retrospective cohort study. *Gastroenterology* **124**(1), 9–17.

132. Moskovitz, D.N., Bodian, C., Chapman, M.L., Marion, J.F., Rubin, P.H., Scherl, E., *et al.* (2004) The effect on the fetus of medications used to treat pregnant inflammatory bowel-disease patients. *Am J Gastroenterol* **99**(4), 656–61.

133. Tendron, A., Gouyon, J.B., and Decramer, S. (2002) In utero exposure to immunosuppressive drugs: experimental and clinical studies. *Pediatr Nephrol* **17**(2), 121–30.

134. Le Ray, C., Coulomb, A., Elefant, E., Frydman, R., and Audibert, F. (2004) Mycophenolate mofetil in pregnancy after renal transplantation: a case of major fetal malformations. *Obstet Gynecol* 103(5 Pt 2), 1091–4.

135. Sifontis, N.M., Coscia, L.A., Constantinescu, S., Lavelanet, A.F., Moritz, M.J., and Armenti, V.T. (2006) Pregnancy outcomes in solid organ transplant recipients with exposure to mycophenolate mofetil or sirolimus. *Transplantation* **82**(12), 1698–702.

136. Kyle, P.M. (2006) Drugs and the fetus. *Curr Opin Obstet Gynecol* **18**(2), 93–9.

137. Cooper, W.O., Hernandez-Diaz, S., Arbogast, P.G., Dudley, J.A., Dyer, S., Gideon, P.S., *et al.* (2006) Major congenital malformations after first-trimester exposure to ACE inhibitors. *N Engl J Med* **354**(23), 2443–51.

138. Mackillop, L.H., Germain, S.J., and Nelson-Piercy C. (2007) Systemic lupus erythematosus. *BMJ* **335**(7626), 933–6.

139. Ostensen, M., Lockshin, M., Doria, A., Valesini, G., Meroni, P., Gordon, C., *et al.* (2008) Update on safety during pregnancy of biological agents and some immunosuppressive anti-rheumatic drugs. *Rheumatology (Oxford)* **47** Suppl 3, iii28–31.

Chapter 12

The treatment of severe proliferative lupus nephritis

Richard J. Glassock

Introduction

In a chapter entitled "Natural history and treatment of lupus nephritis" published in the first edition (1999) of this book, Edmund Lewis stated that "lupus nephritis, its clinical course, prognosis and optimal therapy are subjects which are plagued by a surfeit of authoritative opinion, however there is limited scientifically valid information."[1] More than a decade later, the plague of "authoritative opinion" has not lessened, but the availability of "scientifically valid information" has certainly increased, largely thorough the design and execution of expensive and time-consuming prospective, randomized, controlled clinical trials (RCT) involving the volunteerism of countless brave subjects suffering from lupus nephritis.[2–9] If the magnitude of "scientifically valid information" has increased, as it has, why then are we still plagued by "a surfeit of authoritative opinions?" The answer to this daunting question lies in the vagaries of lupus nephritis itself—its unpredictability, its diversity, its pathogenetic heterogeneity—and in the inherent limitations of RCT, however well designed and executed, to address the critical questions posed by individual patients with lupus nephritis. A large gap exists between the body of scientific evidence and the achievement of a universal strategy for optimally effective and safe treatment of lupus nephritis. Much progress has been made in narrowing this gap, but much still needs to be done. Preliminary expert opinions and evidence-based guidance have been developed[5–8] and more are anticipated. In many respects the future for treatment of lupus nephritis is bright, as we learn more about the intricate details of pathogenesis and design more targeted, "rational" approaches to treatment, while at the same time diminish the risk of adverse consequences of our therapy.

This chapter builds on the base developed by Dr. Lewis and his colleagues in the landmark 1999 contribution,[1] and will focus primarily on new developments in the last decade. In addition, it will deal primarily with "severe," proliferative lupus nephritis, as defined elsewhere in the book (see also Chapter 6). The treatment of membranous lupus nephritis is covered in Chapter 7, lupus podocytopathy in Chapter 8 and thrombotic microangiopathy complicating lupus nephritis in Chapter 9. Milder forms of lupus nephritis, such as the mesangial and mild focal proliferative forms (Class I, II, and III <50%, see also Chapter 6), often respond to steroids alone and do not require aggressive therapy, unless they transform to more severe proliferative lupus nephritis.

In keeping with the theme of this monograph and its predecessor, both "authoritative opinion" and "scientifically valid evidence" will be carefully and separately identified. It is hoped that a proper balance of evidence-based and opinion-based therapeutic strategies for severe lupus nephritis can be achieved.

General considerations in developing a therapeutic plan for severe lupus nephritis

There are four critical elements (questions) that need to be addressed in the development of a strategy for treatment of severe lupus nephritis: (i) What are the short-and long-term goals of therapy?; (ii) What is the nature of the lupus nephritis present in the patient (pathological classification, severity, reversibility, likely responsiveness)?; (iii) What is the extent of systemic (extrarenal) disease and organ involvement?; and (iv) What are the short- and long-term risks of treatment, depending on the strategy chosen?

In designing a therapeutic approach for an individual patient it is best to separate the induction phase (the first 3–12 months of treatment) and the maintenance phase (after successful induction and lasting for many years, perhaps a lifetime).[1] For those patients who do not experience a successful induction (i.e. no remission), one must examine "rescue" strategies for refractory (treatment-resistant) disease. It is not possible to define "refractoriness" in a rigid, uncompromising, and evidence-based manner, as it depends on the original goals of treatment and the intrinsic reversibility of the underlying pathological lesions.

The goals of the induction phase and the maintenance phases of therapy differ. The goal of the induction phase is to produce as rapid a remission of abnormal renal and extrarenal clinical features (complete or partial, see below) at the least risk for serious adverse drug-related events, using an intense, often multi-drug regimen. The goal of the maintenance phase is to avoid relapses of the systemic and renal manifestations of disease at the lowest intensity of therapy achievable and to prevent progression of disease into an irreversible form. Failure to achieve the goals of the maintenance phase (which is all too common) also means that exacerbations of disease will have to be managed by periodic re-induction of remissions. Early response and a complete remission are important factors contributing to a favorable long-term outcome.[10,11] Relapse of renal disease in severe lupus nephritis is also a major factor in determining the long-term course of renal function.[12–14] If relapses can be avoided, the prospects for renal survival are very good, even in severe lupus nephritis, unless treatment has been started at a stage when irreversible renal lesions are already well established. Unfortunately, a delay in the recognition of serious renal involvement also results in a delay of treatment. It is important to recognize that irreversible damage to the kidneys (glomerulosclerosis and interstitial fibrosis) can substantially influence the degree of response to both induction and maintenance therapy.

At present, renal biopsy occupies a central role in the development of treatment strategies for severe lupus nephritis. As is pointed out in Chapter 6, the assessment of the morphological features of lupus nephritis and assignment to a classification category (either World Health Organization (WHO) or International Society for Nephrology/ Renal Pathology Society (ISN/RPS)), helps immeasurably in the approach to designing a rational treatment regimen (both for induction and maintenance phases). But, as clearly pointed out in Chapter 6, certain caveats regarding current classification schemata for lupus nephritis also need to be kept in mind, including sampling error and the vagaries of classifying the severe focal and segmental necrotizing lesions (Class III >50% lupus nephritis), which may have a differing pathogenesis from the diffuse proliferative lesions (Class IV lupus nephritis) (see also Chapter 5).[15–17] Information from renal biopsy can give useful hints as to the likely responsiveness of the lesion to induction therapy, to long-term prognosis, and to the need for tailoring of the treatment regimen to the specific nuances of renal pathology (such as complicating thrombotic microangiopathies, severe glomerular crescentic disease, severe focal and segmental necrotizing (vasculitic) lesions, interstitial nephritis, acute tubular necrosis, and combinations of membranous and proliferative lesions) (see also Chapter 6).[18–22] Re-biopsy may also be necessary from time to time in order to determine the evolution of disease and to determine its reversibility, but there are no evidence-based rules to guide the clinician when such a re-biopsy is needed and would contribute materially to decision making about future management. A repeat renal biopsy may be particularly useful when the patient exhibits a sudden change in clinical features (e.g. a sudden decline in renal function, a dramatic increase in proteinuria, or a reactivation of a previously normal urinary sediment).[23,24]

As pointed out by Edmund Lewis in the previous edition,[1] and also in this volume, some of the differences in the outcomes of treatment reported in RCTs of lupus nephritis could be due to the vagaries of classification of the morphology of lupus nephritis (see also Chapter 6).

Reports of efficacy and safety of regimens for lupus nephritis from RCT (and many observational studies as well) need to be interpreted with great caution as they may have been underpowered to examine the primary endpoints (they are also nearly always underpowered to examine important adverse events), they are often of rather short-duration (3–12 months for induction trials, 1–5 years for maintenance trials), and the definitions used for defining complete and partial remission or renal and systemic relapses vary widely. Inclusion and exclusion criteria are not uniform among RCT and the ancestry of the enrolled patients may be too diverse to make any evidence-based statements regarding efficacy or safety for a particular regimen in a particular ancestral group. Thus, it is often difficult to relate the reports of RCT to individual patients with lupus nephritis of diverse ancestry, social class, and disease severity.[25–29] In addition, differences in the pharmacokinetic, pharmacodynamic, or pharmacogenomic behavior of drugs used in these patients can contribute to the eventual outcome (efficacy and safety). Nevertheless, despite these caveats, the body of evidence from RCT serves as the basis for currently recommended approaches to both induction and maintenance phases of therapy for severe lupus nephritis. Unfortunately, some drugs advocated for treatment of lupus nephritis have not yet been extensively studied in RCT and published in peer-reviewed journals (e.g. anti CD-20 monoclonal antibodies), so evidence-based statements have to be replaced (temporarily, at least) by authoritative opinion. Differences in outcomes using specific drug regimens have also been observed in different ancestral groups, further compounding the difficulty in interpreting extant RCT that enrolled very heterogeneous or more homogeneous ancestral populations.

Although this chapter will focus on treatment of renal disease, it is obvious that the nonrenal manifestations of systemic lupus erythematosus (such as cutaneous, mucous membrane, joint, hematological, lung, cardiac, and neuropsychiatric disorders) be concomitantly managed. Many, but not all, patients with severe lupus nephritis will have such manifestations, of varying severity, and some will have solely renal involvement (see Chapter 1). Oral steroids and nonsteroidal anti-inflammatory agents are often quite effective in controlling these extrarenal manifestations, but often require intolerably high doses and thus result in long-term undesirable adverse events. Immunosuppressive agents, such as cytotoxic drugs (see below) often exert a "steroid-sparing" effect, and allow for better control of the systemic features at lower, better tolerated, doses of steroids. Antimalarials, hydroxychloroquine in particular, are very useful in calming the joint and skin manifestations of the disease, but are not very effective for the renal aspects of the disease.

Induction therapy for severe proliferative lupus nephritis

Here we will examine the efficacy and safety of various regimens for severe, proliferative lupus nephritis. The treatment of membranous lupus glomerulonephritis (Class V lupus nephritis) is covered in Chapter 7. Included in this category are severe focal and segmental necrotizing lesions (Class III >50%), diffuse proliferative lesions (Class IV), and combinations of membranous and proliferative lesions (Class V + Class III or Class IV) (see also Chapter 6). Each of these lesions may exhibit superimposed extensive crescentic disease, thrombotic microangiopathy (see Chapter 9) or severe interstitial nephritis. The degree of activity (fibrinoid necrosis, active intraglomerular or extraglomerular hypercellularity) and chronicity (tubular-interstitial fibrosis, tubular atrophy, fibrotic crescents, arteriolonephrosclerosis) may vary considerably from subject to subject, and assessment of these parameters may have limited reliability, especially if the biopsy sample size is small.

The overall goal of induction therapy is to induce a remission. A complete remission of all of the features of renal involvement is most desirable, but a partial remission is also associated with a better outcome than no response at all.[30] The definition of complete and partial remission have not been universally agreed on, and the use of different definitions of remission leads to different response rates when applied to RCT and observational studies. Table 12.1 gives summary of some widely used definitions of complete and partial remission for severe lupus nephritis.[30–38] Induction therapy has utilized a number of regimens, nearly always an immunomodulating agent (such as cyclophosphamide, azathioprine, calcineurin inhibitors (CNI), mycophenolate mofetil (MMF), intravenous polyclonal immunoglobulins, anti-CD20 monoclonal antibodies, or tumor necrosis factor (TNF)α antagonists) in combination with various dosage levels of glucocorticoids (intravenous or oral). During the induction phase, the doses of glucocorticoids are usually high. Indeed, nearly every regimen for severe lupus nephritis includes glucocorticoids, either intravenous or oral or a combination of the two, but the comparative efficacy and safety of intravenous or oral glucocorticoid regimens for induction is unknown. High-dose oral prednisone may be just as effective as "pulses" of intravenous methylprednisolone. Starting therapy with a 3-day

Table 12.1 Definitions of complete and partial remissions following induction therapy of diffuse proliferative lupus nephritis

Author/study (year)	Renal function	Proteinuria	Urine sediment
Complete remission			
Illei (2002)	<130% of lowest Scr during therapy	UP<1.0 g/day	<10 rbc/hpf (>20ml sample)
Illei (2004)	Absence of failure of therapy (↑Scr to no cellular casts)	UP<1.0 g/day	<10 rbc/hpf
Contreras (2004)	Improvement from BL[a] Scr by >25% with BL[a] of >3 (*CR+PR) or stable Scr or a >50%↓ if within 25% of BL[a]	UP/Cr[b] <3	Not stated
Chan (2005)	Improved or stable RF	UP <0.3 g/day	Normal urine sediment
Ginzler (2005)	Return of Scr to within 10% of normal	Return of proteinuria to within 10% of normal	Return of urine sediment to within 10%
ACR (2006)	>25% ↑ of eGFR from BL	UP/Cr<0.2	<5 rbc and<1 cellular cast/hpf
Chen (LNCSG) (2008)	Scr ≤1.4 mg/dl	UP<0.33 g/day	Not stated
LUNAR (2009)	"Normalization" of Scr	UP/Cr[b]<0.5	<10 rbc/hpf
ALMS (2009)	Normal Scr	UP<500 mg/day	"Inactive" (no abnormal rbc, wbc, or casts)
Partial remission			
Illei (2002)	Stable level of Scr (<150% of lowest level during therapy)	No change in UP	No change
Chan (2004)	Stable or improving Scr	↓ in UP by 50% with values of 0.3–3.0 g/day	Not stated
Contreras (2004)	(Complete and partial remissions combined)		
Illei (2004)	(Complete and partial remissions combined)		
Ginzler (2005)	Improvement of at least 50% in abnormal Scr	Improvement of at least 50% in abnormal proteinuria	Improved by at least 50%
	+ no worsening of any parameter (Scr, proteinuria of urinary sediment)		

(*Continued*)

Table 12.1 (continued) Definitions of complete and partial remissions following induction therapy of diffuse proliferative lupus nephritis

Author/study (year)	Renal function	Proteinuria	Urine sediment
Partial remission			
ACR (2006)	Not stated	UP/Cr[b] >50% lower than BL[a] and 0.2–2.0	Not stated
Chen (LNCSG) (2008)	≤ 25% ↑ BL Scr	≥50% ↓ in BL UP to <1.5 g/day but >0.33 g/day	Not stated
LUNAR (2009)	eGFR <10% above BL[a]	>50% improved UP/Cr from BL (If BL <3.0, then <1.0 and if BL[a]>3.0 then <3.0)	>50% improvement
	+ without worsening of any parameter (eGFR, UP/Cr or urinary sediment)		

ACR, American College of Rheumatology; BL, baseline values; CR, complete remission; eGFR, estimated glomerular filtration rate by the MDRD formula; LNCSG, Lupus Nephritis Collaborative Study Group; PR, partial remission; RF, renal function; Scr, serum creatinine in mg/dl; UP, urine protein excretion rate in g/day; UP/Cr, urine total protein to creatinine ratio in g/g.

course of mega-dose, "pulse" intravenous methylprednisolone (IVMP) (500–1000 mg per dose) is not uncommon, but oral prednisone (1 mg/kg/day; 80 mg/day maximum dose) may be as effective. Pulses of intravenous methylprednisolone repeated on a monthly basis, combined with low-dose oral prednisone is commonly employed for the glucocorticoid component of the regimen for induction.[39] Intravenous pulses of methylprednisolone followed by moderate doses of oral prednisone have the advantage of reducing side effects when compared to high-dose oral prednisone alone. However, repeating IVMP every month or so can increase the steroid-related side effects and dissipate the advantage of IVMP over oral administration. Combinations of pulses of IVMP and intravenous cyclophosphamide (CP) may be superior to either given alone, in terms of both efficacy and toxicity.[40] There is a paucity of RCT comparing intravenous mega-dose and lower dose oral glucocorticoids for induction therapy. Sustained high-dose glucocorticoids (intravenous or oral) can contribute materially to the incidence of serious adverse events (mainly infections), so tapering of dosage on a schedule that will minimize exposure to the cumulative effects of excess steroids is important. The schedule for tapering of steroids has not been standardized by an evidence base from RCT. A schedule similar to that described by the Lupus Nephritis Collaborative Study Group (LNCSG) is a reasonable choice (Table 12.2).[1] Here the initial dose of prednisone (or another glucocorticoid at equivalent dosage) is tapered to about 40 mg/day by 10 weeks and to 30 mg every other day by 20 weeks from the start of induction. More rapid steroid-tapering may be acceptable in certain high-risk patients who exhibit a prompt response to induction treatment, but too

Table 12.2 Suggested regimen for tapering dosage of prednisone after initiation of induction therapy for severe lupus nephritis (adapted from LNCSG, see[1])

Weeks	Patients <80kg	Patients >80kg
1–4	60 mg daily (qd)*	80 mg qd*
5–6	50 mg qd	70 mg qd*
7–8	50 mg qd	60 mg qd
9–10	40 mg qd	50 mg qd
11–12	40 mg qd	40 mg qd
13–14	30 mg qd	40 mg qd
15	30–25 on alternate days (ad)	40–35 ad
16	30–20 ad	40–30 ad
17	30–15 ad	40–15 ad
18	30–10 ad	40–20 ad
19	30–5 ad	40–15 ad
20	30–0 ad	40–10 ad
21	25–0 ad	40–5 ad
22	20–0 ad	40–0 ad
23	20–0 ad	30–0 ad
23–52	20–0 ad	25–0 ad

* In two equally divided doses. qd, as a single dose in the morning; ad, as a single dose on alternate days in the morning.

rapid tapering of steroids can result in an early exacerbation (renal or systemic relapse) of disease. It is also worth recalling that older systematic reviews and meta-analyses of combinations of steroids and cytotoxic agents for severe lupus nephritis have shown beneficial effects on renal survival but not patient survival, with many mortal events linked to opportunistic serious infections.[41] The risk for opportunistic infections can be linked to a profound, persistent deficit in CD4+ T cells and an absolute lymphopenia,[42] but this has not been specifically examined in severe lupus nephritis. No comparable information for glucocorticoids combined with newer treatments, such as CNI or anti-CD20 monoclonal antibodies, exists presently, but it is reasonable to suppose that these regimens will also carry risks of opportunistic infections, although the pattern or organisms and organ systems involved may differ. High-dose, sustained glucocorticoid therapy represents a very real hazard for serious, sometimes fatal, infections, and is a frequent cause of poor compliance in adolescents and young women because of the many side effects, including obesity and esthetic disfigurement.

A proposed definition of a complete and partial remission of severe proliferative lupus nephritis that encompasses the definitions used by the authors/studies listed in Table 12.1 is given in Table 12.3.

Table 12.3 Proposed definitions for a complete and partial remission in diffuse proliferative lupus nephritis (as assessed within 24 weeks of initiation of "induction" therapy)

Complete remission (all four must be present)
Renal function: normalization of Scr to within 10% of the range of normal for laboratory and ≤1.4 mg/dl
Proteinuria: UP/Cr < 0.3g/g
Urine sediment: <10 rbc/hpf, <1 cellular cast, no rbc casts (using a sample size of at least 20 ml of urine)
Normalization of serum albumin (if abnormal at BL)
Partial remission (all four must be present)
Renal function: >50% improvement in Scr from BL
Proteinuria: >50% improvement in UP/Cr; if BL UP/Cr is <3.0 then UP/Cr must be <1.0 and if BL UP/Cr is >3.0 then UP/Cr must be less than 3.0
Urine sediment: >50% improvement in rbc/hpf and no rbc casts (using a sample size of at least 20 ml of urine)
Serum albumin increased to >3.0 g/dl

Estimation of glomerular filtration rate by Cockcroft–Gault or MDRD is not recommended for assessment of remission. The volume of urine used to determine urine sediment changes must be specified. Abbreviations as for Table 12.1.

Cyclophosphamide-based regimens

Oral CP, combined with steroids, began to be used in the therapy of severe lupus nephritis in the early 1970s, and by the 1980s small prospective trials began to appear.[43] Regimens involving either orally administered (daily) CP or intravenously administered (intermittent) CP were examined, often in comparison to steroids alone or some other regimen (such as azathioprine (AZA) plus steroids). A landmark trial published in 1986 of intermittent (monthly) intravenous "pulses" of CP (750–1000 mg/m^2 over 2–4 hours), conducted by the National Institutes of Health (NIH), suggested that this approach was safer and more effective than steroids alone in severe lupus nephritis.[43,44] The data from this trial did not demonstrate superiority of the IVCP regimen compared to other cytotoxic agent-containing treatment regimens, including oral AZA + oral CP, oral CP plus steroids and AZA + steroids, in part because of the paucity of subjects followed for 7 years or more (<20 in each group) (see Edmund Lewis' comments in the first edition of this book for a more detailed critique of the NIH trials).[1] For the first 5 years all the treatments were roughly equivalent in overall efficacy (preventing end stage renal disease (ESRD)). However, because of suggestions that the safety profile for the intermittent IVCP regimen was superior (never formally proven), this IVCP regimen quickly became very popular (in the USA, less so in Europe and in the UK). Except for this initial NIH trial, IVCP has never been formally compared (for both efficacy and safety) in a head-to-head RCT fashion with an oral CP regimen in severe lupus nephritis. However, Mok and colleagues compared IVCP to oral CP in a prospective but uncontrolled fashion.[45] The overall efficacy of CP in severe lupus nephritis was more related to total cumulative dosage than to the route of administration—but the findings suggested that the oral route might be more toxic.[45] Some highly experienced clinicians still hold to the view that oral CP given in short courses (usually 3–6 months, averaging about 4 months) are both useful and safe as induction therapy in patients with severe lupus nephritis, with 70% of patients so treated achieving remissions with low frequency of adverse events.[46] Nevertheless, because of lower cumulative dosage, and the relative freedom from serious (life-threatening) adverse events, the NIH-style IVCP-based regimen for the induction phase of severe lupus nephritis quickly became adopted as the "standard of care" for severe lupus nephritis (at least in the majority of the USA).

However, more recently the Euro-Lupus collaboration has shown, with long-term follow-up, that a less intense regimen involving 500 mg doses of IVCP + steroids every 2 weeks for 3 months followed by AZA (compared to the NIH IVCP regimen of 6 monthly doses of 750–1000 mg/m^2 and two quarterly IVCP doses + steroids) provides equivalent results, in terms for renal and patient survival and frequency of relapses, even after 10 years of follow-up.[47,48] Adverse events are quite similar for the NIH IVCP and the Euro-Lupus regimens. The main caveat about the Euro-Lupus trial findings is that they may not be applicable to a group of subjects with different ancestry (such as African Americans or Hispanics). Importantly, these studies have shown that a less intense regimen with partial sparing of CP dosage (total cumulative dose of CP = 3.0 g) can achieve very acceptable results.

Cyclophosphamide may cause bladder irritation (hemorrhagic cystitis) and predispose to bladder cancer over the long term. For this reason it should be administered in the morning hours, with frequent voidings and under adequate hydration and urine flow (a water diuresis). Some investigators use concomitant MESNA (an acronym for 2-mercapto-ethane-sulfonate sodium) administration when the intravenous route is used and when larger CP doses are prescribed, in order to protect the bladder from the adverse effects of the main metabolite of CP excreted in the urine (acrolein).[49] MESNA neutralizes the toxic metabolites of CP by binding through its sulfhydryl moieties. Whether such MESNA treatments are needed when one uses the lower dose Euro-Lupus protocol is not clear.[47,48] Mild nausea from the IVCP infusion can usually be controlled by co-administration of parenteral anti-emetics.

The IVCP-based regimens are capable of inducing remissions (complete and partial) in between 60% and 85% of patients with severe lupus nephritis, depending on the stage of disease (as assessed by serum creatinine), when treatment is begun, the nature of the disease (morphological classification), the definitions used for remissions, and the ancestry of the patient. The initial level of serum creatinine is a powerful predictor of responsiveness to induction therapy, and is a good surrogate for the delay in recognition and initiation of treatment.[1] Differences in overall remission rates would be expected in trials enrolling patients with normal or near-normal serum creatinine levels, compared to those trials in which the serum creatinine level was distinctly abnormal ($\geq$ 1.4 mg/dl) at the onset of induction therapy. Poorer responses to induction with this regimen can also be expected in African Americans and Hispanics, and those with mixed membranous and proliferative lesions.[25–27] Superimposed extensive crescentic disease (especially if concomitant antineutrophil cytoplasmic antibody (ANCA) is present), although rather uncommon, may respond better, and thrombotic microangiopathies poorer, to these regimens, based on anecdotal observations (see Chapter 9).[50,51] The best responses to induction therapy are usually seen in the diffuse proliferative lesions (Class IV), with poorer responses in the severe focal proliferative lesions (Class III >50%) or the mixed membranous and proliferative lesions (Class V + Class III or Class IV).[16,20,21] Class III >50% + Class V lesions are more common in patients of African American ancestry, which may, in part, explain their poorer response to induction therapy as a group.[28] Patients who are refractory to induction will be discussed below (see Refractory lupus nephritis).

Oral (daily) CP regimens, combined with steroids, may also be quite effective for the induction phase of therapy. The LNCSG treated 86 patients with severe lupus nephritis (as a part of a RCT of the effect of plasma exchange, see below) with oral CP daily (1–2 mg/kg/day) plus oral steroids for 8–9 weeks, and showed a remission rate (at 1 year) of about 45%, if the serum creatinine concentration was initially less than 1.2 mg/dl, much less if serum creatinine concentration was elevated.[1,30] This observational study demonstrates again that delays in initiation of induction therapy, allowing for irreversible damage to occur (manifested by a persistently elevated serum creatinine), are a very important factor determining the eventual outcome of aggressive induction therapy in severe lupus nephritis. As stated above, there are no RCT directly comparing the efficacy and safety of the oral versus the intravenous CP regimens in severe lupus nephritis (other than the small NIH trial), but observational studies have suggested that they are of equivalent efficacy.[45,46] The use of prolonged courses of IVCP (750–1000 mg/m^2 monthly for 3–6 months and every 3 months for up to 4 years) can result in total cumulative exposure to CP much higher (about 35 g) than that used in the LNCSG trial (about 7 g), and much greater risk of toxicity (ovarian failure, serious infections, bone marrow failure, cytogenetic damage, risk of late-onset myelogenous leukemia or bladder cancer).[1] If the NIH IVCP or the Euro-Lupus treatment strategies achieve remission more quickly and completely than the short-term LNCSG oral CP regimen (when evaluated at 6 months to 1 year), then these IVCP regimens might be preferred for very aggressive disease, but this has never been formally proven.

Mycophenolate mofetil-based regimens

This topic is extensively reviewed in Chapter 10, and only a few brief comments will be included here. All RCT examining the effects of MMF-based induction regimens have used a CP-based regimen (either intravenous or oral) as the comparator group, usually the NIH-style IVCP regimen or an oral CP-based regimen of defined duration such as that used by the LNCSG.[1,34–38,52–57] The results have been mixed. Some studies, particularly those from Asia or in populations enriched for African Americans or Hispanics, have shown favorable results, with a lower profile of adverse effects for MMF (less serious infections and ovarian failure).[38] On the other hand, the largest RCT of induction therapy for severe lupus nephritis conducted to date (the Aspreva Lupus Management Study, ALMS) showed that MMF and NIH-style IVCP were equivalent (about a 65% total remission rate in each group) and comparable to the remission rate with the Euro-Lupus regimen (70%).[38,58] In addition, there was no decided advantage of one treatment over the other in terms of total adverse events, including death, although the profile of individual adverse events were different. The ALMS induction trial enrolled a significant percentage of patients (about 25%) of African American, Hispanic, or mixed ancestry. In a secondary analysis there was a suggestion that MMF was more beneficial (or IVCP less effective) in non-Caucasian subjects.[58] The optimum dosage of MMF (most effective with least side effects) is not clear from these studies, but Asians may tolerate less daily dosage of MMF than non-Asians.[59] A proportion of patients cannot tolerate the recommended MMF maximal dose of 3.0 g/day, mainly due to gastrointestinal effects and leukopenia. Thus, under some circumstances, MMF can be regarded as equivalent to CP-based treatment regimens for induction of a remission in severe lupus nephritis. Whether MMF offers superior efficacy and safety in non-Caucasians (Asians, African Americans, or Hispanics) needs to be tested in a properly designed prospective RCT, but post hoc analysis suggests that this may be the case. The profile of side effects and cost may be a deciding factor regarding the choice of agent.[60] The desire for maintenance of reproductive capacity and the risk of the drug for fetal development needs to be taken into consideration in sexually active women of childbearing age (see also Lupus nephritis in pregnancy, Chapter 11).

Calcineurin inhibitor-based regimens

Much less information is available regarding efficacy and safety of regimens using CNI (cyclosporine or tacrolimus) for induction of remissions in severe lupus nephritis.[1,61,62,63] Most of the studies are anecdotal and observational, and many used CNI as "rescue" therapy for unresponsive patients rather than *de novo* for induction. The data show a tendency for improvement in proteinuria, but long-term studies of outcomes (renal and patient survival) are lacking. There are very few RCT comparing CNI with "standard therapy" (e.g. CP-based regimens for induction). However, one small and short-term RCT (from China) has examined, in 40 patients, the efficacy and safety of a "multi-target" approach to severe lupus nephritis due to mixed membranous and diffuse proliferative disease (Class V plus Class IV lupus nephritis) using a combination of tacrolimus, MMF, and steroids compared to an IVCP-based regimen.[64] Tacrolimus was given in a dose of 3–4 mg/day and titrated according to blood levels, MMF was given in doses of 1.5–2.0 g/day titrated according to mycophenolic acid blood levels, and steroids were given in doses of 0.5 g of methylprednisolone intravenously for three consecutive days followed by oral prednisone at 0.6–0.8 mg/kg/day followed by rapid tapering. After 6 months, complete remissions developed in 50% of the "multi-target"-treated patients compared to only 5% in the IVCP-treated patients. Partial remissions occurred in an equal fraction of the two treatment groups (total remissions in "multi-target" therapy of 90% versus only 45% with the IVCP-based regimen). The "multi-target" therapy was well tolerated. Transient increases in serum creatinine, as have been seen in observational studies of CNI therapy of lupus nephritis, were not seen in this study. Although this RCT is very short term (maximum observation period 9 months), small, limited to Asian (Chinese) subjects, and not yet independently confirmed, it does again demonstrate the poor outcome of mixed membranous and severe proliferative lupus nephritis with "standard" IVCP-based therapy and does offer some new hope for control of this very serious and often devastating form of lupus nephritis.

Azathioprine-based regimens

Azathioprine, combined with steroids, is now seldom used as induction therapy in severe lupus nephritis, whereas it is commonly incorporated into maintenance regimens (see below).[1] Retrospective, uncontrolled studies conducted over many years consistently suggested modest beneficial effects of AZA on lupus nephritis and a low level of undesirable side effects.[1] A steroid-sparing effect was also noted. Until recently, no large-scale RCT comparing AZA to standard IVCP-based regimens were available. This deficiency was corrected in 2006 by the publication of an open-label RCT from the Netherlands in severe proliferative lupus nephritis.[65] Eighty-seven patients were randomized to receive either IVCP (750 mg/m^2; 13 doses over 2 years) combined with oral prednisone, or AZA (2 mg/kg/day for 2 years and nine FVMP pulses) combined with similar doses of oral prednisone. After a follow-up of almost 6 years, progressive renal failure (doubling of baseline serum creatinine) was nonsignificantly increased and relapses were more frequent in the AZA group. All relapses responded well to intensification of therapy. Infections (particularly herpes zoster) were more common in the AZA group. The frequency of complete and partial remission was equal in the two groups, and at last follow-up the median serum creatinine and proteinuria were equivalent. This study was underpowered to examine the potential benefit of the drugs on long-term outcomes; but, at last follow-up, almost 90% of the AZA group was free of CP treatment. Serial renal biopsies demonstrated that CP was superior to AZA in terms of avoidance of progressive chronic lesions.[66] This study has been interpreted as showing that AZA is not the first choice for induction therapy of severe lupus nephritis, but that it could be viewed as an alternative in patients who choose not to receive CP (or possibly MMF or CNI). The overall treatment burden perceived by patients is greatest with CP-based regimens.[67] It is likely that mizoribine (a drug similar to AZA and available in Japan) would have similar effects on lupus nephritis.[68] The main drawback of an AZA plus prednisone regimen for induction is the high likelihood of relapse (relative risk 4.9 compared to IVCP in the study cited above). This tendency for relapse in AZA plus prednisone-treated patients for induction of remission would likely translate to a poorer long-term outcome and a greater frequency of progressive chronic lesions.[66] These reservations about the use of AZA plus prednisone induction regimens should not indicate that AZA-based maintenance regimens would be ineffective (see below).

Other agents used for induction of remission

Not surprisingly, a variety of agents and techniques has been studied as possible alternatives to intravenous or oral CP, MMF, or AZA for induction of a remission in severe lupus nephritis. These regimens include chimeric or humanized anti-CD20 monoclonal antibodies, other B cell directed therapies, leflunomide, intravenous immunoglobulin (IVIg), TNFα antagonism, abetimus (B cell toleragen), proteasome inhibitors, artesunate, and inhibition of complement activation and effect.[37,69–86] With a few exceptions, these studies have been observational rather than randomized and controlled, and thus the role for these regimens in treatment of severe lupus nephritis remains unknown. However, recent preliminary findings of RCT for some of these agents have become available, and still others are in progress. The observational studies of these agents have been largely conducted in patients unresponsive to standard therapy (see Refractory lupus nephritis, below), or in patients with special features such as a superimposed necrotizing vasculitis (ANCA+).[79,81,87]

Intravenous immunoglobulin

Preparations of polyclonal immunoglobulin suitable for parenteral use (IVIg) have been employed in treatment of lupus nephritis for many years.[81] The doses used are generally in the range of 2 g/kg over a 5-day period by slow infusion. The putative mechanism of action of IVIg is not well known, but might be due to a potent anti-inflammatory action of a highly glycosylated subfraction of the polyclonal Ig.[88] The response rate is thought to be between 33% and 100%, but no RCT have been conducted. Anecdotes have suggested particular efficacy of IVIg in rapidly progressive (crescentic) disease and in the situation of complicating thrombotic microangiopathy (possibly related to autoantibodies to ADAMTS13, complement factor H or antiphospholipid antibody) (see Chapter 9).[81,89] Intravenous immunoglobulin therapy is generally well tolerated, but episodes of acute renal failure have frequently been reported with the use of the sucrose- or maltose-stabilized forms of IVIg.[90] Only preparations devoid of sucrose or maltose should be used. In addition, high-dose polyclonal IVIg preparations with high titers of red cell isoagglutinins (anti-A, anti-B) can induce an acute immune hemolytic anemia in susceptible persons.[91]

Monoclonal antibodies to CD20 (B cell)

The use of monoclonal antibodies to CD20, a differentiation antigen present on the surface of maturing B cells, but not on plasma cells, is a rapidly growing strategy for management of a wide variety of autoimmune diseases, including lupus nephritis.[37,70–75,79–81] Preliminary, largely observational or pilot case–control studies suggest that this class of biological immunomodulating agents (exemplified by the mouse–human chimeric monoclonal hybridoma, rituximab) may have a role in the treatment of severe lupus nephritis, both for induction and maintenance of remissions, as well as for "rescue" therapy of subjects failing to respond to "standard" therapy (see Refractory lupus nephritis, below).[37,70–75,79–81] These agents also have the potential to exert a "steroid-sparing" effect. Rituximab and its successors all display potent ability to eliminate B cells (CD19+/CD20+) from the circulation and have variable effects on B cells in germinal centers of lymphoid tissue. The fundamental putative mechanism of action in lupus nephritis is unknown, but may involve an effect on antigen-processing or T–B cell interactions. Treatment has a variable effect on anti-dsDNA antibody levels, relapses can occur without return of circulating B cells, and remission can develop with no or minimal decreases in anti-dsDNA antibody levels. It is possible that anti-CD20 monoclonal antibodies selectively deplete subsets of B cells that are involved in promoting production of specific nephritogenic autoantibodies. Rituximab is administered intravenously by slow infusion in doses of 375 mg/m^2 weekly for four doses (total dose of 2500 mg for an average body surface area of 1.73 m^2), or more commonly as 1000 mg doses every 2 weeks for two doses (2000 mg) in autoimmune diseases (like SLE and rheumatoid arthritis). The schedule may be repeated at 6 months, depending on serial measurements of CD19+ cells in the peripheral blood. Anecdotal published reports indicate a complete and partial remission rate of 40–90%, but most reported cases have been refractory to prior treatments.[37,70–72,79–81] Induction therapy for severe lupus nephritis using rituximab has been examined in the recently completed LUNAR Trial,[37] which compared rituximab plus MMF plus steroids, to MMF plus steroids. Analysis of the data is ongoing, but the primary endpoint of a renal response (complete or partial remission) was not achieved. There was no difference in complete remissions (26% in rituximab versus 30% in control), but there was a trend toward a greater number of partial remissions (31% in rituximab versus 15% in controls) at 1 year. The overall remission rate in the MMF-treated subjects was lower (43%) than that observed in the MMF arm of the ALMS induction trial (65%) (see above and Chapter 10), possibly related to differences in the inclusion and exclusion criteria, the definitions of criteria for remission, and/or the ancestry of the enrolled patients (5% Asian, 36% Hispanic and 27% Black in LUNAR versus 33% Asian, 35% Hispanic and 27% Black and mixed in the ALMS Trial). Rituximab therapy was generally well tolerated, with some possible excess of viral infections. Occasional hypersensitivity reactions (e.g. serum sickness-like reactions) can occur. No case of progressive multifocal leukoencephalopathy (PML) was observed, but instances of this fatal reactivation of the polyoma JC virus (JCV) has been observed in other heavily immunosuppressed patients with autoimmune disease, including those treated with anti-CD20 antibody.

Thus, the exact role of anti-CD20 monoclonal antibody therapy for induction (and maintenance) therapy of severe lupus nephritis remains very uncertain at this juncture. The drug may have value in rescue of refractory cases, but this has not yet been demonstrated in a rigorously designed RCT. In addition, if this class of agents can be demonstrated, in a RCT, to spare steroids in the long-term management of lupus nephritis, then they may yet become a part of the routine armamentarium, particularly in promoting freedom from relapse in steroid-free maintenance regimens (see below).[92] Newer humanized monoclonal antibodies directed to CD20 (ocreluzimab), CD22 (epratuzumab), cytotoxic T lymphocyte antigen (CTLA)4-Ig (abatacept, belatacept), or other functional antigens of B cells (e.g. belimumab; anti-B cell activating factor (BAFF) or B lymphocyte stimulator (BlyS)) are also under intense investigation in systemic lupus erythematosus, including lupus nephritis,[93,94] and the final results of these trials are eagerly awaited (see www.clinicaltrials.gov). It is presently unclear if these biological immunomodulating agents will provide superior control of the renal disease with equal or fewer side effects compared to "standard" induction or maintenance regimens in severe lupus nephritis effects, but observational studies in small series have suggested efficacy as "rescue therapy" in refractory or multiple relapsing cases (see Refractory lupus nephritis, below).

Tumor necrosis factor antagonists

The use of TNFα antagonists in the induction of a remission in severe lupus nephritis has been limited so far to observational studies of small size and limited duration, and largely confined to refractory disease (see below).[95,96] No RCT have yet been performed, so the role of this class of agents in primary induction of a remission in severe lupus nephritis is not well established. It is known, however, that these agents can induce a picture resembling lupus nephritis in patients with other autoimmune diseases (such as rheumatoid arthritis).[97] Also, an increased risk of opportunistic infection (including tuberculosis) is found in patients treated with these agents.[98] The role of TNFα antagonists for the treatment of severe lupus nephritis may be limited because of adverse events in this susceptible group of subjects, and enthusiasm for development of this class of agents for treatment of severe lupus nephritis appears to be waning.

Intensive plasma exchange

Although the rationale for the use of intensive plasma exchange (4 litres per session in adults; plasmapheresis) appears sound on the surface (removal of immune complexes, decrease in procoagulant factors, removal of complement components, immunomodulation),[99] the only RCT of this form of therapy was negative when intensive plasma exchange therapy was compared to standard treatment with oral cyclophosphamide and prednisone (the LNCSG study of plasmapheresis).[1,100] Theoretically, synchronization of plasma exchange therapy with IVCP therapy might be better, but this has never been proven to be the case in a well-designed RCT.[101] It also remains possible that plasma exchange could provide some additive benefits in subjects with severe lupus nephritis presenting with extensive crescentic disease and rapidly progressive glomerulonephritis, particularly with dialysis-dependent renal failure,[101] but this has never been formally tested in a RCT. Due to the rarity of this event, the value of plasma exchange is not likely to be tested in a RCT any time soon. Also, intensive plasma exchange with fresh frozen plasma replacement could be helpful in those uncommon subjects with severe lupus nephritis and complicating thrombotic microangiopathy (due to antibody to ADAMTS13, complement factor H or antiphospholipid antibodies) (see Chapter 9). This has not been, and is not likely to be, tested in a RCT any time soon.

Maintenance therapy for severe proliferative lupus nephritis

As indicated above, the prevention of renal relapses (renal flares) in patients who have achieved a complete or partial remission following induction therapy is an extremely important objective in the overall management of severe lupus nephritis.[12–14] Indeed, the frequency and severity of such relapses are among the most powerful determinants of long-term outcome. Renal relapses of severe lupus nephritis can be described as nephritic or nephrotic (also known as proteinuric relapses) (see Table 12.4).[102–105] Nephritic renal relapses are the more common variety and are characterized by an increase in excretion of red cells and formed elements (including red cell casts) in the urine, accompanied by an increase in protein excretion and a diminution of renal function (falling glomerular filtration rate (GFR) and rising serum creatinine).[102–105] Nephrotic (proteinuric) renal relapses are less common than nephritic renal relapses and are characterized predominantly by an increase in protein excretion, often to "nephrotic" ranges (greater than 3.5 g/day in an adult) with a variable change in renal function. Renal function may often be stable in nephrotic renal relapses. A change in red cell excretion is not required. A nephrotic renal relapse may also herald a transformation of the underlying lesion from a proliferative one (Class IV lupus nephritis) to a membranous pattern (Class V lupus nephritis) (see also Chapter 7). Nephritic relapses occur more often after a partial remission to induction therapy, when maintenance therapy is inadequate, and in patients with persistently low levels of C4 complement at the time that remission occurs with induction.[12–14,102–105] Nephritic relapses, when frequent, also indicate a much higher risk of ESRD (Table 12.4).[61–63,65]

As the risk of relapse extends for many years after the initial remission is attained, the regimens for maintenance of remission must not only be effective but also have a very low profile of cumulative toxicity and adverse events. High-dose glucocorticoids are very effective in preventing relapses, but they cannot be used for maintenance therapy due to unacceptable risks of side effects (cosmetic, psychological, diabetes, osteoporosis, skin atrophy, ulcers, weight gain, muscle atrophy, etc.). On the other hand, low-dose alternate-day prednisone can be quite effective for maintaining remission, as was shown in the long-term follow-up of the LNCSG trial of plasma exchange (see above).[1]

Table 12.4 Definition of relapse ("renal flare") in severe lupus nephritis*

Nephritic relapse
Mild
Urine sediment: ↑ cellular casts by one category (rated 0–4+) or ≥rbc/hpf if BL <10 rbc/hpf or doubling of rbcv/hpf if BL ≥10 rbc/hpf
Proteinuria: ↑ UP by <2.0 g/day
Renal function: ↑ in Scr by <30% over BL
Moderate
Urine sediment: ↑ in number of cellular cast or rbc
Proteinuria: ↑ by ≥ 2.0 g/day
Renal function: ↑in Scr by ≤30% from BL
Severe
Urine sediment: ↑ in number of cellular casts or rbc
Proteinuria: ↑ in UP by ≥2.0 g/day
Renal function: ↑ Scr by >30% (regardless of the change in UP)
Proteinuric relapses
Urine sediment: no change from BL
Proteinuria: ↑ in UP by >2.0gm/d
Renal function: ↑ in Scr by ≤ 30% from BL

* From Illei et al.[40]

Similarly, agents that are effective for induction may be unsuitable for maintenance (e.g. cyclophosphamide) for the same fundamental reasons. Thus, maintenance therapeutic regimens span a narrower range of drugs. The optimal duration of maintenance therapy that balances efficacy with safety in severe lupus nephritis in complete (or partial) remission is not well known. In patients treated with intravenous or oral CP or MMF-based regimens for induction, and who achieve a complete or partial remission, the rate of relapse is about 6–10 relapses per 100 patient years for the first 5 years of follow-up, although there is considerable variability in this risk from study to study (Glassock RJ, unpublished observations) (see also Table 12.4). The regimen chosen for induction may have an important influence on the risk of relapse (e.g. AZA- and CNI-induced remissions may have a higher risk of relapse compared to MMF- or CP-induced remissions).[61–63] A partial instead of a complete remission after induction greatly increases the risk for relapses, as does a persistently low C4 level (<11 mg/dl).[102–105] Patients who remain free from relapse for 5 years seldom relapse subsequently,[106] thus maintenance therapy may not be required indefinitely in very stable patients in remission. The treatment of relapses is outlined below (see Treatment of relapses in severe lupus nephritis).

Cyclophosphamide-based maintenance regimens

As alluded to above, oral or intravenous CP is not suitable for long-term relapse-free maintenance therapy of severe lupus nephritis. This is due to its cumulative toxicity (ovarian failure, bone marrow hypoplasia, cytogenetic damage, oncogenesis, opportunistic infections). Early experience with CP utilized prolonged treatment regimens. These have now largely been abandoned and replaced by sequential therapy regimens (see below). Indeed, in this author's opinion, patients with severe lupus nephritis should seldom (if ever) be exposed to CP for more than 1 year (cumulatively, including re-treatment of relapses), and the great majority should not be exposed for more than 6 months of therapy (total dose of 300 mg/kg orally or 85 mg/kg intravenously)—many will require much less exposure for induction of a remission. Nearly all subjects induced into remission with a CP-based regimen (intravenous or oral) should be converted to a less toxic regimen (such as AZA or MMF) combined with low-dose alternate-day glucocorticoid regimens, see below) for maintenance of remission.

Azathioprine-based maintenance regimens

Azathioprine-based maintenance regimens have a long history of use in severe lupus nephritis. Long-term treatment with AZA is well tolerated (except for macrocytic anemia, cervical and vulvar carcinoma (in papilloma virus antibody-positive nonvaccinated women), skin cancer, cholestatic jaundice, leukopenia and opportunistic infections, and rarely hypersensitivity reactions (either to the imidazole ring or the parent 6-MP compound)).[107] Uncommonly, a genetic trait, thiopurine methyltransferase (TPMT) deficiency, can promote leukopenic reactions to conventional doses of AZA (1–2 mg/kg/day).[108] This occurs in <1% of the population at large.

A RCT of maintenance therapy in severe lupus nephritis has definitively shown that AZA (plus low-dose steroids) is superior to CP-based therapy in terms of relapse-free survival.[34] Conversion to AZA therapy can be achieved after a partial or complete remission is obtained, usually after 3–6 months, occasionally up to a year, after start-ing induction therapy. The optimum duration of AZA maintenance therapy is not known, but it should be at least 2 years and probably 5 years at a minimum. Some patients will require even longer periods of therapy, if frequent relapses still occur. The persistence of frequent relapses, more than three per year, while on AZA therapy should lead to consideration of a change in the maintenance therapy regimen.

Mycophenolate mofetil-based maintenance regimens

Oral MMF has been shown to be an effective agent both for induction and mainte-nance of remission in severe lupus nephritis (see also Chapter 10). Formal comparison of MMF, AZA, and IVCP therapy for maintenance of remission has been conducted in a RCT in which all subjects were induced to a remission by IVCP.[34] In this compari-son, MMF was equivalent to AZA and superior to IVCP for preventing relapses (a group maintained on glucocorticoids only was not included in this trial). Less is known about the efficacy of MMF compared to AZA when a remission has been induced by MMF. This is being tested in the ALMS maintenance phase trial. The pre-liminary results of this landmark trial suggest that MMF is superior to AZA for main-tanence of relapse-free survival at an acceptable level of adverse effects.[109] Due to cost differences, it is important to determine the overall efficacy and safety for these two regimens at dosages deemed to be pharmacologically equivalent. Azathioprine is more likely to be associated with leukopenia and MMF is more likely to be associated with gastrointestinal disturbances, but both can result in an increased risk of infections. There may be differences in the pharmacodynamic and pharmacokinetic behavior of MMF between Asians and non-Asians.[110] Enterohepatic recirculation of MMF may give rise to potential drug interactions (e.g. bile acid binding resins).[111] At the present time, the duration of MMF maintenance therapy for severe lupus nephritis in remis-sion is unknown but is probably in excess of two to three years.

Calcineurin inhibitor-based maintenance regimens

The use of CNI, cyclosporine (CSA) or tacrolimus, for maintenance of remission of severe lupus nephritis has not been extensively studied.[61,111] However, a RCT was conducted in 75 patients with severe diffuse proliferative lupus nephritis comparing the effects of CSA and AZA on maintenance of remission induced by oral CP plus prednisone.[111] The primary endpoint was incidence of disease relapses over 4 years of follow-up. Renal relapse developed in seven of 36 patients (4.9 per 100 patient years) receiving CSA and eight of 33 (6.0 per 100 patient years) in the AZA group ($P = NS$). Adverse events requiring discontinuation of therapy were equal in the two groups (about 12%). Protein excretion and renal function were also not different in the two groups during follow-up. The average dose of CSA was only 2 mg/kg/day, and that of AZA was about 1.5 mg/kg/day. Low-dose prednisone was used in both groups (about 10–12 mg/day). Thus, low-dose CSA combined with low-dose steroids is an acceptable alternative to AZA plus steroids or MMF plus steroids for maintenance therapy of patients with severe lupus nephritis in remission. Long-term outcome in patients main-tained on CNI plus low-dose steroids in terms of prevention of ESRD is not known.

Glucocorticoid only maintenance regimens

High doses of oral prednisone are not suitable for long-term maintenance of remission for obvious reasons of cumulative toxicity (iatrogenic Cushing syndrome). Low-dose, alternate-day regimens (10–20 mg prednisone or its equivalent on alternate days) can be effective in subjects exhibiting a stable post-induction course (freedom from relapses for 6 months or longer), as was shown in the LNCSG experience stated above.[1] Low-dose steroids are often combined with AZA, MMF, or CNI, as indicated above, on the presumption that these drugs will permit lowering of the doses of prednisone without unleashing relapses (steroid-sparing effect). Until now, a long-term, adequately powered, RCT comparing a steroid-alone maintenance regimen with an AZA, MMF, or CNI plus steroid maintenance regimen has not been conducted. Many RCT of maintenance therapy in severe lupus nephritis have not included a steroid-only arm, most likely because of the presumption that patients with severe lupus nephritis, particularly those with only a partial remission following induction, require some adjunctive treatment with an immunomodulating agent (AZA, MMF, or CNI), in addition to glucocorticoids. Limited observational studies have also shown that intermittent IVMP pulses (e.g. quarterly) can prolong remission and lower the frequency of relapses.[113] No RCT have been conducted to examine the efficacy or safety of this approach.

Other maintenance regimens

No RCT of regimens other than AZA, MMF, or CSA have been conducted, with the exception of abetimus (Riquent; Jolla Pharmaceuticals).[114] Despite earlier encouraging results, this interesting "B cell toleragen" was unable to reduce the incidence of renal flares and is not currently approved for use in lupus nephritis.[114] A desirable goal, not yet achieved, would be to maintain a remission, or avoid frequent and serious relapses, without resorting to any glucocorticoid administration (steroid-free maintenance). Preliminary data from observational cohorts using rituximab induction and MMF maintenance may permit complete steroid withdrawal without any increase in renal relapse, at least in some patients.[71,92] It is possible that regimens involving judicious use of anti-CD20 monoclonal antibody (rituximab or another biologic B-cell modulating agent) might be able to make "steroid-free" maintenance a reality, but no RCT have yet demonstrated this possibility.

Treatment of refractory severe lupus nephritis

About 15–40% of patients with severe lupus nephritis will fail to respond to initial attempts to induce a complete or partial remission, and are thus labeled as refractory to treatment. This wide variation in the fraction of refractory patients is due to a number of factors: (i) the delay between the onset of renal disease and presentation for treatment; (ii) the extent of loss of renal function at the time treatment is begun; (iii) the underlying severity of disease and classification of disease; (iv) complicating lesions (such as crescents and thrombotic microangiopathy); (v) possibly ancestral and societal (e.g. poverty) factors; and (vi) different definitions of what constitutes a "refractory" patient. The specific regimen used for induction of remission (e.g. intravenous or oral CP, MMF) does not contribute greatly to the variation in "refractoriness." Isolated persistence of proteinuria, with improvement in all other features of renal disease, is not a very useful definition of "refractoriness," as the improvement in protein excretion may be delayed for many months or even years after the successful initial induction of a remission. Nevertheless, these patients constitute a difficult challenge for the clinician, in part because there are no RCT to guide their therapeutic decisions, and, in part, because such patients represent a high risk for complications (or even death) from overly aggressive immunosuppressive therapy. The initial and/or repeat renal biopsy findings can help, in that advanced irreversible changes (fibrous crescents, glomerulosclerosis, interstitial fibrosis) augur a poor response to any treatment, whereas persistent active lesions (proliferation, necrosis, cellular crescents) indicate a potentially responsive lesion. At present, the choice of a specific regimen for "rescue" of a refractory patient is more directed by expert opinion than by evidence. If a patient has failed induction therapy after a reasonable attempt with adequate doses of effective agents and a long-enough period of observation (at least 6 months and perhaps as long as a year), then the designation "refractory" is appropriate. If induction was with intravenous or oral CP, a conversion to MMF might be chosen, or if MMF was the induction regimen, then a change to intravenous or oral CP might be used. A trial of a repeat of the "pulse" IVMP used for induction can also be tried. A response to these kinds of treatment modifications is difficult to predict. A more common approach would be to introduce another agent, such as rituximab, a TNF antagonist, or even IVIg. Anecdotes attest to the success of this approach but no RCTs are available, and the risk of over-immunosuppression and its attendant hazards of opportunistic infections are great, so caution and vigilant follow-up are needed.

Treatment of renal and systemic relapses in severe lupus nephritis

As mentioned previously, renal relapses (exacerbations) are to be expected in the majority of patients who achieve a complete or partial remission during induction phase. These exacerbations are more common following a partial remission from induction therapy and may vary somewhat according to the agents used for induction and maintenance (Glassock, unpublished observations). Also see Table 12.5. The severity of relapses varies widely, from a minor increase in hematuria (and formed elements such as casts) and/or proteinuria with stable renal function to fulminant renal failure. One must be careful to distinguish exacerbations from *de novo* diseases due to a complication of therapy, such as an acute hypersensitivity interstitial nephritis from a drug (antimicrobial, diuretic, NSAID). Serological findings (rising anti-dsDNA, falling C3/C4) may be somewhat helpful and renal biopsy may be required for definitive diagnosis. A low level of C1q or a high level of anti-C1q auto-antibodies seem particularly valuable to detect renal relapses,[115] and when all serological values (anti-dsDNA, C3/C4) are normal, the likelihood of a renal relapse is quite remote.[115]

For mild exacerbations, without any change in renal function, a temporary increase in oral prednisone to 1 mg/kg/day may suffice. For more severe relapses, accompanied

Table 12.5 Relationship of complete or partial remission and renal relapses in severe lupus nephritis after induction therapy*

Remission status after induction therapy	Total relapses	Nephritic relapses	Time to relapse	ESRD after relapse
Complete remission	39%	79%	36 months	10%
Partial remission	64%	83%	18 months	67%

* From Ilei et al.[40]

by a significant reduction in renal function, re-introduction of the induction regimen, perhaps at a reduced dosage, is the usual treatment regime advised, particularly if the exacerbation was connected to too rapid tapering or discontinuance of immunosuppression. The response to treatment for an exacerbation, unless it is very severe, is usually quite favorable, and a tapering regimen can be started soon after improvement is in evidence, although at a slower rate than used prior to the exacerbation. Frequent exacerbations (e.g. more than three per year) should occasion a consideration of a change to another maintenance regimen (e.g. from AZA to MMF or CSA).

Special issues in treatment of severe lupus nephritis

Pregnancy and fertility

Many patients with severe lupus nephritis are concerned about fertility and procreation. As lupus affects mostly young women of childbearing age, these concerns revolve around the possible adverse effects of a pregnancy on their disease, the expected outcome of a pregnancy (live births, fetal malformations, prematurity), and the effects of drugs used in the treatment of their disease on long-term fertility and upon a fetus *in utero*. This topic is extensively reviewed in Chapter 11, and will not be discussed further here. Careful collaboration with an obstetrician–gynecologist experienced in managing patients with lupus nephritis should be encouraged in pregnant patients with lupus nephritis. A pregnancy test should be performed in all female patients (sexually active) of childbearing age prior to the initiation of any cytotoxic drug (including CP, AZA, or MMF).

The preservation of fertility is a major issue in both males and females with severe lupus nephritis undergoing treatment with immunosuppressive agents. This concern is limited to those patients receiving CP-based regimens (intravenous, oral). Cyclophosphamide has adverse effects on gonadal function (ovulation and spermatogenesis) and these effects are related to the total cumulative dosage. For oral CP the "threshold" for adverse gonadal effects is about 200 mg/kg. The "threshold" for IVCP is not as well understood. Older subjects appear to be an increased risk for these adverse events. Prolonged amenorrhea and ovulatory failure (or azoospermia) can be seen in 50% or more of patients receiving prolonged CP therapy. Leuprolide (3.75 mg intramuscularly every 4–6 weeks) in women or testosterone (100 mg intramuscularly every 2 weeks) in men for the duration of CP therapy can be used to reduce the risk of gonadal failure, but the evidence for efficacy is weak.[116] In a study of short-term oral CP (cumulative dosage of CP around 10 g; approximately 150 mg/kg) in which leuprolide was used, only 2.2% of treated patients developed amenorrhea, but in the absence of a leuprolide-untreated group one cannot be sure whether this was related to the low cumulative dosage of CP or to the leuprolide therapy.[117] In patients desiring to have children, and in whom a prolonged course of CP is anticipated, gonadal-sparing therapy with leuprolide (females) or testosterone (males) may be indicated, but proof of efficacy and safety is lacking. Prolonged cryogenic preservation of semen in males may be utilized as well. If the course of CP is expected to be short, these steps are usually not necessary.

Advanced renal failure

Unfortunately, a fraction of patients with severe lupus nephritis may progress to advanced renal failure (Stage 4 and 5 chronic kidney disease). In a minority this is due to rapidly progressive renal failure unresponsive to aggressive induction therapy (see above). This may be due to underlying extensive crescentic disease or a severe complicating thrombotic microangiopathy (see also Chapter 9). Treatment of such patients is not well established due to the expected lack of RCT, but very intense regimens of intravenous or oral CP, high doses of potential steroids, perhaps intensive plasma exchange, IVIg, or anticoagulation might be of some benefit.[118,119] The decision of when to abandon therapy of the nephritis and rely on renal replacement therapy (dialysis and transplantation) is a difficult one, and revolves around the balance of possible benefit and the risks (especially the burden of excessive immunosuppressive therapy) and futility of further treatment of the nephritis. No evidence-based recommendations can be proposed, as this is a highly individualized situation. Evidence of irreversibility of the lesions from repeat renal biopsy analysis may be helpful in concluding that further treatment is futile and excessively risky.

More often, patients with severe lupus nephritis gradually develop impaired renal function, often associated with persistent heavy proteinuria and/or repeated renal relapses (nephritic or proteinuric) unresponsive to maintenance therapy. In such patients, it is worthwhile attempting to slow the rate of progression by use of angiotensin II inhibition and rigorous control of blood pressure (to <130/80 mmHg or lower if urine protein excretion is >1.0 g/day), while focusing on minimization of immunosuppression for control of extrarenal manifestations only. Initiation of dialysis or pre-emptive renal transplantation when the estimated GFR reaches levels less than about 8 ml/min/1.73 m^2 would be appropriate.

Maintenance dialysis and renal transplantation

Patients with severe lupus nephritis who reach ESRD are perfectly acceptable candidates for both forms of renal replacement therapy.[120–122] Because of the usual age of the subjects with severe lupus nephritis, renal transplantation is preferred and pre-emptive renal transplantation is ideal unless the patient has been over-immunosuppressed to prevent progressive renal failure, where pre-emptive renal transplant may be too risky. Recurrences of the original disease may develop in the transplanted kidney, but this is relatively uncommon using standard post-transplant immunosuppressive therapy.[122,123] The long-term outcome for lupus nephritis patients receiving living or deceased donor transplants is not greatly different from those patients with nonlupus-related renal disease.[123,124] Both hemo- and peritoneal dialysis are effective renal replacement therapy regimens. Patients with ESRD often enter into a remission of their extrarenal manifestation of disease, despite discontinuance of all immunosuppressive therapy, but exceptions to this general rule have been described.[125,126] Continuation of the lowest possible dose of an immunosuppressant drug (MMF, AZA, CSA or tacrolimus) sufficient to control the extrarenal manifestation to a tolerable level is indicated in these uncommon patients. Attempts to withdraw therapy in such patients should be conducted at regular intervals.

Thrombotic microangiopathy

The development of a thrombotic microangiopathy (TMA), often with moderate thrombocytopenia, microangiopathic hemolytic anemia, severe hypertension, and neurological manifestations, is a not uncommon event associated with severe lupus nephritis.[118,119,127,128] This topic is covered in detail in Chapter 9 and will not be discussed extensively here. Briefly, such a complication greatly worsens the prognosis and alters the approach to therapy of the disease, depending on the specifics of the underlying pathogenesis. Uncommonly, the complication is due to the development of autoantibodies to ADAMTS13 (von Willebrand factor cleaving enzyme) and the disorder can resemble thrombotic thrombocytopenic purpura (TTP). These patients are best treated with intensive plasma exchange and replacement with fresh frozen plasma in addition to standard immunosuppression.[128] More commonly, the complication is due to the presence of an antiphospholipid autoantibody (lupus anticoagulant) that promotes both venous and arterial thrombi and the microvascular lesions of a TMA.[127–129] Neurological manifestations in these patients may be due to "ischemic" (microthrombotic) strokes rather than a "cerebral vasculitis." These patients may be best managed by a combination of anticoagulants (initially heparin, fractionated or unfractionated) followed by warfarin, often with a relatively high internationalized ratio (INR) for prothrombin time of 2.5–3.0.[127,128] Intravenous immunoglobulin can also be life-saving in severe cases, and intensive plasma exchange might also be beneficial but this is not well documented.[130] Finally, it is theoretically possible that a hemolytic uremic syndrome (HUS)-like picture might ensue if an autoantibody to the complement factor H (CfH) develops.[131] These patients would be expected to have very low C3 levels, due to dysregulation of the alternative complement pathway, and low activity but normal protein levels of CfH in the circulation. Treatment with fresh frozen plasma infusions and intensive plasma exchange might be indicated. Eculizumab (a monoclonal antibody to C5) is undergoing a trial in similar patients (atypical HUS due to CfH deficiency).[132]

Summary of the therapy of severe lupus nephritis

It should be abundantly clear from the foregoing review that the ideal therapy for patients with severe lupus nephritis involves the consideration of a large number of variables. It is not surprising that experts differ on the recommendations for treatment of individual patients with severe lupus nephritis, due to the wide diversity of presentations and courses pursued by such patients. Therefore, it is not appropriate to make generalizations or prepare algorithms, as treatment has to be highly individualized. Although the "scientific evidence" underlying the choices of therapy has certainly increased (since the last edition of this book in 1999),[1] "authoritative opinion" still remains as a factor in choosing one specific regimen over another, and many uncertainties regarding rational (evidence-based) choices of therapeutic approaches remain. Filling these gaps is likely to result in a substantial modification of the current recommendations. A summary of existing information for induction of remission, maintenance of remission, therapy of renal relapses, and treatment of refractory disease follows.

Induction therapy in severe lupus nephritis

Fundamentally, four choices are available: (i) oral CP plus oral (or intravenous) steroids; (ii) high-dose (NIH) IVCP plus oral (or intravenous) steroids; (iii) low-dose (Euro-Lupus) IVCP plus oral (or intravenous) steroids; or (iv) oral MMF plus oral (or intravenous) steroids. Concomitant administration of diuretics (e.g. furosemide) and IVMP should be avoided. Oral prednisone at 1 mg/kg once daily in the morning (maximum dose 80 mg/day) can be started simultaneously. Prednisone can be tapered beginning at 2–4 weeks depending on the response and by 10 weeks the patient should on about 40–50 mg/day. One can then commence a gradual shift to alternate-day regimen or continue to taper the single daily dose regimen. The goal is to have the patient on the equivalent of 15–20 mg/day by 20 weeks and 10–12.5 mg/day by 26 weeks (barring any relapses during the tapering phase). Oral prednisone (1 mg/kg, maximum dose 80 mg/day) can also be used for induction, in the absence of IVMP, apparently without any loss of efficacy, although the benefits and safety of the IVMP and the oral prednisone regimens have never been compared in a RCT.

The choices for the cytotoxic/immunosuppressive component of treatment are mainly based on toxicity, as they all appear to be roughly equivalent in efficacy. The high-dose course (NIH protocol) of IVCP (750–1000 mg/m^2 CP intravenously as a slow infusion monthly for 6 months) is no more effective than the low-dose course (Euro-Lupus protocol) of IVCP (fixed dose of 500 mg CP intravenously every 2 weeks for six doses) at least in European Caucasians. The low-dose IVCP regimen has not been evaluated for efficacy in patients with severe lupus nephritis of African, Hispanic or Asian ancestry. Oral CP (1–2 mg/kg/day once a day in the morning with adequate hydration and frequent voiding) for 2–4 months can be used instead of IVCP, in compliant and dependable patients, without loss of efficacy or any increase in toxicity. Patients in whom concern is raised about the adverse effects of CP on fertility might be offered leuprolide (females) or testosterone (males). Those patients who receive high-dose IVCP can be concomitantly treated with MESNA, if desired, to minimize bladder toxicity. This is usually not necessary in the low-dose IVCP regimen. In all cases, CP should not be given if the total leukocyte count is <4000/μl or the absolute neutrophil count is <1500/μl. White blood cell counts should be monitored weekly during induction therapy involving CP, irrespective of the specific regimen. Patients with severely impaired renal function (serum creatinine over 2.0–2.5 mg/dl) should receive reduced doses (50% of the usual dose) of CP and the high-dose IVCP regimen may be risky in such cases. Prophylactic trimethoprim-sulfamethoxazole is often recommended for prevention of *Pneumocystis juvei* infections during induction therapy, especially if the CD4 lymphocyte count is <350/mm^3.

Oral MMF (initially 2–3 g/day, divided into two equal doses daily) is a satisfactory alternative to the CP-based regimens described above (see also Chapter 10). It might be more effective in individuals of African or Hispanic ancestry and is as effective as intravenous or oral CP in Caucasians and Asians; however, this evidence has been gleaned primarily from secondary analysis of RCT. Asians may not tolerate the higher doses of MMF and a starting dose of 2.0 g/day is preferred in this group. Monitoring of hemoglobin levels and leukocyte counts at 2-week intervals is suggested. Patients may require temporary reduction in dosage if gastrointestinal complaints ensue (abdominal pain, diarrhea).

All female patients with severe lupus nephritis who are in their reproductive years, and who are about to undergo induction therapy, should have a negative pregnancy test before commencing therapy (unless treatment is initiated on an emergency basis). At least two methods of contraception should be used.

With the above induction regimens, between 60% and 85% of patients with severe lupus nephritis, and reasonably normal renal function (serum creatinine level <1.4 mg/dl) can be expected to achieve a complete or partial remission (see above for definitions) within 3–6 months of beginning treatment. The response to induction is likely to be less complete in those subjects with more severe impairment of renal function at the beginning of treatment.

Conversion to maintenance therapy can be commenced no sooner than 3 months and usually by 6 months, depending on the severity of the disease and the rapidity of the response to treatment.

Maintenance therapy in severe lupus nephritis

For patients who received a CP-based induction regimen, several choices are available for maintenance of remission. A commonly used regimen for maintenance therapy is AZA (2 mg/kg/day, maximum dose 200 mg/day), but MMF may be of equivalent or even superior efficacy and safety. In addition, a small subset of patients with severe lupus nephritis in stable complete remission can be maintained satisfactorily on low-dose (10–20 mg), alternate-day prednisone alone. If AZA is selected, it can be started about 4 weeks after the last dose of high-dose IVCP (NIH) when the total leukocyte count is >4000/μl and the absolute neutrophil count is >1500/μl. Azathioprine may be started sooner when a low-dose IVCP (Euro-Lupus) regimen is used. Azathioprine may be started 2 weeks after the last dose, so long as the white blood cell count meets the criteria noted above. With oral CP, the AZA can be started within 1 week after the last CP dose. Patients should be monitored for renal and systemic relapses (serum C3/C4 complement, urinalysis, urine protein excretion, serum creatinine), and the hemoglobin and white blood cell counts measured frequently to assure the absence of bone-marrow toxicity. It is not necessary to screen AZA-treated patients for TPMT deficiency. Contraceptive methods should be continued until the patient is stable (free from relapses for at least 1 year). The optimum duration of AZA maintenance therapy is not known, but some treat patients for about 5 years and for at least 1 year from the last relapse, if no limiting toxicity occurs. Females with prior papilloma virus infection (or who have not been vaccinated against this virus) may be at increased risk for cervical (or vulvar) cancer, so routine pelvic examinations and cervical cytology (at least once yearly) are desirable. Cyclosporine (2–4 mg/kg/day) may also be used for maintenance therapy instead of AZA. This may be especially true in those with persistent nephritic-range proteinuria. Such patients may have undergone a transformation to pure membranous lupus nephritis (a repeat renal biopsy may be indicated; see Chapter 7).

If MMF is chosen for maintenance of remission, in patients who have achieved a complete or partial remission, the same guidelines that have been suggested for AZA apply. The preferential use of MMF for maintenance of remission is based on the results of the ALMS trial. Patients who were induced into a partial or complete remission with MMF should remain on this therapy (unless toxicity occurs). In the absence of a relapse, the dose of MMF may be gradually reduced from 2 to 3 g/day to 1.5g/day in the first year, 1.25 g/day in the second year, and 1.0 g/day in the third and subsequent years. The optimum duration of MMF maintenance therapy is unknown, but stable patients (no relapses for 1 year) may be weaned from MMF after 3 years. Monitoring of patients during maintenance therapy is the same for MMF and AZA. Patients on MMF should use at least two methods of contraception for as long as they are on the drug.

Prednisone dosage should be slowly tapered during maintenance therapy with either AZA or MMF. During the early phases of maintenance therapy, dosage can be slowly tapered to 0.02–0.20 mg/kg/day as a single dose in the morning or 0.04–0.40 mg/kg every other day (usual dose 5–7.5 mg daily or 10–15 mg every other day). Rarely (at least in my experience), patients may be tapered to "zero" prednisone. Patients with multiple relapses may require somewhat higher doses, but if prolonged treatment with >0.3–0.4 mg/kg/day is required, the patient will be susceptible to the adverse consequences of iatrogenic Cushing syndrome (diabetes, obesity, hypertension, osteoporosis, striae, infection, cataracts, skin and muscle atrophy) and require adjunctive therapy (e.g. antihypertensives, insulin, bisphosphonates, vitamin D). Persistent proteinuria should be treated with angiotensin II inhibitory agents (angiotensin converting enzyme inhibitors (ACEI) or angiotensin receptor blockers (ARB)).

During maintenance therapy the average patient can be expected to have one or more renal relapses (see below). The relapse rate is about eight relapses per 100 patient years of follow-up (range 6–12) for the first 5 years, much lower after that period.

Therapy for renal relapses

Renal relapses are common during maintenance therapy and can even occur during induction therapy, most notably in patients with a partial remission. Nephritic and proteinuric relapses are defined above (see Renal relapses), and nephritic relapses are more common and more ominous in terms of long-term prognosis. Very mild renal relapses can often be managed by a brief increase in oral prednisone dosage or a short course of IVMP. More severe relapses often require re-institution of a modified induction protocol. Patients who are on AZA after induction with CP-based regimen can have the relapse treated with MMF (1–3 g/day) and discontinuance of AZA. A switch to cyclosporine can also be considered, especially in proteinuric renal relapses. Repeat re-induction with CP (intravenous or oral) is generally not advised due to an effect on the cumulative dose of CP. In patients on MMF maintenance therapy after MMF-based induction, a trial of the Euro-Lupus low-dose IVCP induction or oral CP could also be considered. If repeated renal relapses continue (three or more a year), a course of rituximab 1000 mg on days 1 and 15 can be tried, but the benefits and risks of this approach have not been well studied. The maintenance dose of AZA or MMF can often be reduced, but not discontinued, with the addition of rituximab. It may also be possible to reduce or eliminate the prednisone dosage in rituximab-treated patients. A switch to cyclosporine maintenance may also be considered in patients with relapses on MMF maintenance, especially in proteinuric relapses.

Therapy of refractory severe lupus nephritis

There is no strict definition for treatment-resistant or refractory severe lupus nephritis. However, most would agree that a patient who fails to achieve a complete or partial remission within 6 months to 1 year after starting any induction therapeutic regimen would qualify as "refractory" to treatment. Such patients are more likely to have significant renal functional impairment at the onset of induction therapy. The management of these patients is difficult, challenging, and risky, especially as many will have varying degrees of renal functional impairment and there are no RCT to guide "evidence"-based treatment. For those patients refractory to MMF induction, a course of CP (oral or intravenous) is often used (see CP-based induction therapy above). For those patients refractory to a CP-based induction (oral or intravenous), a course of MMF is frequently utilized (see MMF-based induction therapy above), but few data are available to assess the benefits and risks of these approaches. For patients intolerant to or refractory to both CP and MMF, a course of rituximab (1000 mg intravenous) on days 1 and 15, repeated at 6 months, or cyclosporine 4–5 mg/kg/day, has been tried with varying degrees of success. Cyclosporine may be contraindicated if renal function is greatly impaired, due to the risk of nephrotoxicity. Cyclosporine, or tacrolimus, based regimens (combined with MMF) may be of particular value in mixed membranous and proliferative lupus nephritis (Class V + Class IV or Class III >50%) and in those patients with persistent heavy proteinuria during induction. Extensive crescentic glomerulonephritis with rapidly progressive renal failure (an uncommon presentation for severe lupus nephritis) can be managed by a combination of IVMP and oral or intravenous CP. The value of additional plasma exchange in these subjects is not known but, by analogy to ANCA+ crescentic glomerulonephritis, might be considered in unusual circumstances.

Excessive immunosuppression of these "refractory" patients can be very risky, and opportunistic infections may arise, which are sometimes lethal. A high degree of vigilance for these infections is absolutely necessary, and, if the burden of immunosuppression is too high, then discontinuance of all therapy except for the minimum to control extrarenal symptoms and signs of lupus erythematosus while awaiting dialysis and transplantation may be the better course.

References

1. Lewis, E.J. (1999) The natural history and treatment of lupus nephritis. In: *Lupus Nephritis* (Lewis, E.J., Schwartz, M.M., Korbet, S.M., eds), pp. 185–218. Oxford University Press, Oxford.

2. Lewis, E.J. (2001) The treatment of lupus nephritis: Revisiting Galen. *Ann Intern Med* **135**, 296–8.

3. Ponticelli, C. (2006) New therapies for lupus nephritis. *Clin J Am Soc Nephrol* **1**, 863–8.

4. Houssiau, F.A., and Ginzler, E.M. (2008) Current treatment of lupus nephritis. *Lupus* **17**, 426–30.

5. Bertsias, G., Gordon, C., and Boumpas, D.T. (2008) Clinical trials in systemic lupus erythematosus (SLE): lessons from the past as we proceed to the future–the EULAR recommendations for the management of SLE and the use of end-points in clinical trials. *Lupus* **17**, 437–42.

6. Bertsias, G., Ioannidis, J.P., Boletis, J., Bombardieri, S., Cervera, R., Dostal, C., *et al.*; Task Force of the EULAR Standing Committee for International Clinical Studies Including Therapeutics (2008) EULAR recommendations for the management of systemic lupus erythematosus. Report of a Task Force of the EULAR Standing Committee for International Clinical Studies Including Therapeutics. *Ann Rheum Dis* **67**, 195–205.

7. Gordon, C., Bertsias, G., Ioannidis, J.P., Boletis, J., Bombardieri, S., Cervera, R., *et al.* (2009) EULAR points to consider for conducting clinical trials in systemic lupus erythematosus. *Ann Rheum Dis* **68**(4), 470–6.

8. Ponticelli, C., Glassock, R.J., and Moroni, G. (2010) Induction and maintenance therapy in proliferative lupus nephritis. *J Nephrol* **23**, 9–16.

9. Lee, Y., Woo, J.H., Choi, S., Ji, J., and Song, G. (2010) Induction and maintenance therapy for lupus nephritis: a systematic review and meta-analysis. *Lupus* [Epub ahead of print].

10. Fraenkel, L., MacKenzie, T., Joseph, L., Kashgarian, M., Hayslett, J.P., and Esdaile, J.M. (1994) Response to treatment as a predictor of long-term outcome in patients with lupus nephritis. *J Rheumatol* **21**, 2052–7.

11. Houssiau, F.A., Vasconcelos, C., D'Cruz, D., Sebastiani, G.D., de Ramon Garrido, E., Danieli, M.G., *et al.* (2004) Early response to immunosuppressive therapy predicts good renal outcome in lupus nephritis: lessons from long-term followup of patients in the Euro-lupus nephritis Trial. *Arthritis Rheum* **50**, 3934–40.

12. Goulet, J.R., MacKenzie, T., Levinton, C., Hayslett, J.P., Ciampi, A., and Esdaile, J.M. (1993) The longterm prognosis of lupus nephritis: the impact of disease activity. *J Rheumatol* **20**, 59–65.

13. Moroni, G., Quaglini, S., Maccario, M., Banfi, G., and Ponticelli, C. (1996) 'Nephritic flares' are predictors of bad long-term renal outcome in lupus nephritis. *Kidney Int* **50**, 2047–53.

14. Barber, C.E., Geldenhuys, L., and Hanly, J.G. (2006) Sustained remission in lupus nephritis. *Lupus* **15**, 94–101.

15. Hill, G.S., Delahousse, M., Nochy, D., and Barity, J. (2005) Class IV-S versus class IV-G lupus nephritis: clinical and morphologic differences suggesting different pathogenesis. *Kidney Int* **68**, 2288–97.

16. Schwartz, M.M., Korbet, S.M., and Lewis, E.J. (2008) The prognosis and pathogenesis of severe lupus glomerulonephritis. *Nephrol Dial Transplant* **23**, 1298–306.

17. Schwartz, M.M., Korbet, S.M., Katz, R.S., and Lewis, E.J. (2009) Evidence of concurrent immunopathological mechanisms determining the pathology of severe lupus nephritis. *Lupus* **18**, 149–58.

18. Esdaile, J.M., Levinton, C., Federgreen, W., Hayslett, J.P., and Kashgarian, M. (1989) The clinical and renal biopsy predictors of long-term outcome in lupus nephritis: a study of 87 patients and review of the literature. *Q J Med* **72**, 779–833.

19. Esdaile, J.M., Federgreen, W., Quintal, H., Suissa, S., Hayslett, J.P., and Kashgarian, M. (1991) Predictors of one year outcome in lupus nephritis: the importance of renal biopsy. *Q J Med* **81**, 907–18.

20. Lewis, E.J., Schwartz, M.M., and Korbet, S.M. (2001) Severe lupus nephritis: importance of re-evaluating the histologic classification and the approach to patient care. *J Nephrol* **14**, 223–7.

21. Najafi, C.C., Korbet, S.M., Lewis, E.J., Schwartz, R., and Evans, J for the Collaborative Study Group (2001) Significance of histologic patterns of glomerular injury upon long-term prognosis in severe lupus glomerulonephritis. *Kidney Int* **59**, 2156–63.

22. Kim, Y.G., Kim, H.W., Cho, Y.M., Oh, J.S., Nah, S.S., Lee, C.K., and Yoo, B. (2008) The difference between lupus nephritis class IV-G and IV-S in Koreans: focus on the response to cyclophosphamide induction treatment. *Rheumatology* **47**, 311–4.

23. Moroni G, Pasquali S, Quaglini S, Banfi G, Casanova S, Maccario M, *et al.* (1999) Clinical and prognostic value of serial renal biopsies in lupus nephritis. *Am J Kidney Dis* **34**, 530–9.

24. Ponticelli, C., and Moroni, G. (1998) Renal biopsy in lupus nephritis—what for, when and how often? *Nephrol Dial Transplant* **13**, 2452–4.

25. McAlindon, T., Giannotta, L., Taub, N., D'Cruz, D., and Hughes, G. (1993) Environmental factors predicting nephritis in systemic lupus erythematosus. *Ann Rheum Dis* **52**, 720–4.

26. Barr, R.G., Seliger, S., Appel, G.B., Zuniga, R., D'Agati, V., Salmon, J., and Radhakrishnan, J. (2003) Prognosis in proliferative lupus nephritis: the role of socio-economic status and race/ethnicity. *Nephrol Dial Transplant* **16**, 2039–46.

27. Adler, M., Chambers, S., Edwards, C., Neild, G., and Isenberg, D. (2006) An assessment of renal failure in an SLE cohort with special reference to ethnicity, over a 25-year period. *Rheumatology* **45**, 1144–7.

28. Korbet, S.M., Schwartz, M.M., Evans, J., Lewis, E.J., for the Collaborative Study Group (2007) Severe lupus nephritis: Racial differences in presentation and outcome. *J Am Soc Nephrol* **18**, 244–54.

29. Contreras, G., Lenz, O., Pardo, V., Borja, E., Cely, C., Iqbal, K., *et al.* (2006) Outcomes in African Americans and Hispanics with lupus nephritis. *Kidney Int* **69**, 1846–51.

30. Chen, Y.E., Korbet, S.M., Katz, R.S., Schwartz, M.M., Lewis, E.J., for the Collaborative Study Group (2008) Value of a complete or partial remission in severe lupus nephritis. *Clin J Am Soc Nephrol* **3**, 46–53.

31. Classification and Response Criteria Subcommittee of the American College of Rheumatology Committee on quality measures (2006) Development of classification and response criteria for rheumatic diseases. *Arthritis Rheum* **55**, 348–52.

32. Renal Disease Subcommittee of the American College of Rheumatology Ad Hoc Committee on Systemic Lupus Erythematosus Response Criteria (2006) The American College of Rheumatology response criteria for proliferative and membranous renal disease in systemic lupus erythematosus clinical trials. *Arthritis Rheum* **54**, 421–32.

33. Petri, M., Kasitanon, N., Lee, S.S., Link, K., Magder, L., Bae, S.C., *et al.*; Systemic Lupus International Collaborating Clinics (2008) Systemic lupus international collaborating clinics renal activity/response exercise: development of a renal activity score and renal response index. *Arthritis Rheum* **58**, 1784–8.

34. Contreras, G., Pardo, V., Leclercq, B., Lenz, O., Tozman, E., O'Nan, P., and Roth, D. (2004) Sequential therapies for proliferative lupus nephritis. *N Engl J Med* **350**, 971–80.

35. Chan, T.M., Li, F.K., Tang, C.S.O., *et al.* (2000) Efficacy of mycophenolate mofetil in patients with diffuse proliferative lupus nephritis. *N Engl J Med* **343**(16), 1156–62.

36. Ginzler, E.M., Dooley, M.A., Aranow, C., Kim, M.Y., Buyon, J., Merrill, J.T., *et al.* (2005) Mycophenolate mofetil or intravenous cyclophosphamide for lupus nephritis. *N Engl J Med* **353**(21), 2219–28.

37. Furie, R., Looney, J., Rovin, B., Latinis, K., Sanchez-Guerro, J., Fervenza, F., *et al.* (2009) *Efficacy and safety of Rituximab in patients with proliferative lupus nephritis: Results from the randomized, double-blind Phase III LUNAR (Lupus Nephritis Assessment with Rituximab) Study.* Abstract presented at the American College of Rheumatology Meeting 2009.

38. Appel, G.B., Contreras, G., Dooley, M.A., Ginzler, E.M., Isenberg, D., Jayne, D., *et al.*, for the Aspreva Lupus Management Study Group (2009) Mycophenolate mofetil versus cyclophosphamide for induction treatment for lupus nephritis. *J Am Soc Nephrol* **20**, 1103–12.

39. Boumpas, D.T., Austin, H.A., III, Vaughn, E.M., Klippel, J.H., Steinberg, A.D., Yarboro, C.H., and Balow, J.E. (1992) Controlled trial of pulse methylprednisolone versus two regimens of pulse cyclophosphamide in severe lupus nephritis. *Lancet* **340**, 741–5.

40. Illei, G.G., Austin, H.A., Crane, M., Collins, L., Gourley, M.F., Yarboro, C.H., *et al.* (2001) Combination therapy with pulse cyclophosphamide plus pulse methylprednisolone improves long-term renal outcome without adding toxicity in patients with lupus nephritis. *Ann Intern Med* **135**, 248–57.

41. Felson, D.T., and Anderson, J. (1984) Evidence for the superiority of immunosuppressive drugs and prednisone over prednisone alone in lupus nephritis. Results of a pooled analysis. *N Engl J Med* **311**, 1528–33.

42. Gautam, H., Bhalla, P., Saini, S., Uppal, B., Kaur, R., Baveja, C.P., and Dewan, R. (2009) Epidemiology of opportunistic infections and its correlation with CD4 T-lymphocyte counts and plasma viral load among HIV-positive patients at a tertiary care hospital in India. *J Int Assoc Physicians AIDS Care* **8**, 333–7.

43. Austin, H.A., III, Klippel, J.H., Balow, J.E., le Riche, N.G., Steinberg, A.D., Plotz, P.H., and Decker, J.L. (1986) Therapy of lupus nephritis. Controlled trial of prednisone and cytotoxic drugs. *N Engl J Med* **314**, 614–9.

44. Carette, S., Klippel, J.H., Decker, J.L., Austin, H.A., Plotz, P.H., Steinberg, A.D., and Balow, J.E. (1983) Controlled studies of oral immunosuppressive drugs in lupus nephritis. A long-term follow-up. *Ann Intern Med* **99**, 1–8.

45. Mok, C.C., Ying, K.Y., Ng, W.L., Lee, K.W., To, C.H., Lau, C.S., *et al.* (2006) Long-term outcome of diffuse proliferative lupus glomerulonephritis treated with cyclophosphamide. *Am J Med* **119**, e25–e33.

46. McKinley, A., Park, E., Spetie, D., Hackshaw, K.V., Nagaraja, S., Hebert, L.A., and Rovin, B.H. (2009) Oral cyclophosphamide for lupus glomerulonephritis: an underused therapeutic option. *Clin J Am Soc Nephrol* **4**, 1754–60.

47. Houssiau, F.A., Vasconcelos, C., D'Cruz, D., Sebastiani, G.D., Garrido Ed Ede, R., Danieli, M.G., *et al.* (2002) Immunosuppressive therapy in lupus nephritis: the Euro-lupus nephritis Trial, a randomized trial of low-dose versus high-dose intravenous cyclophosphamide. *Arthritis Rheum* **46**, 2121–31.

48. Houssiau, F.A., Vasconcelos, C., D'Cruz, D., Sebastiani, G.D., de Ramon Garrido, E., Danieli, M.G., *et al.* (2010) The 10-year follow-up data of the Euro-lupus nephritis Trial comparing low-dose and high-dose intravenous cyclophosphamide. *Ann Rheum Dis* **69**, 61–4.

49. Gøransson, L.G., Brodin, C., Ogreid, P., Janssen, E.A., Romundstad, P.R., Vatten, L., *et al.* (2008) Intravenous cyclophosphamide in patients with chronic systemic inflammatory diseases: morbidity and mortality. *Scand J Rheumatol* **37**, 130–4.

50. Nasr, S.H., D'Agati, V.D., Park, H.R., Sterman, P.L., Goyzueta, J.D., Dressler, R.M., *et al.* (2008) Necrotizing and crescentic lupus nephritis with antineutrophil cytoplasmic antibody seropositivity. *Clin J Am Soc Nephrol* **3**, 682–90.

51. Pan, H.F., Fang, X.H., Wu, G.C., Li, W.X., Zhao, X.F., Li, X.P., *et al.* (2008) Anti-neutrophil cytoplasmic antibodies in new-onset systemic lupus erythematosus and lupus nephritis. *Inflammation* **31**, 260–5.

52. Li, L., Wang, H., Lin, S., *et al.* (2002) Mycophenolate mofetil treatment for diffuse proliferative lupus nephritis: a multicenter clinical trial in China. *Zhonghua Nei Ke Za Zhi* **41**, 476–9.

53. Chan, T.-M., Tse, K.-C., Tang, C. S.-O., Mok, M.-Y., Li, F.-K., Hong Kong Nephrology Study Group (2005) Long-term study of mycophenolate mofetil as continuous induction and maintenance treatment for diffuse proliferative lupus nephritis. *J Am Soc Nephrol* **16**, 1076–84.

54. Ong, L.M., Hooi, L.S., Lim, T.O., Goh, B.L., Ahmad, G., Ghazalli, R., *et al.* (2005) Randomized controlled trial of pulse intravenous cyclophosphamide versus mycophenolate mofetil in the induction therapy of proliferative lupus nephritis. *Nephrology (Carlton)* **10**, 504–10.

55. F L, Y T, X P, L W, H W, Z S, H Z, Z H; MMF in Induction Therapy for Active lupus nephritis in Mainland China Study Group. (2008) A prospective multicentre study of mycophenolate mofetil combined with prednisolone as induction therapy in 213 patients with active lupus nephritis. *Lupus* **17**, 622–9.

56. Appel, A.S., and Appel, G.B. (2009) An update on the use of mycophenolate mofetil in lupus nephritis and other primary glomerular diseases. *Nat Clin Pract Nephrol* **5**, 132–42.

57. Walsh, M., James, M., Jayne, D., Tonelli, M., Manns, B.J., and Hemmelgarn, B.R. (2007) Mycophenolate mofetil for induction therapy of lupus nephritis: a systematic review and meta-analysis. *Clin J Am Soc Nephrol* **2**, 968–75.

58. Isenberg, D., Appel, G.B., Contreras, G., Dooley, M.A., Ginzler, E.M., Jayne, D., *et al.* (2010) Influence of race/ethnicity on response to lupus nephritis treatment: the ALMS study. *Rheumatology* **49**, 128–40.

59. Yau, W.P., Vathsala, A., Lou, H.X., and Chan, E. (2007) Is a standard fixed dose of mycophenolate mofetil ideal for all patients? *Nephrol Dial Transplant* **22**(12), 3638–45.

60. Tse, K.C., Tang, C.S., Lam, M.F., Yap, D.Y., and Chan, T.M. (2009) Cost comparison between mycophenolate mofetil and cyclophosphamide-azathioprine in the treatment of lupus nephritis. *J Rheumatol* **36**, 76–81.

61. Moroni, G., Doria, A., and Ponticelli, V. (2009) Cyclosporine (CsA) in lupus nephritis: assessing the evidence. *Nephrol Dial Transplant* **24**, 15–20.

62. Mok, C.C., Tong, K.H., To, C.H., Siu, Y.P., and Au, T.C. (2005) Tacrolimus for induction therapy of diffuse proliferative lupus nephritis: an open-labeled pilot study. *Kidney Int* **68**, 813–7.

63. Politt, D., Heintz, B., Floege, J., and Mertens, P.R. (2004) Tacrolimus- (FK 506) based immunosuppression in severe systemic lupus erythematosus. *Clin Nephrol* **62**, 49–53.

64. Bao, H., Liu, Z.H., Xie, H.L., Hu, W.X., Zhang, H.T., and Li, L.S. (2008) Successful treatment of class V+IV lupus nephritis with multitarget therapy. *J Am Soc Nephrol* **19**, 2001–10.

65. Grootscholten, C., Ligtenberg, G., Hagen, E.C., van den Wall Bake, A.W.L., de Glas-Vos, J.W., Bijl, M., et al., Dutch Working Party on Systemic Lupus Eerythematousus (2006) Azathioprine/methylprednisonlone versus cyclophosphamide in proliferative lupus nephritis. A randomized controlled trial. *Kidney Int* **70**, 732–42.

66. Grootscholten, C., Bajema, I.M., Florquin, S., Steenbergen, E.J., Peutz-Kootstra, C.J., Goldschmeding, R., et al.; Dutch Working Party on Systemic Lupus Erythematosus. (2007) Treatment with cyclophosphamide delays the progression of chronic lesions more effectively than does treatment with azathioprine plus methylprednisolone in patients with proliferative lupus nephritis. *Arthritis Rheum* **56**, 924–37.

67. Grootscholten, C., Snoek, F.J., Bijl, M., van Houwelingen, H.C., Derksen, R.H., Berden, J.H.; Dutch Working Party of SLE (2007) Health-related quality of life and treatment burden in patients with proliferative lupus nephritis treated with cyclophosphamide or azathioprine/methylprednisolone in a randomized controlled trial. *J Rheumatol* **34**(8), 1699–707.

68. Kawasaki, Y. (2009) Mizoribine: a new approach in the treatment of renal disease. *Clin Dev Immunol* E Pub December 2009.

69. Favas, C., and Isenberg, D.A. (2009) B-cell-depletion therapy in SLE—what are the current prospects for its acceptance. *Nat Rev Rheumatol* **5**, 711–16.

70. Lateef, A., Lahiri, M., Teng, C.G., and Vasoo, S. (2010) Use of Rituximab in the treatment of refractory systemic lupus erythematosus: Singapore experience. *Lupus* **19**(6), 765–70.

71. Jayne, D. (2010) Role of Rituximab therapy in glomerulonephritis. *J Am Soc Nephrol* **21**, 14–17.

72. Melander, C., Sallee, M., Troillet, P., Candon, S., Belenfant, X., Daugas, E., et al. (2009) Rituximab in severe lupus nephritis: early B-cell depletion affects long-term outcome. *Clin J Am Soc Nephrol* **4**, 579–87.

73. Jin, O., Zhamng, H., Gu, Z., Zhao, S., Xu, T., Zhou, K., et al. (2009) A pilot study of the therapeutic efficacy and mechanism of artesunate in the MRL/lpr murine model of systemic lupus erythematosus. *Cell Mol Biol* **6**, 461–7.

74. Levesque, M.C. (2009) Translational Mini-Review Series on B Cell-Directed Therapies: Recent advances in B cell-directed biological therapies for autoimmune disorders. *Clin Exp Immunol* **157**, 198–208.

75. Robak, E., and Robak, T. (2009) Monoclonal antibodies in the treatment of systemic lupus erythematosus. *Curr Drug Targets* **10**, 26–37.

76. Boletis, J.N., Marinaki, S., Skalioti, C., Lionaki, S.S., Iniotaki, A., and Sfikakis, P.P. (2009) Rituximab and mycophenolate mofetil for relapsing proliferative lupus nephritis: a long-term prospective study. *Nephrol Dial Transplant* **24**, 2157–60.

77. Cambridge, G., Leandro, M.J., Teodorescu, M., Manson, J., Rahman, A., Isenberg, D.A., and Edwards, J.C. (2006) B cell depletion therapy in systemic lupus erythematosus: effect on autoantibody and antimicrobial antibody profiles. *Arthritis Rheum* **54**, 3612–22.

78. Gunnarsson, I., Sundelin, B., Jónsdóttir, T., Jacobson, S.H., Henriksson, E.W., and van Vollenhoven, R.F. (2007) Histopathologic and clinical outcome of rituximab treatment in patients with cyclophosphamide-resistant proliferative lupus nephritis. *Arthritis Rheum* **56**, 1263–72.

79. Smith, K.G., Jones, R.B., Burns, S.M., and Jayne, D.R. (2006) Long-term comparison of rituximab treatment for refractory systemic lupus erythematosus and vasculitis: Remission, relapse, and re-treatment. *Arthritis Rheum* **54**, 2970–82.

80. Cambridge, G., Isenberg, D.A., Edwards, J.C., Leandro, M.J., Migone, T.S., Teodorescu, M., and Stohl, W. (2008) B cell depletion therapy in systemic lupus erythematosus: relationships among serum B lymphocyte stimulator levels, autoantibody profile and clinical response. *Ann Rheum Dis* **67**, 1011–6.

81. Arahata, H., Migita, K., Izumoto, H., Miyashita, T., Munakata, H., Nakamura, H., *et al.* (1999) Successful treatment of rapidly progressive lupus nephritis associated with anti-MPO antibodies by intravenous immunoglobulins. *Clin Rheumatol* **18**, 77–81.

82. Zhang, F.S., Nie, Y.K., Jin, X.M., Yu, H.M., Li, Y.N., and Sun, Y. (2009) The efficacy and safety of leflunomide therapy in lupus nephritis by repeat kidney biopsy. *Rheumatol Int* **29**, 1331–5.

83. Wang, H.Y., Cui, T.G., Hou, F.F., Ni, Z.H., Chen, X.M., Lu, F.M., *et al.*; China Leflunomide Lupus Nephritis Study Group (2008) Induction treatment of proliferative lupus nephritis with leflunomide combined with prednisone: a prospective multi-centre observational study. *Lupus* **17**, 638–44.

84. Neubert, K., Meister, S., Moser, K., Weisel, F., Maseda, D., Amann, K., *et al.* (2008) The proteasome inhibitor bortezomib depletes plasma cells and protects mice with lupus-like disease from nephritis. *Nat Med* **14**(7), 748–55.

85. van der Vlag, J., and Berden, J.H.M. (2008) Proteasome inhibition: a new therapeutic option in lupus nephritis. *Nephrol Dial Transplant* **23**, 3771–2.

86. Bao, L., Haas, M., Kraus, D.M., Hack, B.K., Rakstang, J.K., Holers, V.M., and Quigg, R.J. (2003) Administration of a soluble recombinant complement C3 inhibitor protects against renal disease in MRL/lpr mice. *J Am Soc Nephrol* **14**, 670–9.

87. Tang, Z., Wang, Z., Zhang, H.T., Hu, W.X., Zeng, C.H., Chen, H.P., *et al.* (2009) Clinical features and renal outcome in lupus patients with diffuse crescentic glomerulonephritis. *Rheumatol Int* Apr 23 E Pub.

88. Nimmerjahn, F., and Ravetch, J.V. (2008) Anti-inflammatory actions of intravenous immunoglobulin. *Annu Rev Immunol* **26**, 513–33.

89. Zhang, W., Shi, H., Ren, H., Shen, P.Y., Pan, X.X., Li, X., *et al.* (2009) Clinicopathological characteristics and outcome of Chinese patients with thrombotic thrombocytopenic purpura-hemolytic uremic syndrome: a 9-year retrospective study. *Nephron Clin Pract* **112**, c177–83.

90. Vo, A.A., Cam, V., Toyoda, M., Puliyanda, D.P., Lukovsky, M., Bunnapradist, S., *et al.* (2006) Safety and adverse events profiles of intravenous gammaglobulin products used for immunomodulation: a single-center experience. *Clin J Am Soc Nephrol* **1**, 844–52.

91. Kahwaji, J., Barker, E., Pepkowitz, S., Klapper, E., Villicana, R., Peng, A., *et al.* (2009) Acute hemolysis after high-dose intravenous immunoglobulin therapy in highly HLA sensitized patients. *Clin J Am Soc Nephrol* **4**, 1993–7.

92. Pepper, R., Griffith, M., Kirwan, C., Levy, J., Taube, D., Pusey, C., *et al.* (2009) Rituximab is an effective treatment for lupus nephritis and allows a reduction in maintenance steroids. *Nephrol Dial Transplant* **24**, 3717–23.

93. Anolik, J.H., and Aringer, M. (2005) New treatments for SLE: cell-depleting and anti-cytokine therapies. *Best Pract Res Clin Rheumatol* **19**, 859–78.

94. Ding, C., Foote, S., and Jones, G. (2008) B-cell-targeted therapy for systemic lupus erythematosus. *BioDrugs* **22**, 239–49.

95. Aringer, M., and Smolen, J.S. (2008) Efficacy and safety of TNF-blocker therapy in systemic lupus erythematosus. *Expert Opin Drug Saf* **7**, 411–9.

96. Aringer, M., Houssiau, F., Gordon, C., Graninger, W.B., Voll, R.E., Rath, E., *et al.* (2009) Adverse events and efficacy of TNF-alpha blockade with infliximab in patients with systemic lupus erythematosus: long-term follow-up of 13 patients. *Rheumatology* **48**, 1451–4.

97. Ramos-Casals, M., Brito-Zerón, P., Muñoz, S., Soria, N., Galiana, D., Bertolaccini, L., *et al.* (2007) Autoimmune diseases induced by TNF-targeted therapies: analysis of 233 cases. *Medicine (Baltimore)* **86**, 242–51.

98. Dixon, W.G., Hyrich, K.L., Watson, K.D., Lunt, M., Galloway, J., Ustianowski, A., and Symmons, D.P. (2010) Drug-specific risk of tuberculosis in patients with rheumatoid arthritis treated with anti-TNF therapy: Results from the British Society for Rheumatology Biologics Register (BSRBR). *Ann Rheum Dis* **69**(3), 522–8.

99. Leaker, B.R., Becker, G.J., Dowling, J.P., and Kincaid-Smith, P.S. (1986) Rapid improvement in severe lupus glomerular lesions following intensive plasma exchange associated with immunosuppression. *Clin Nephrol* **25**, 236–44.

100. Lewis, E.J., Hunsicker, L.G., Lan, S.P., Rohde, R.D., Lachin, J.M. for the Lupus Nephritis Collaborative Study Group (1992) A controlled trial of plasmapheresis therapy in severe lupus nephritis. *N Engl J Med* **326**, 1373–9.

101. Yamaji, K., Kim, Y.J., Tsuda, H., and Takasaki, Y. (2008) Long-term clinical outcomes of synchronized therapy with plasmapheresis and intravenous cyclophosphamide pulse therapy in the treatment of steroid-resistant lupus nephritis. *Ther Apher Dial* **12**, 298–305.

102. Illei, G.G., Takada, K., Parkin, D., Austin, H.A., Crane, M., Yarboro, C.H., *et al.* (2002) Renal flares are common in patients with severe proliferative lupus nephritis treated with pulse immunosuppressive therapy: long-term followup of a cohort of 145 patients participating in randomized controlled studies. *Arthritis Rheum* **46**, 995–1002.

103. El Hachmi, M., Jadoul, M., Lefèbvre, C., Depresseux, G., and Houssiau, F.A. (2003) Relapses of lupus nephritis: incidence, risk factors, serology and impact on outcome. *Lupus* **12**, 692–6.

104. Mok, C.C., Ying, K.Y., Tang, S., Leung, C.Y., Lee, K.W., Ng, W.L., *et al.* (2004) Predictors and outcome of renal flares after successful cyclophosphamide treatment for diffuse proliferative lupus glomerulonephritis. *Arthritis Rheum* **50**, 2559–68.

105. Ponticelli, C., and Moroni, G. (1998) Flares in lupus nephritis: incidence, impact on renal survival and management. *Lupus* **7**, 635–8.

106. Moroni, G., Gallelli, B., Quaglini, S., Banfi, G., Rivolta, E., Messa, P., and Ponticelli, C. (2006) Withdrawal of therapy in patients with proliferative lupus nephritis: long-term follow-up. *Nephrol Dial Transplant* **21**, 1541–8.

107. Nagy, F., Molnar, T., Szepes, Z., Farkas, K., Nyari, T., and Lonovics, J. (2008) Efficacy of 6-mercaptopurine treatment after azathioprine hypersensitivity in inflammatory bowel disease. *World J Gastroenterol* **14**, 4342–6.

108. Stassen, P.M., Derks, R.P., Kallenberg, C.G., and Stegeman, C.A. (2009) Thiopurinemethyltransferase (TPMT) genotype and TPMT activity in patients with anti-neutrophil cytoplasmic antibody-associated vasculitis: relation to azathioprine maintenance treatment and adverse effects. *Ann Rheum Dis* **68**, 758–9.

109. Wofsy, D., Appel, G.B., Dooley, M.A., Ginzler, E.M., Isenberg, D., Jayne, D., *et al.* (2010) Aspreva Lupus Management Study: Maintenance Results. *Lupus* **19**, (Abstract) (Supplement): **27** (Abstract #CS12.5).

110. Zhou, P.J., Xu, D., Yu, Z.C., Wang, X.H., Shao, K., and Zhao, J.P. (2007) Pharmacokinetics of mycophenolic acid and estimation of exposure using multiple linear regression equations in Chinese renal allograft recipients. *Clin Pharmacokinet* **46**, 389–4.

111. Kuypers, D.R. (2008) Influence of interactions between immunosuppressive drugs on therapeutic drug monitoring. *Ann Transplant* **13**, 11–8.

112. Moroni, G., Doria, A., Mosca, M., Alberighi, O.D., Ferraccioli, G., Todesco, S., *et al.* (2006) A randomized pilot trial comparing cyclosporine and azathioprine for maintenance therapy in diffuse lupus nephritis over four years. *Clin J Am Soc Nephrol* **1**, 925–32.

113. Ponticelli, C., Zucchelli, P., Banfi, G., Cagnoli, L., Scalia, P., Pasquali, S., and Imbasciati, E. (1982) Treatment of diffuse proliferative lupus nephritis by intravenous high-dose methylprednisolone. *Q J Med* **51**, 16–24.

114. Cardiel, M.H., Tumlin, J.A., Furie, R.A., Wallace, D.J., Joh T, Linnik, M.D.; LJP 394-90-09 Investigator Consortium (2008) Abetimus sodium for renal flare in systemic lupus erythematosus: results of a randomized, controlled phase III trial. *Arthritis Rheum* **58**, 2470–80.

115. Moroni, G., Radice, A., Giammarresi, G., Quaglini, S., Gallelli, B., Leoni, A., *et al.* (2009) Are laboratory tests useful for monitoring the activity of lupus nephritis? A 6-year prospective study in a cohort of 228 patients with lupus nephritis. *Ann Rheum Dis* **68**, 234–7.

116. Blumenfeld, Z., Shapiro, D., Shteinberg, M., Avivi, I., and Nahir, M. (2000) Preservation of fertility and ovarian function and minimizing gonadotoxicity in young women with systemic lupus erythematosus treated by chemotherapy. *Lupus* **9**, 401–5.

117. Dooley, M.A., and Nair, R. (2008) Therapy Insight: preserving fertility in cyclophosphamide-treated patients with rheumatic disease. *Nat Clin Pract Rheumatol* **4**, 250–7.

118. Zheng, T., Chunlei, L., Zhen, W., Ping, L., Haitao, Z., Weixin, H., *et al.* (2009) Clinical-pathological features and prognosis of thrombotic thrombocytopenic purpura in patients with lupus nephritis. *Am J Med Sci* **338**, 343–7.

119. Yu, F., Tan, Y., and Zhao, M.H. (2010) Lupus nephritis combined with renal injury due to thrombotic thrombocytopaenic purpura-haemolytic uraemic syndrome. *Nephrol Dial Transplant* **25**, 145–52.

120. Rietveld, A., and Berden, J.H. (2008) Renal replacement therapy in lupus nephritis. *Nephrol Dial Transplant* **23**, 3056–60.

121. Tang, H., Chelamcharla, M., Baird, B.C., Shihab, F.S., Koford, J.K., and Goldfarb-Rumyantzev, A.S. (2008) Factors affecting kidney-transplant outcome in recipients with lupus nephritis. *Clin Transplant* **22**, 263–72.

122. Bunnapradist, S., Chung, P., Peng, A., Hong, A., Chung, P., Lee, B., *et al.* (2006) Outcomes of renal transplantation for recipients with lupus nephritis: analysis of the Organ Procurement and Transplantation Network database. *Transplantation* **82**, 612–8.

123. Burgos, P.I., Perkins, E.L., Pons-Estel, G.J., Kendrick, S.A., Liu, J.M., Kendrick, W.T., *et al.* (2009) Risk factors and impact of recurrent lupus nephritis in patients with systemic lupus erythematosus undergoing renal transplantation: data from a single US institution. *Arthritis Rheum* **60**, 2757–66.

124. Lionaki, S., Kapitsinou, P.P., Iniotaki, A., Kostakis, A., Moutsopoulos, H.M., and Boletis, J.N. (2008) Kidney transplantation in lupus patients: a case-control study from a single centre. *Lupus* **17**, 670–5.

125. Kimberly, R.P., Lockshin, M.D., Sherman, R.L., Beary, J.F., Mouradian, J., and Cheigh, J.S. (1981) 'End-stage' lupus nephritis: clinical course to and outcome on dialysis. Experience with 39 patients. *Medicine (Baltimore)* **60**, 277–87.

126. Coplon, N.S., Diskin, C.J., Petersen, J., and Swenson, R.S. (1983) The long-term clinical course of systemic lupus erythematosus in end-stage renal disease. *N Engl J Med* **308**, 186–90.

127. Tincani, A., Andreoli, L., Chighizola, C., and Meroni, P.L. (2009) The interplay between the antiphospholipid syndrome and systemic lupus erythematosus. *Autoimmunity* **42**, 257–9.

128. Palomo, I., Segovia, F., Ortega, C., and Pierangeli, S. (2009) Antiphospholipid syndrome: a comprehensive review of a complex and multisystemic disease. *Clin Exp Rheumatol* **27**, 668–77.

129. Cervera, R., Bucciarelli, S., Plasín, M.A., Gómez-Puerta, J.A., Plaza, J., Pons-Estel, G., *et al*; Catastrophic Antiphospholipid Syndrome (CAPS) Registry Project Group (European Forum On Antiphospholipid Antibodies) (2009) Catastrophic antiphospholipid syndrome (CAPS): descriptive analysis of a series of 280 patients from the 'CAPS Registry'. *J Autoimmun* **32**, 240–5.

130. Bao, L., and Quigg, R.J. (2007) Complement in lupus nephritis: the good, the bad, and the unknown. *Semin Nephrol* **27**, 69–80.

131. Scheiring, J., Rosales, A., and Zimmerhackl, L.B. (2010) Clinical practice. Today's understanding of the hemolytic uraemic syndrome. *Eur J Pediatr* **169**, 7–13.

132. www.ClinicalTrials.gov. Identifier # NCT00844844, 2010.

Index

Page numbers in *italics* indicate figures and tables.

abatacept 187, 294
abetimus 299
ACE inhibitors
  lupus membranous nephropathy 181
  pregnancy 271
acute interstitial nephritis 19
acute myocardial infarction 180
acute pulmonary hemorrhage 20
acute renal failure 18–19, 203–4
ADAMTS13 221, 303
advanced renal failure 302
African Americans
  anti-Sm antibodies 4
  C1QA gene 6
  cyclophosphamide induction therapy 289, 290
  kidney disease 8
  lupus nephritis 7
  mortality rates 1
  mycophenolate mofetil
    response 241–42, 298
  prevalence of SLE 7
age 9
agrin 63
AKT 63
aliskiren 181
alkylating agents 183–4
allogeneic reactions 61
alopecia 10, 19, 238
α3(IV)NC1 109–10
alpha-actinin 42
American College of Rheumatology diagnostic
    criteria 3–4
amyloidosis 23
ANCA-associated crescentic
    glomerulonephritis 111–12
anemia 21
anergy 59, *60*, *61*
angiotensin converting enzyme (ACE) inhibitors
  lupus membranous nephropathy 181
  pregnancy 271
angiotensin receptor blockers
  lupus membranous nephropathy 181
  pregnancy 271
antenatal care *265*, 266–70
anti-alpha-actinin antibodies 42
anti-B cell activation factor (BAFF) 70, 294
anti-β_2 GPI ELISA 49
anti-C1q antibodies 48, 72, 87, 300

anticardiolipin antibodies *37*, 224
anticardiolipin ELISA 48–9
anti-CD20 monoclonal antibody therapy 69,
    293–4
anticoagulation
  APL antibodies/APS 226, 303
  lupus membranous nephropathy 181
  pregnancy 264, 270
anti-DNA antibodies 72
  glomerular damage 39–44
  historical perspective 3
  lupus nephritis 37–9
anti-double-stranded DNA antibodies
  alpha-actinin interaction 42
  clinicopathological correlates 23
  drug-induced 4
  glomerular damage 41, 42–4
  heparan sulfate binding 44–5
  lupus nephritis 4, 36–9
  pre-eclampsia 267
  prevalence in SLE patients 36, *37*
anti-elastase antibodies 47
anti-GBM glomerulonephritis 110–11
antigen cross-reactivity 72
antigen presenting cell 60
anti-histone antibodies 45–6
anti-HMG-17 antibodies 46
anti-La antibodies 4, *37*, 46, 262
antilactoferrin antibodies 47
antilysozyme antibodies 47
antineutrophil cytoplasmic antibodies
    (ANCA) 10, 47, 152, 218
  c-ANCA 47
  p-ANCA 10, 47
antinuclear antibodies 4, 16–17, *37*
  ANA negative patients 4, 46–7
antinucleosome antibodies 40, 71
antiphospholipid antibodies 3, 5, 48–9, 88, 224,
    303
  clinical detection tests 48–9
  end-stage renal disease 225–6
  pregnancy 264, 268
  renal transplantation 2, 226
antiphospholipid nephropathy 224–5
antiphospholipid syndrome 5, 48, 224–6
  acute renal failure 19
  pregnancy 264, 268
anti-Ro antibodies 4, *37*, 46–7, 262

anti-single-stranded DNA antibodies 36, *37*, 38
anti-Sm antibodies 4, *37*, 46, 47
anti-TNF monoclonal antibody 188
anti-ubiquitin antibodies 46
anti-U$_1$RNP antibodies *37*, 47
apoptosis 44, 49–50, *62*, 92
arthralgia 19
arthritis 19–20
Arthrotec 268
Asians
  lupus nephritis severity 7
  mycophenolate mofetil response 240, 242, 298
  outcome 8
  prevalence of SLE 7
aspirin
  APL antibodies 226
  pregnancy 264, 266
Aspreva Lupus Management Study
  (ALMS) 248, *285*, 290–91, 294, 298, 306
autoimmune response 59–64
azathioprine
  induction therapy 292
  lupus membranous nephropathy 182–3
  maintenance therapy 297–8, 305–6
  pregnancy *269*, 270

B10 cells 70
B cell depletion therapy 69
B cells
  abnormalities in lupus 5, 63
  immune complexes 73
  lupus nephritis 69–73
  self-reactivity 59
B lymphocyte stimulator (BLyS) 70, 188, 294
B-lymphoid tyrosine kinase 61
BAFF *62*, *65*, 70, *71*, 294
BCA-1 70
bead assays 4
belatacept 294
belimumab 188, 294
betamethasone, pregnancy 270
Black patients 155–6, 177;
  see also African Americans
bone marrow 3, 21–2
bowel, vasculitis 22
brain imaging 21
brainstem lesions 21
breast-feeding 271–72
bromocriptine 259
butterfly rash 19

C-reactive protein 21, 84
C1-inhibitor (C1-INH) 86, 94
C1q 6, 48, 72, 83–4, 87, 88, 300
C1q receptors 84
C1QA gene 6
C1qr$_2$s$_2$ complex 84
C3 6, 86, 87, 89, 93, 148
C3a anaphylatoxin 85, 92

C3aR 85, 92–3
C3b opsonins 85
C3d 86
C4 86
C4bp 86, 91
C4d 87, 88
C5a anaphylatoxin 85, 92
C5aR 85, 92
C5b-9 85, 86, 92, 172–3
calcineurin inhibitors
  induction therapy 291–92
  lupus membranous nephropathy 184–5
  maintenance therapy 298
calcium/calmodulin-dependent protein kinase
  (CaMKIV) 63
calcium response 63
cardiac murmurs 20
cardiac tamponade 20
cardiopulmonary features 20
cardiovascular events 180
Carolina Lupus Study 10, *11*
casts *15*, 17
catastrophic APL syndrome 19
cbl-b 63
CCR5 112
CD4–CD8– T cells 65, 68
CD4+ T cells 5, 65, 67–8, 106–8
CD8+ T cells 65, 67–8
CD11a/CD18 63
CD11c/CD18 63
CD21 86
CD25+ T cells 5
CD28 60
CD40 60, *61*, 112
CD40L 9, 60, 63
CD44 63, 110
CD46 85
CD59 86, 93, 94
CD68 117
CD70 63
CD80 60, 64
CD152 66
cellular immunity 64–8
cerebral blood flow 21
cerebrospinal fluid 21
cerebrovascular accidents 180
CH$_{50}$ 84
Charcot arthropathy 9
children
  clinical presentation of lupus nephritis 12, *13*
  family history of lupus 5
  incidence of SLE 8
  minimal change glomerulopathy (MCG) 199, 207
  mycophenolate mofetil treatment 248
  neonatal lupus syndromes 262
  neonatal membranous nephropathy 170, 172
  neurological lupus 21
  Th1 and Th2 112
chlorambucil 183, *190*

chorea 21
chromatin 40, 45–6, 60, 88
chronic fibrosing alveolitis 20
chronic kidney disease, pregnancy
    outcomes 263
cigarette smoking 7
classification systems 2–3, 129–31, 135, *135*,
    145–8, 157–9, 170, 282–3
clearance hypothesis 88
cold sores 6
collagen, type V 41
coma 21
complement 4, 38, 39, 61, 72, 82–104
    activation pathways 83–5
    alternative pathway 84–5
    classical activation pathway 83–4
    functional studies in experimental lupus
        models 89–93
    human SLE 86–3
    inherited deficiencies 6
    mannose-binding lectin pathway (MBL) 83, 85
    mouse models of SLE 88–9
    regulatory proteins 85–6
complement factor H 85, 86, 90–2, 303
complement factor I 85
complement receptors (CR1–4) 85;
    see also individual receptors
complementarity determining regions 43–4
complete remission 284, *285*, *288*
computed tomography (CT) 21, 219
concordance rate 5
congenital heart block 262
coronary artery disease 180
corticosteroids
    cyclophosphamide and 238
    inducing psychosis 21
    induction therapy 284, 286–7, 304
    lupus membranous nephropathy 182
    maintenance therapy 296, 299, 305
    pregnancy 270
    tapering doses 286–7, 304, 306
costs of treatment 246–7
COX-2 63
COX-2 inhibitors, pregnancy 268, *269*
CR1 6, 86, 87, 91
    soluble 90, 93
CR1-related gene/protein y 86, 90–1
CR2 86, 87, 91, 93
CR3 86
CR4 86
cranial nerve palsy 21
creatinine, remission 156
crescentic glomerulonephritis
    acute renal failure 18
    adaptive immunity 105–6
    ANCA-associated 111–12
    crescentic lesions 143
    dendritic cells 116
    mycophenolate mofetil treatment 247–8

T helper cells 106–10
T regulatory cells 113–14
toll-like receptors 117–18
crescentic lesions
    crescentic glomerulonephritis 143
    lupus membranous nephropathy 175
    surrogate for glomerular necrosis 138, 143
Crry 84, 90–1
CTLA4 5, 66
CTLA4-Ig 294
Cushing syndrome 299, 306
Cutaneous Lupus Erythematosus Disease Area
    and Severity Index (CLASI) 4
cutaneous neonatal lupus 262
CXCL13 70
CXCR5 68
cyclophosphamide 238
    adverse effects 238
    bladder irritation 289
    ethnicity and response 289, 290
    fertility 257–8, 301–2
    induction therapy 288–90, 304–5
    lupus membranous nephropathy 183–4,
        185
    maintenance therapy 297
    MESNA co-administration 289, 304
    pregnancy 268, *269*
    refractory severe lupus nephritis 300, 307
cyclosporine
    induction therapy 291
    lupus membranous nephropathy 184–5
    maintenance therapy 298, 306
    pregnancy *269*, 270
    severe lupus nephritis 307

decay accelerating factor 85, 89–90
dehydroepiandrosterone (DHEA) 259
dendritic cells 73, 116–17, 118
deoxyribonuclease (DNase) 40
    DNase1 88
dermatological features 4, 19
dexamethasone, pregnancy 268
diagnostic criteria for lupus 3–4
dialysis 2, 303
    pregnancy 270
diastolic murmurs 20
differential diagnosis 9–10
diffuse global glomerulonephritis (DGGN)
    classification 129–30, 131–32, 135
    glomerular pathology 141, 143–4
    pathogenesis 148, 149–50
    plasmapheresis 153
    prognosis 154–5
diffuse proliferative
    glomerulonephritis 130–1
diffuse proliferative lupus nephritis 130
digital subtraction venography 220
discoid lupus 19
DNA–histone complexes 44–5

Dnmt1 60
Doppler ultrasonography 219
double-stranded RNA 60
drug-induced anti-dsDNA antibodies 4
drug-induced lupus 6, 45, 67

E-C4d 87
E-CR1 87
eculizumab 94–5, 188, 303
editing 59
elastase 47
end stage renal disease (ESRD) 1, 302
  APL antibodies 225–6
  risk factors 155–6
endocarditis 20
environmental factors 6–7, 60–1
epratuzumab 188, 294
Epstein–Barr virus 5, 6
ERK 63
erythrocyte C4d 87
erythrocyte CR1 87
erythropoiesis 87
estrogen 8–9, 258–9
ethnicity
  cyclophosphamide induction therapy 289, 290
  lupus nephritis incidence and prevalence 7–8
  mycophenolate mofetil response 240, 241–2,
    248, 291, 298
  outcome in severe lupus nephritis 155–6
  prognosis in lupus membranous
    nephropathy 179–80
  renal involvement in lupus 1
Euro-Lupus trial 10, 11, 283
extracellular signal-related kinase 63
extrarenal flare in pregnancy 260, 268
eyes 18, 21

Fc receptors 6, 61, 72, 118
female sex 8–9
fertility 257–8, 301–3
fetal loss 261
flare (relapse) 295–6, 300–1, 306–7
  in pregnancy 8, 257–8, 264, 265–6
focal adhesion kinase 63
focal proliferative glomerulonephritis 130, 131
focal segmental glomerulonephritis (FSGN)
  classification 129–32, 136
  glomerular pathology 136–41
  pathogenesis 148, 150–2
  plasmapheresis 153
  prognosis 154–5
focal segmental glomerulosclerosis 199, 202,
  207
foot process fusion 199, 201
Foxp3 5, 67, 106
"full house" 14, 86

gadolinium exposure 21
gastrointestinal tract 22
gender differences 8–9

genetic factors 5, 61–2
germinal centers, ectopic 70
glomerular epithelial foot process fusion 199, 201
glomerular filtration rate (GFR) 23
  pregnancy 252
glomerular necrosis 88, 137–8, 143, 151–2
glomerular scars 137, 199, 202
glucocorticoids, see corticosteroids
glutathione S transferase M1 7
glycolipid therapy 66
β_2 glycoprotein I 48
gold 61
Goodpasture's disease 111
granular casts 15, 17
GRO-γ 207
GSTM1 7

hair dyes 6
headache 21
heart murmurs 20
hematological features 21–2
hematuria 15, 17
hemiparesis 21
hemodialysis 303
  pregnancy 270
hemolytic uremic syndrome (HUS) 303
Henoch–Schönlein purpura 10
heparan sulfate (HS) 41, 42, 44
heparin 264, 270, 302
hepatic features 22
hereditary angio-edema (HAE) 94
high-mobility group protein 17 (HMG-17) 46
Hispanics
  C1QA gene 6
  cyclophosphamide induction therapy 289
  lupus nephritis severity 7
  prognosis in lupus membranous
    nephropathy 179
histones 40
  DNA–histone complexes 44–5
historical issues 1–3, 169–70
HMG C0-A reductase inhibitors 180
hormone replacement therapy 258
hormones 8–9, 258–9
humanized monoclonal antibodies 94–5, 188,
  294
humoral immunity 69–73
hyaline thrombi 139, 143, 144, 149, 151, 152
hydralazine-induced lupus 6, 60
hydrocarbon oil 61
hydroxychloroquine, pregnancy 269, 270
hypercholesterolemia 15
hyperkalemia 16
hyperlipidemia 180
hypertension 18, 216
  pregnancy 257
hypoxemia 20

ICOS (ICOSL) 60, 63, 68
idiopathic glomerulonephritis 14–15

idiopathic membranous
    nephropathy 95, 170, 172
idiopathic thrombocytopenia 14
Ig-producing B cells 70
immune complex deposition 39–41, 86–7, 148,
    211–13, *214*
    diffuse global glomerulonephritis 149–50, *152*
    lupus membranous nephropathy 170
    mechanism 70, 72–3
    necrotizing vasculopathy 216
    severe focal segmental
        glomerulonephritis 138–40, 151, *152*
    staging 174–5
immunodeficiency 6
immunofluorescence assays 4
immunoglobulin A deficiency 6
immunoglobulin G antibodies 38, 39, 72
immunotherapy *71*
incidence figures 7, 257
incomplete remission 208
inducible co-stimulator (ligand) (ICOSL/
    ICOS) 60, 63, 68
induction therapy 238–42, 282, 284–95, 304–5
inflammation 59
inflammatory bowel disease 22
inflammatory vasculitis 216–18
infliximab 188
inherited immunodeficiency 6
inosine monophosphate dehydrogenase
    (IMPDH) 237
β_2 integrins 63
intensive plasma exchange 295, 303
interferon α 87, 118
interferon α blockade 188
interferon γ 64, 107, 108, 112
interferon regulatory factor (IRF-5) 61
interferons, type I 117, 118
interleukin-1 5
interleukin-1β 108
interleukin-2 63
interleukin-4 107, 112
interleukin-6 106
interleukin-10 107, 112
interleukin-12 107, 108
interleukin-17 68, 106, 108–10, 112–13
interleukin-18 107, 112
interleukin-21 68, 106
interleukin-23 106
interleukin-27 68
International Society of Nephrology and Renal
    Pathology Society (ISN/RPS)
    classification 2–3, 135, *136*, 144–8, 157–9,
    170, 282–3
intestinal vasculitis 22
intravenous immunoglobulin
    induction therapy 293
    pregnancy 268, *269*
    thrombotic microangiopathies 302
intravenous urography 219
invariant NKT cells 114

Jaccoud's arthropathy 9
JAK2 62
joint pain 19
juvenile-onset SLE 67

kidney transplantation
    APL antibodies 2, 226
    fertility 257
    lupus patients 2, 302–3
    mycophenolate mofetil 237–8
Klinefelter's syndrome 9

La antigen 46
lactoferrin 47
laminin 42, 72
Langerhans cells 116
LE-cell preparations 2, 4
leukocyte function-associated antigen-1
    (LFA-1) 60, 62
leuprolide 301–2
Libman–Sachs endocarditis 20
light chain excretion 16
lipid-lowering drugs 180
lipid rafts 63
lipopolysaccharide 60, 116
livedo reticularis 19
local immune responses 63–4
low molecular weight heparin (LMWH) 264, 270
LUNAR trial 294
lung involvement 20
lupus, historical use of term 1–2
lupus anticoagulant *37*, 224, 303
lupus anticoagulant test 49
lupus erythemateux 2
lupus erythematosus-cell preparations 2, 4
"lupus frizz" 19
lupus membranous nephropathy 169–97
    clinical presentation 177–8
    early clinical signs 177
    experimental therapies 187–9
    historical perspective 169–70
    immunosuppressive therapies 182–7
    morphology 169
    mycophenolate mofetil treatment 186–7, 245
    nephrotic syndrome 179, 180–1
    pathogenesis 170–74
    prognosis 178–80
    renal biopsy 174–5, *176*
    secondary membranous nephropathy 169
    supportive therapies 180–91
    survival estimates *178*
    treatment recommendations 189, *190*
Lupus Nephritis Collaborative Study
    Group *134*, 135, 145, 153–6
lupus podocytopathy 199–210
    nephrotic syndrome 203–4
    prevalence 205
    renal biopsy 199, *200*
lupus vasculitis 211, 215

lymphocyte activation 59, *61*
lymphoma 20
Lyn kinase 63
lysozyme 47

Mac-1 63
macroscopic hematuria 17
magnetic resonance angiography 21
magnetic resonance imaging 21
magnetic resonance venography 219
maintenance therapy 242–4, 282, 295–9, 305–6
major histocompatibility complex 5
  Class II 61, 111
mannose-binding lectin pathways 83, 85
MAP kinase 63
maternal death 255
MBL-associated serine proteases (MASP) 85
membrane attack complex (C5b-9) 85, 86, 92, 172–3
membrane cofactor protein 85
mercuric chloride 61
mesangial pattern 138–9, *140*, 205–6
MESNA co-administration 289, 304
methylprednisolone 286
MHC Class II 59, 111
32-microglobulin 16
β2-microglobulin 66
microRNAs 62–3
microscopic hematuria 17
minimal change glomerulopathy 199, *202*,
  204–5, 207
miRNAs 62–3
misoprostol preparations and pregnancy 268
mitogen activated protein kinase 63
mixed connective tissue disease 9
mixed membranous and proliferative lupus
  nephropathy 170, *174*, *176*
mizoribine 292
monoclonal antibodies 69, 94–5, 188, 293–4
monoclonal anti-dsDNA antibodies 42–3
monozygotic twins 5
mood disorder 21
mortality rates 1, 35, *36*
mouth ulcers 19
mTOR 63
musculoskeletal features 19–20
myalgia 20
mycophenolate mofetil 237–55
  cost of treatment 246–7
  crescentic lupus nephritis 247–8
  ethnicity and response 240, 231–42, 248, 291, 298
  impact on renal and patient survival 243–5
  induction therapy 238–42, 290–1, 303
  kidney transplantation 237–8
  lupus membranous nephropathy 186–7, 245
  maintenance therapy 242–4, 298, 305, 306
  pediatric patients 248
  pharmacokinetic variability 249
  pregnancy *269*, 270–1
  refractory severe lupus nephritis 300, 307
  therapeutic drug monitoring 249

mycophenolic acid 237, 246
myeloperoxidase 111
myeloperoxidase ELISA 10
myocardial infarction 180
myocarditis 20
myositis 20

N-acetyltransferase (NAT) 5, 6, 7
nasal ulcers 19
National Institutes of Health trial 288
natural killer cells 114–15
natural killer T cells 65, 115
  invariant 115
nausea 22
necrosis, glomerular 88, 137–8, 1431, 151–2
necrotizing vasculopathy *212*, 213–16
neonatal lupus syndromes 262
neonatal membranous nephropathy 170, 172
nephritic renal relapses 295–6
nephrogenic fibrosing dermopathy 21
nephrotic renal relapses 295, 296
nephrotic syndrome 15
  complications 17
  lupus membranous nephropathy 179, 180–1
  lupus podocytopathy 203–5
  prevalence *16*
  thrombosis 181
neuropsychiatric lupus 21
neutrophils 5
NFκB 63
NKG2D 67
noninflammatory necrotizing
  vasculopathy 213–16
non-iNKT cells 115
non-steroidal anti-inflammatory drugs
  minimal change glomerulopathy 199, 204
  pregnancy 268, *269*

ocreluzimab 294
oligonucleosomes 43
ophthalmoplegias 21
opportunistic infections 287
oral contraceptives 258–9
oral ulcers 19

p65 86
pattern associated molecular patterns (PAMPs) 117
papilloma virus 306
paracetamol, pregnancy 268, *269*
paroxysmal nocturnal hemoglobulinuria 94–5
partial remission 284, 286, 288
pattern associated molecular patterns 117
pauci-immune pattern 138, 139, *141*, 151–2
pediatrics, *see* children
perforin 63
pericarditis 20
peritoneal dialysis 303
PET scan 21
pexelizumab 94
phosphorylated ERM 63

photosensitivity 19
PKCα 63
plasma exchange 295, 303
plasmablasts 70
plasmacytoid dendritic cells 116, 117
plasmapheresis 18–19, 153, 295
pleuritis 20
Pneumocystis juvei infection 305
podocytes 42
  lupus membranous nephropathy 172–3
  see also lupus podocytopathy
positron emission tomography 21
poverty 179
pp125FAK 63
PR3 111, 112
prednisolone, pregnancy 268, *269*, 270
prednisone
  induction therapy 286, 304
  lupus membranous nephropathy 182
  maintenance therapy 296, 299, 304
  renal relapses 300
  tapering doses 286, *287*, 304, 306
pre-eclampsia 261, 267–8
pregnancy 257–79
  antenatal care *266*, 266–70
  anticoagulation 264, 270
  antiphospholipid antibodies 264, 268
  chronic kidney disease 263
  diagnosis of lupus nephritis during
      pregnancy 264–5
  disease activity at conception 262
  disease flare 8, 259–60, 266, 267–8
  erythropoietin requirements 270
  extrarenal flare 260, 268
  features of pregnancy mimicking
      SLE *266*
  fetal loss 261
  glomerular filtration rate 258
  hemodialysis 270
  histological class of lupus 263–4
  hormones 257–9
  hydronephrosis 258
  hypertension 263
  lupus activity 259–60
  maternal death 261
  medication safety 268, *269*, 270–1
  neonatal lupus syndromes 262
  normal renal physiology 258
  post-partum monitoring 270–72
  pre-eclampsia 261, 267–8
  pre-pregnancy counseling 265
  pre-term delivery 262
  progression of renal disease 260–1
  proteinuria 258, 263
  pulmonary hypertension 264
  renal biopsy 266
  renal flare 259–60, 267–8
  renal impairment 270
  small for gestational age 262
  thromboprophylaxis 268, 270

urinary tract infection 258
vitamin D supplements 270
pre-pregnancy counseling 265
pre-term delivery 262
prevalence of lupus 7
primary antiphospholipid syndrome 48
pristane 61
procainamide 60, 61
prognosis
  lupus membranous nephropathy 178–80
  severe lupus nephritis 154–6
programmed death 1 (PD-1) 60
proinflammatory cytokines 108, 114
prolactin 259
protein-losing enteropathy 22
protein phosphatase 2A (PP2A) 63
protein tyrosine phosphatase, nonreceptor
      type 22 (Ptpn22) 60–1
proteinase 3 (PR3) 111, 112
proteinase 3 ELISA 10
proteinuria 15
  predictive value 177–9
  pregnancy 258, 262
proteinuric renal relapses 295, 296
proteoglycan 62
psychosis 21
PTEC–T cell interactions 64
pulmonary arterial hypertension 20
pulmonary embolism 20
pulmonary hypertension 20, 224, 265, 272
pulmonary–renal syndrome 20

race, *see* ethnicity
Ras 63
rashes 19
Raynaud's phenomenon 20, 22
red cell casts 15, 17
refractory severe lupus nephritis 299–80, 307
regulators of complement activation (RCA)
      gene family 85–6
regulatory B cells 70
regulatory T cells (Treg) 5, 64, 66–7, 106, 108,
      113–14
relapse, *see* renal flare
remission
  complete/partial 284, *285–6*, *288*
  incomplete 208
  predictive features 155, *157*
renal amyloid 23
renal arterial thrombosis 19
renal biopsy
  first report of lupus nephritis 129
  lupus membranous nephropathy 174–5, *176*
  lupus podocytopathy 199, *200*
  misclassification 140–1, *142*
  pregnancy 267
  refractory severe lupus nephritis 300
  repeated 283
  silent lupus nephritis 12
  therapeutic plan 282–3

renal dialysis 2, 303
  pregnancy 270
renal flare (relapse) 295–6, 300–1, 306–7
  pregnancy 259–60, 267–8
renal replacement therapy 302–3
renal scintigraphy 219–20
renal transplantation
  APL antibodies 2, 226
  fertility 257
  lupus patients 2, 302–3
  mycophenolate mofetil 237–8
renal tubular dysfunction 16
renal vasculitis 212, 213, 216–18
renal vasculopathy, lesion types and
    pathology 211, 212;
    see also specific lesions
renal vein thrombosis 17, 19, 218–20
renal venography 219
renin inhibitors 181
retinoblastoma protein 63
retinopathy 18
rheumatic fever 9
rheumatoid arthritis 9–10, 20
rheumatoid factor 3, 37, 72
rituximab
  induction therapy 293, 294
  lupus membranous nephropathy 187
  pregnancy 268, 269
  refractory severe lupus nephritis 300, 307
  renal relapses 307
Ro antigen 46
RORγt 106

scarred glomeruli 137, 199, 202
secondary membranous nephropathy 169
seizures 21
self-reactive T and B cells 59
severe focal segmental glomerulonephritis 135
  glomerular pathology 136–41
  immune deposits 138–40, 151, 152
  pathogenesis 148, 150–52
  plasmapheresis 153
  prognosis 154–7
severe (proliferative) lupus nephritis
  classification 129–32, 135, 136, 145–8
  clinical features and prognosis 153–5
  definition 129–36
  glomerular pathology 136–45
  induction therapy 282, 284–95, 304–5
  maintenance therapy 282, 295–9, 305–6
  pathogenesis 148–53
  plasmapheresis 153
  refractory to treatment 299–81, 307
  remission 156, 157
  renal relapses 295–6, 300–1, 306–7
  risk factors for progression 155–6
  therapeutic plan 282–4
severe segmental proliferative lupus
    nephritis 132, 133
sex differences 8–9

sex hormones 8–9, 258–9
shingles 6
sicca symptoms 10
signal transducer and activator transcription 4
  (STAT4) 61, 106
signal transducer and activator transcription 5
  (STAT5) 63
silent lupus nephritis 12, 14
Sjögren's syndrome 10, 46
skin involvement 4, 19
Sm antigen 46
small for gestational age 262
smoking 7
socieconomics 179
splenomegaly 20
SS-A and SS-B 4, 46, 262
standardized mortality ratio 1
statins 180
sterile pyuria 19
steroid-free maintenance 299
steroids, see corticosteroids
stroke 180
subendothelial immune deposits 149–50,
  151, 152
subepithelial immune deposits 170
sulfasalazine 269
sun exposure 5, 7
Syk 63
symptoms, onset of SLE 10
systemic vasculitides 151
systolic murmurs 20

T cell effectors 66–8
T cells
  abnormalities in lupus 63, 64–8
  α/β T cells 108
  cytotoxic response 67
  DNA hypomethylation 60
  self-reactivity 59
T follicular helper cells 68, 106
T helper cells 66, 106
  autoimmune human
    glomerulonephritis 110–13
  experimental crescentic
    glomerulonephritis 106–10
T regulatory cells (Treg) 5, 64, 66–7, 106, 108,
  113–14
tacrolimus
  induction therapy 291
  maintenance therapy 298
  pregnancy 269, 270
  refractory severe lupus nephritis 307
TCR signaling 63
TCRα/β T cells 65, 66, 68
TCRγ/δ T cells 65, 66
testosterone 259
testosterone therapy 301–32
Th1 68, 106–8, 112, 173
Th2 68, 106–8, 112, 173
Th3 113

Th17 68, 106, 109–10, 112–13
therapeutic drug monitoring 249
therapeutic plan 282–4
thiopurine methyltransferase (TPMT)
      deficiency 297
thromboprophylaxis
   lupus membranous nephropathy 181
   pregnancy 268, 270
thrombosis 17, 19, 20, 22, 48, 49, 88, 181,
      218–19
thrombotic microangiopathies 88, *212*, *213*,
      220–24, 303
thrombotic thrombocytopenic purpura-like
      syndrome 18, 220–24, 303
"tickover" 84
tolerance 59–60, *61*
toll-like receptors 60, 117
   TLR3 118
   TLR7 5, 118
   TLR9 5, 117–18
TP10 94
transforming growth factor β 106
transverse myelitis 23
treatment delay, remission 156
trimethoprim-sulfamethoxazole 305
tubulointerstitial injury 19
tumor necrosis factor 5, 108
tumor necrosis factor antagonists 295
tumor necrosis factor apoptosis-inducing ligand
      (TRAIL) 64

twins, monozygotic 5
type II NKT cells 115
type V collagen 41

ubiquitin 46
United Kingdom National Renal Pathology
      External Quality Assessment Scheme 147
unmethylated CpG DNA 60
urine abnormalities 15

vasculitic process 151–52
vasculitis
   differential diagnosis of lupus 10
   intestinal 22
   rash 19
   renal *212*, *213*, 216–18
vena caval thrombosis 17, 20

warfarin
   APL antibodies/APS 226, 303
   pregnancy 264
Wasserman reaction, false-positive 3
Wegener's granulomatosis 47, 112
West Africa(ns) 5, 7
wire-loops 143, *144*, 148, 150, 151, *152*
World Health Organization (WHO) classification
      130–32, 135, *136*, 170, 282–3

X chromosome 9